THE ENCYCLOPEDIA OF

DENTAL AND ORAL HEALTH

THE ENCYCLOPEDIA OF

DENTAL AND ORAL HEALTH

Carol Ann Rinzler

Foreword by
Mark S. Wolff, D.D.S., Ph.D.

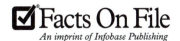

☑ Facts On File
An imprint of Infobase Publishing

The Encyclopedia of Dental and Oral Health

Facts On File, Inc.
An imprint of Infobase Publishing, Inc.
132 West 31st Street
New York NY 10001

Library of Congress Cataloging-in-Publication Data

Rinzler, Carol Ann.
The encyclopedia of dental and oral health / Carol Ann Rinzler ; foreword by Mark S. Wolff.
p. ; cm.—(Library of health and living)
Includes bibliographical references and index.
ISBN-13: 978-0-8160-7403-7 (hardcover : alk. paper)
ISBN-10: 0-8160-7403-8 (hardcover : alk. paper) 1.   Dentistry—Encyclopedias.
2.   Teeth—Care and hygiene—Encyclopedias. 3.   Mouth—Care and hygiene—Encyclopedias.
I. Title. II. Series: Facts on File library of health and living.
[DNLM: 1.   Oral Health—Encyclopedias—English. 2.   Dental Care—methods—Encyclopedias—English. 3.   Mouth Diseases—Encyclopedias—English. 4.   Tooth Diseases—Encyclopedias—English.   WU 13 R584e 2010]
RK27.R56 2010
617.6003—dc22   2009053597

Facts On File books are available at special discounts when purchased in bulk quantities for businesses, associations, institutions, or sales promotions. Please call our Special Sales Department in New York at (212) 967-8800 or (800) 322-8755.

You can find Facts On File on the World Wide Web at http://www.factsonfile.com
Excerpts included herewith have been reprinted by permission of the copyright holders; the author has made every effort to contact copyright holders. The publishers will be glad to rectify, in future editions, any errors or omissions brought to their notice.

Text design by Cathy Rincon
Illustrations by Sholto Ainslie
Composition by Hermitage Publishing Services
Cover printed by Sheridan Books, Ann Arbor, Mich.
Book printed and bound by Sheridan Books, Ann Arbor, Mich.
Date printed: November 2010
Printed in the United States of America

10 9 8 7 6 5 4 3 2 1

This book is printed on acid-free paper.

For my husband,
Perry Luntz,
always.

CONTENTS

FOREWORD

A Smile Is Contagious

A smile, though contagious, is not a classic infectious disease. A smile is a clear view into our moods and emotions. We communicate with a smile. A smile is welcoming. A smile can say thank you. What makes that smile attractive and inviting is a combination of teeth (their shape, color, and position) and lips (their color, shape, and muscle tone). A good smile does not happen by accident and teeth are not only important for a smile.

Dental health has become increasingly important as the health professions recognize an oral-systemic health connection. Recent research has linked dental disease, specifically the presence of gum disease, to elevated risk of developing heart disease and stroke. Patients with periodontal disease have greater difficulty managing their diabetes and patients with diabetes have increased problems with gum health and healing after dental procedures. Multiple medications reduce the flow of saliva and saliva in large part is responsible for protecting teeth from decay.

The oral cavity is clearly the gateway to the body. This world is filled with foods that can cause cavities and stain teeth. We are born with genetics that may make a tooth susceptible to gum disease. Caring for your teeth may mean doing the hard work to maintain them for a lifetime. Unfortunately, 52 percent of children ages six to eight had one or more dental cavities in their primary and/or permanent teeth and 61 percent of adolescents at age 15 years had cavities in their permanent teeth. Sixty-nine percent of adult Americans age 35 to 44 years have had at least one permanent tooth extracted because of dental caries or periodontal disease. By age 70, the average adult has fewer than 20 teeth.

Each year less than 50 percent of the public see the dentist for an annual checkup. What are the reasons people fail to see the dentist regularly? The expense of dental care is clearly one (but not always the actual reason, as many people have insurance and government assistance they do not utilize). Are there less expensive alternative treatments available for dental care? How do we start looking for the answer? Is it possible to invest in prevention and reduce the cost of future care? How do we even know what these technologies are?

Fear is a common explanation for why many people do not see their dentist. Fear of dental care may be considerably deeper than worries about pain (which can be well managed by the dentist). Fear is commonly caused by the unknown. By having a better understanding of what the dentist is going to do, what they are talking about as they speak with you, and even having an idea of what they should be suggesting to you works to reduce fear. Consumers need considerable education both in the terminology used by the dental profession and about the conditions that exist in their mouths. Unfortunately the mouth does not come with an owner's manual.

The availability of resources to help translate the complex dental language and explain conditions in an easily understandable form may be difficult to find. *The Encyclopedia of Dental and Oral Health* provides a comprehensive A-to-Z (literally) description of dentistry. It is a simple to use resource for consumers to better understand dentistry for themselves and their family.

—Mark S. Wolff, D.D.S., Ph.D.
Professor and Chair
Department of Cariology and Comprehensive Care
Associate Dean Pre-doctoral Clinical Education
New York University College of Dentistry

PREFACE

About This Book

The information in the main part of this book is conveniently arranged in the easily accessible, classic A-to-Z format covering three distinct types of entries; after that, there are appendixes, a glossary, and a bibliography.

Conditions entries. The first type of entry in the A-to-Z section of the book is a group of individual entries for specific dental or oral health conditions such as *cavities, herpes (oral)*, and *periodontal disease.* Each of these entries starts with a brief description of the condition, followed by a listing of the symptoms and diagnostic path explaining how the dental professional identifies the specific condition. Then each condition's entry lays out the possible treatment options and the results one may hope to achieve if the treatment is successful. The entry concludes with a list of the known risk factors and preventive measures.

Procedures entries. The second type of A-to-Z entry is the list of entries for specific dental and oral treatment procedures such as *accelerated orthodontia, guided bone regeneration,* and *tongue reconstruction.* Again, each entry begins with a brief description, in this case including the conditions in which the procedure may be useful. Next comes a detailed explanation of the procedure, followed by the possible risks and/or complications. The entry concludes with a list of the lifestyle changes (if any) that may result.

General entries. Third, as with any encyclopedia, this book presents a series of general entries. In this case, that means detailed descriptions of various dental and oral structures such as the lips, teeth, and tongue, as well as descriptions, and often the history, of dental appliances, dental tools, and other paraphernalia common to the dental office and practice such as the dental laser, dental drill, or the continually evolving dental chair.

Appendixes. Fifth, a series of appendixes provides practical information, such as a list of accredited dental schools in the United States, state dental societies (the best place to check out your dentist's credentials or look for a new dentist), and Web sites that will prove useful when looking for more information about dental and oral health.

Glossary. Fourth, there is a glossary of common dental terms from A (*abscess*) through Z (*zone*) used throughout the book in the conditions, procedures, and general entries.

Bibliography. Finally, there is a complete bibliography listing every source used in writing this book. Wherever possible, the bibliographical reference includes an Internet site for the source.

ACKNOWLEDGMENTS

I am grateful to Mark S. Wolff, D.D.S., Ph.D., who was kind enough to read and comment on the manuscript, a sometimes tedious task to which he brought not only professionalism but also a perfectly delightful sense of humor. My thanks also to Greg Diamond, D.D.S., for his comments and for his skill over the years.

As always, I appreciate the editorial guidance of James Chambers, my editor at Facts On File, and his associate Matt Anderson, who handles details (even the crisis ones) with calm efficiency.

Finally, my gratitude to The Women—Erica Bell, Louise Dankberg, Patricia Dolan, Minna Elias, Barbara Kloberdanz, Carolyn Maloney, Carol Schachter, and Phyllis Westberg—for their support at a difficult time.

INTRODUCTION

Over the centuries, human beings have exercised their customary ingenuity in an effort to beautify their smiles and solve their dental problems.

The Egyptians made tooth powders of brushed eggshells; the British, of powdered bricks. Others sweetened their breath with herbal mouthwashes, and—depending on the century and social class—used fingers or twig "chewsticks" to clean the mouth or crafted false teeth of ivory and wood. Contrary to common belief, George Washington's teeth were not made of wood, but rather, as University of Pittsburgh forensic anthropologist Jeffrey Schwartz discovered in 2005 via laser scanning, they were made of gold, ivory, lead, and human and unidentified animal teeth with springs to open them and bolts to hold them together.

Modern dentistry has more effective tools. Fluoride dentifrices reduce the risk of cavities while they clean. Durable porcelain and plastic dentures sit comfortably on gums or are anchored to implants. The electric toothbrush relieves the tedium of brushing. Antimicrobial mouthwashes cure as well as sweeten. And lasers and bleaches work magic in cosmetic dentistry.

But dental beauty is more than tooth-deep. Or, as an impressive number of the articles that pop up on screen when you search the phrases "cosmetic dentistry" or "good oral health" are likely to put it, "Dental health is more than a pretty smile."

While shiny, even, white teeth are nice to look at, the more salient fact is that the condition of one's teeth, tongue, gums, and palate is often an important and reliable reflection of one's general health. Many systemic illnesses and conditions such as cancer, diabetes, heart disease, HIV/AIDS, kidney disease, leukemia, and osteoporosis, to name a few, are likely to make their first appearance as dental symptoms such as swollen or infected gums, mouth ulcers, or dry mouth. At the same time, untreated dental problems such as decay or periodontal disease may trigger illness elsewhere in the body as microorganisms flow from the mouth through the bloodstream to other organs and systems. For example, several studies link periodontal disease to an increased risk of infection of the lining of the heart in susceptible patients. Others suggest that pregnant women with serious periodontal disease are several times more likely than other women to give birth to premature or low birth weight infants. And as the Mayo Clinic notes on its Web site, untreated tooth decay can lead to abscess and infection, as well as broken or lost teeth.

Given all that, Americans might well be expected to be brushing and flossing with enthusiasm every single day with resulting excellent dental health. But according to the *Oral Health in America: A Report of the Surgeon General* (2000), a major catalog of dental health at the turn of the 21st century:

Tooth decay among American children five to 17 years old was five times as common as asthma and seven times as common as hay fever.

Eighteen percent of all two-to-four-year-old American children had at least one cavity; 16 percent went untreated. By age 17, the number of American children with one cavity climbed to 78 percent; 7 percent had lost at least one permanent tooth.

Sixty-nine percent of all Americans aged 35 to 44 years had lost at least one permanent tooth. By age 74, 26 percent had lost all their natural teeth.

Among adults aged 35 to 44, 48 percent had gingivitis (an inflammation of the gums), and 22 percent had destructive gum disease.

To reverse these figures, improve dental and oral health, and reduce the incidence of tooth loss and oral disease, the Surgeon General issued a second report, "A National Call to Action," in 2003. This time the intent was not to tote up the figures but provide the information and programs required to enable Americans to integrate dental care into their general health regimens.

Perhaps as a result, two years later, the Centers for Disease Control and Prevention (CDC) released the *Surveillance Summaries for Dental Caries, Dental Sealants, Tooth Retention, Edentulism, and Enamel Fluorosis,* which had some good news. Compared to the numbers in the 2000 Surgeon General's Report, the CDC found the incidence of tooth decay decreasing among Americans of all ages and more adults retaining their natural teeth.

Three years after that, the agency's *Health United States: 2008* showed a slight uptick in dental visits, with 77 percent of American children aged two to 17 having seen a dentist within the past year. For adults aged 18 to 64, the figure was 63 percent; for adults older than 65, 58 percent. The obvious outcome: Better dental and oral health with fewer cavities left untreated, fewer teeth lost to dental disease, and earlier diagnoses with longer survival times for the most serious oral health problem, oral cancer.

This is important health information, but it is not as available to the general public as one might hope. Face it: Dentistry is simply not as sexy a subject as, say, "How to Make Yourself Look Good Enough to Find Your Dream Partner by Eating Five Special Foods." Obviously, there are textbooks and journals for professionals, but few indeed for the reader who wants to know more about dental treatment—but not necessary everything her dentist knows.

Like other volumes in Facts On File's widely respected *Library of Health and Living* series, this book is designed to meet that need and to provide the information you require to continue to protect your smile—and your health.

What You Need to Know before You See the Dentist

Like all health choices, finding and selecting the appropriate dentist is serious business. The task is made easier, however, with a few simple commonsense rules.

Rule #1   Choose your dentist *before* you need him. Waiting for an emergency is not a good way to choose a dental or medical professional. If you have put off the task and you do experience an emergency such as a broken or knocked-out tooth, the proper place to go is, of course, the emergency room at your local hospital. Some hospitals have dental specialists on call or on site; others depend on oral surgeons or refer to a local dentist.

Rule #2   Ask for references. One tried-and-true way to find a dentist in your area is to ask for references from friends or a doctor who knows your medical history and whose judgment you trust.

Rule #3   Comparison shop. The investment in time and money required to check out two or three dentists before choosing one can pay off dividends in the long run—that is, in the long-term relationship between you and your dental health professional.

Rule #4   Interview the dentist. When you visit the dentist (and his or her staff), begin by checking out these important points:

- Professional credentials. (While you're waiting to be seen, read the diplomas on the wall.)

- The ease with which you were able to make an appointment and the attitude of the office staff: Helpful? Pleasant? Or not? Remember, these are the people with whom you must deal in order to get to the dentist. They count.

- The condition of the office. Is it clean and neat? Is the equipment up-to-date? Are there enough seats in the waiting room and lighting adequate for reading while you wait?

- The dentist's policy for dealing with emergencies. Is the dentist reachable by phone? Does the dentist have someone who covers for her if she is unavailable?

Rule #5   Don't be shy about money. Dental care frequently is not covered by insurance, so it is important to have an idea of your prospective dentist's fees and payment schedule, as well as the types of payment the dentist accepts, and her policy about payment for canceled appointments.

Rule #6   Ask about the proposed treatments for various conditions and the specialists to whom your general dentist sends patients. Then do your research to see if the treatment the dentist proposes meets the current standards for care and the specialists he suggests have the qualifications you require.

Rule #7   Once you have found a dental professional who meets your expectations, follow his advice conscientiously. The teeth you save will be your own.

—Carol Ann Rinzler
December 2009

ENTRIES A TO Z

abrasion, dental The term abrasion comes from the Latin verb *abradere* meaning scrape *(radere)* and off *(ab)*. Dental abrasion is damage to the dental enamel caused by mechanical means such as brushing too hard with a stiff toothbrush or pressing too hard when cleaning between the teeth with a wooden toothpick. Damage may also occur from scratching the surface of the tooth with a metal dental tool or clenching and grinding the teeth so tightly that the biting surface of the tooth chips.

There are two other types of damage to dental enamel: Dental erosion is damage to the enamel surface of a tooth due to a chemical reaction, and dental decay describes damage due to bacterial activity.

Symptoms and Diagnostic Path

Common signs of dental abrasion include scratches on the tooth surface, small notches carved out near the gum line or between the teeth, and chips on the biting surface of the teeth. In the worst cases, the pressure exerted during BRUXISM may actually fracture the tooth, a more serious problem than abrasion.

Treatment Options and Outlook

The treatment for dental abrasion is tailored to the specific damage. For example, minor scratches may be smoothed away with a dental abrasive. Pits or small chips may be filled or restored with a tooth-colored, plastic COMPOSITE material that hardens to form a protective and cosmetically appealing shield. In more severe cases, the tooth may be covered with a VENEER, cap, or CROWN. Depending on the severity of the injury, a fractured tooth may have to be extracted and replaced.

Risk Factors and Preventive Measures

To reduce the risk of mechanical injury to the teeth, the patient is usually advised to use a soft-bristled toothbrush and taught to use dental floss, toothpicks, and instruments with care. To avoid the risk of simple chemical injury, patients should never brush their teeth immediately after consuming a highly acid drink, which intensifies the potential brush-related abrasion. If the damage was caused by bruxism, the patient may be instructed to wear a MOUTH GUARD or seek other treatments to prevent further damage.

See also ENAMEL, DENTAL; EROSION, DENTAL.

abrasive In dentistry, a substance or an instrument such as a disk used to smooth the surface of a tooth or a restoration such as a filling or a cap. For home use, abrasive ingredients that promise to remove stains from teeth may be added to tooth powders, toothpastes, and tooth gels.

In the dentist's office, a variety of dental instruments such as abrasive disks or abrasive drill bits are used to remove dental decay. Diamond-tipped abrasives are used to smooth the surface of a tooth in preparation for a restoration such as a filling, cap, or crown. AIR ABRASION is a dental technique that uses a compressed air instrument to bombard the interior of a cavity with microscopic particles of an abrasive powder, usually aluminum oxide, which cleans and smooths the cavity and prepares it for the filling.

COMMON DENTAL ABRASIVES

Abrasive	Found In/On
Aluminum oxide	Preparation of cavities
Calcium carbonate powders (chalk, whiting)	Stain-removing toothpastes, gels
Diamond particles	Dental instruments for preparing teeth for a restoration and for smoothing porcelain restorations
Rouge (jewelers' rouge, red iron powder)	Dental instruments for smoothing and developing a high polish on gold and other precious metals in restorations such as crowns
Silica	Polishing gels and toothpastes
Tin oxide	Dental polishing instruments

The type of abrasive compound or instrument the dentist chooses varies with the task. The following table lists common abrasive substances and the dental products in which they are found.

See also AIR ABRASION.

accelerated orthodontics Accelerate orthodontics is a technique designed to speed the movement of teeth during orthodontic treatment. Traditional orthodontic treatment may require the patient to wear dental braces for several years. Accelerated orthodontics may reduce the brace-wearing time to months, and may significantly reduce the cost of the treatment as well.

Procedure

The periodontist or oral surgeon administers local anesthetic and peels the gum tissue back from the bone holding the teeth that are to be moved. Next he scores (makes fine indentations in) the exposed bone and applies bone GRAFT material to the bone, filling in the grooves. Once the bone material has been applied, the surgeon replaces the gum tissue and stitches it into place. While it heals, the bone graft expands and the orthodontist can move the teeth more easily into line with dental braces, thus reducing the time required to straighten the teeth.

Commonly, oral surgeons used artificial or bovine bone tissue for this procedure. In 2008, researchers at the University of Southern California School of Dentistry in the advanced education in periodontology program introduced the use of bone fragments taken from the patient's own JAW. Using the patient's own bone is called periodontally accelerated osteogenic orthodontics (PAOO). Autogenous bone transplants (transplant of an individual's own bone from one site to another) is common in periodontic procedures and may become so in this form of orthodontics.

Risks and Complications

Postsurgical discomfort is common; as with any surgical procedure, infection may occur.

If the bone graft material does not expand as planned, excess pressure may damage the root surface of the tooth.

Because some patients are allergic to bovine bone tissue, the orthodist will test the patient for an allergic sensitivity before proceeding.

Outlook and Lifestyle Modifications

Like standard orthodontic treatment, successful accelerated orthodontics corrects irregularities and properly aligns the teeth.

See BONE RECONSTRUCTION; ORTHODONTICS.

acupuncture An Asian healing technique sometimes used to relieve pain and/or anxiety before, during, and after dental treatments.

Acupuncture is the practice of inserting very thin metal (usually stainless steel) needles at one or more of a possible 2,000 specific points on the body in order to stimulate the flow of qi (life force) through a meridian, one of 20 pathways through which qi moves. Acupressure is a similar technique that applies pressure on specific body points rather than needles.

In the West, medical researchers look for a more traditional physical explanation for acupuncture's ability to relieve pain or reduce stress. One possibility lies in data from studies showing that acupuncture may enhance the brain's release of natural hormones and chemicals called neurotransmitters that enable nerve cells to transmit messages from one to another and affect involuntary body processes such as heartbeat, blood pressure, and temperature. The result is an increase in the production of other chemicals called endorphins, which are natural analgesics. While this theory fits well into Western science, the true explanation of acupuncture's effects remains to be shown.

In the United States, acupuncture is practiced by a variety of healthcare providers, including physicians, dentists, chiropractors, and licensed acupuncturists (L.A.), the last being professionals trained in Chinese medical theory, acupuncture, and basic biosciences. The professional association for U.S. physicians trained in acupuncture is the American Academy of Medical Acupuncture. Licensed acupuncturists are tested and certified by the National Certification Commission for Acupuncture and Oriental Medicine. While most states have established training standards for acupuncture certification, the requirements for licensing for nonmedical personnel vary from state to state. For example, in some states, acupuncturists are required to work with an M.D. who may or may not have training in acupuncture.

Acupuncture and Dentistry

In 2002, the World Health Organization published "Acupuncture: Review and Analysis of Reports on Controlled Clinical Trials," a report concluding that acupuncture effectively relieves pain as well as a variety of dental and medical conditions, including temporomandibular disorder (TMD).

As a matter of course, clinical trials to test the effects of drugs are conducted with one group of subjects getting the drug and a second control group getting a placebo (a "look-alike pill"). This technique is difficult if not impossible to accomplish with a physical treatment such as acupuncture in which the patient can clearly see the procedure. Some researchers have theorized that it might work if the control groups were treated with placebo acupuncture (using acupuncture needles to touch but not penetrate the skin).

As a result, as one 2001 report in the *Journal of the American Dental Association* noted, while acupuncture has been studied during endodontic (root canal) treatment, postsurgical dental pain (i.e., after tooth extraction), and as a technique to reduce excess salivation, most accounts of its ability to control dental pain are anecdotal. However, in 2007, researchers at the departments of Anesthesiology, Oral and Maxillofacial Surgery, Biometrics, and Physical Medicine and Rehabilitation, Pain Clinic, at the Hannover Medical School, in Germany, reported in the journal *Anesthesia and Analgesia* that auricular acupuncture (acupuncture in which needles are inserted at points on the ear) appeared as effective as injections of a sedative drug. Acupuncture or sedative injections were more effective than either placebo acupuncture or no treatment at all. In addition, patients given the sedative or the acupuncture were more cooperative in following their dentists' directions during the procedure. The technique's true value in dental situations has remained ambiguous. Future studies may well resolve this issue.

See also TEMPOROMANDIBULAR DISORDER.

adipose tissue *Adipose* comes from the Latin word *adeps,* meaning fat. Adipose tissue is fatty tissue found at various sites on the human body, including the fat pads on the face. These fat pads under the skin of the cheek and under the skin along the jawline are as important as the teeth and jaws in defining the shape of the face. When the adipose tissue is inadequate, due either to a birth defect or to tissue loss related to an injury, disease, or simply advancing age, surgery to reshape the jawline or cheek may require the surgeon to insert an implant under the skin to produce a normal appearance.

The Composition of Adipose Tissue

Adipose tissue is composed of fat cells, cells with a small nucleus (center), very little cytoplasm (the fluid inside cells), and one or more droplets of fat. The fat cells have one important function, to store excess calories as fat. The number and physical activity of fat cells in a person's body depend to some extent on his body type. For example, a lean adult has about 40 billion fat cells. An obese adult may have more than twice as many, and the fat cells in the obese body are larger and more metabolically active than those in a lean body.

The Functions of Adipose Tissue

There are two main types of adipose tissue: white adipose tissue and brown adipose tissue. The first is the fat that insulates the body against heat loss, cushions internal organs, and shapes the body. The second, which appears brown due to a plentiful supply of blood vessels, is the fat that holds stored energy, which is released as heat to warm a shivering body or as energy when a person is starving (or simply eating less than normal). Because the fetus does not develop adipose tissue until late in pregnancy, a premature infant cannot regulate his body temperature and must be kept in a warm environment, such as an incubator.

The Adipose Tissue Body Sites

Where a human being carries adipose tissue is a function of gender and genetics. From the moment they are born, human males commonly have proportionately less adipose tissue and proportionately more muscle tissue than females do. When they reach puberty, the differences in body composition becomes more obvious; as an adult, the average male body is 15 to 20 percent adipose tissue while the average female body may be as much as 25 percent adipose tissue. The extra fat tissue on a woman's body performs several important tasks, among them insulating and protecting her more porous bones and, after menopause, serving as a site where her body can synthesize the female hormone estrogen, which is no longer provided by the ovaries.

A fat pad is a lump of adipose tissue under the skin that contributes to body contours. Fat pads are commonly found on the face, where they shape the eyelid, cheek, and chin. A body site where adipose tissue accumulates is called a fat depot. Fat depots are gender related. For example, women have fat depots at the breasts, hips, and thighs, while men typically have fat depots on the shoulders and upper body. The distribution of female fat depots produces what is commonly known as the pear-shape body. The distribution of male fat depots, the apple-shape, is sometimes linked to a higher risk of heart disease, high blood pressure, and type 2 (non-insulin-dependent) diabetes. The National Institutes of Health suggests that the waist circumference (waist-to-hip ratio) measurement—a number identified by dividing the circumference of the waist by the circumference of the hips—may predict the extent of a person's fat depot–related risk. Women are considered to be at risk if the result is 0.85 or higher; for men the risky ratio is 0.95.

See also CHIN RECONSTRUCTION; GENDER AND ORAL HEALTH; JAW RESTORATION.

age factor   The effect a patient's age may exert on health and/or the success or failure of any treatment. For example, in dentistry, the incidence and severity of several conditions such as tooth DECAY, tooth appearance, and tooth loss may be age-related, with incidence and severity of most dental problems increasing as the patient grows older.

Tooth Decay and Age

Cavities are the most common form of dental disease. They may occur at any age but are most common in childhood. In children and young adults, decay most often occurs on the top (chewing surface) of the tooth. In older people, as the gums recede and leave more of the tooth root exposed, decay more commonly occurs along the line where gum meets tooth. At any age, decay may also occur along the edges of a restoration such as a filling or a CROWN.

The cause of tooth decay is also somewhat age-related. Among young people, decay is commonly linked to bacterial growth in sugary residue on the tooth. In older people, while the same bacteria are also at work, decay is promoted by dry mouth, a condition of having a lower amount of SALIVA, which is the liquid that lubricates the mouth, neutralizes acids, and remineralizes the teeth. The reduction in saliva may be due to the use of medications such as antihistamines, antihypertensives, and antidepressants, or to it may occur due to RADIATION THERAPY to the head or neck.

Tooth Appearance and Age

As one ages, teeth look darker and seem to grow longer. The color change is due to shrinkage of the dental pulp (soft tissue inside the tooth) and a buildup of layers of dentin inside the tooth. DENTIN, a darker material than the dental enamel on the tooth surface, blocks light, making the tooth look dark and yellowish. A similar effect occurs after root canal surgery when the pulp and nerve inside the tooth are removed and the clear fluid inside the root canal is replaced with an opaque filling. While the length of a tooth does not actually change, a natural age-related shrinkage of gum tissue makes the tooth look longer (and increases the risk of decay at the root). Finally, with age, the teeth may simply appear worn from use.

Tooth Loss and Age

In childhood, the most likely cause of tooth loss is an injury or decay. Among older people, the most common causes of tooth loss are PERIODONTAL DISEASE and natural wear-and-tear that weakens the tooth, making it vulnerable to fracture. Although periodontal disease is caused by PLAQUE, age-related factors such as badly fitting dental appliances like DENTURES and systemic disease more common among older people can increase the risk or severity of periodontal disease.

See also CAVITY.

air abrasion A technique, also called "drill-less dentistry," that bombards the tooth with a fine spray of small abrasive particles. This may be done to cut away decay, remove old fillings, or erase minor discoloration on the surface of the tooth. It is also used to roughen the surface of a tooth so that the adhesive used to hold a RESTORATION such as a VENEER in place will attach more firmly. Most patients are likely to find air abrasion less irritating than the vibrations and pressure of the classic dental drill.

Procedure

The dentist will cover the patient's eyes and cover the gums and teeth with a RUBBER DAM. A rubber dam is an appliance that covers areas inside the mouth that are not being treated to prevent irritation from flying sand particles. Then she uses a special instrument that allows her to send compressed air or gas through the dental handpiece that propels the abrasive particles at high speed toward the tooth. When the decay is removed or the stain erased or the surface sufficiently roughened, she rinses the mouth and suctions away any excess particles.

Risks and Complications

Some patients may experience discomfort when air hits exposed areas of the tooth root. The only serious risk during this procedure is injury from the flying particles, which is minimized with the protective covering for eyes and mouth.

Outlook and Lifestyle Modifications

Like dental drilling, air abrasion produces a clean cavity that the dentist seals to reduce the risk of further decay and thus protect the tooth.

alignment   See OCCLUSION.

allergy   A reaction of the body's immune system to an allergen, an otherwise harmless substance such as peanut butter, penicillin, mold, or an airborne particle such as dust or latex. The first step toward an allergic reaction is sensitization, the process by which the body becomes vulnerable to a particular substance known as the allergen. Continued exposure to the allergen causes the body to produce antigens (a.k.a. antibodies). Eventually, as sensitivity rises, the production of antigens increases to the point where specialized body cells in the immune system release histamines, chemicals that cause inflammation that leads to the swelling, redness, and heat associated with an allergic reaction. There is a broad range of treatment available to counter allergic reactions ranging from simple oral and topical antihistamine products to systemic corticosteroids and epinephrine or adrenalines for severe or life-threatening reactions.

The allergens most commonly encountered by dental patients and dental professionals include:

- Materials in dental restorations
  - Metals such as nickel in dental AMALGAM, a rare occurrence, or used in denture plates or restorations such as a CROWN
  - Plastics such as the acrylic resins commonly used in DENTURES
- Medical drugs
  - Local anesthetics
  - Antibiotics
  - Painkillers, including common over-the-counter drugs such as aspirin and other NSAIDs (nonsteroidal anti-inflammatory drugs)
- Dental products
  - MOUTHWASH
  - Toothpaste/tooth powders
  - Protective gear
- Latex products and devices such as gloves, masks, orthodontic elastics, and RUBBER DAMS (a device inserted into the patient's mouth to protect the airway from debris during certain procedures). Most commonly, people who are allergic to latex are sensitive to natural latex, a product derived from the milky sap of the rubber tree. People who are sensitive to plastic may be allergic to the synthetic latex used in many consumer products such as "rubber" gloves.

Once an allergy has been identified, the safest course is to avoid the allergen. Therefore, at the first meeting between patient and dentist, the dentist will obtain a complete medical history for the patient, including notice of any known allergies. Once the dentist is aware of potential allergic reactions, he can adjust treatment plans to avoid potential problems by substituting nonallergenic materials for known allergens in dental restorations and choosing alternate procedures or medicines.

See also EXAMINATION, IMMUNE SYSTEM; RESTORATIONS.

alveolus, alveoli (pl)   An alveolus is a small hollow cavity, a socket; in dentistry, it is the hollow into which a tooth fits and is connected to the jawbone by the periodontal ligament. The alveoli are located in a part of the JAW called the alveolar ridge, also known as the alveolar margin, a ridge behind the teeth that can be felt with the tongue just above the top front teeth and just below the bottom front teeth. The alveolar ridge creates the borders of the upper and lower jaws; its failure to develop in the fetus during pregnancy is one contributing factor to a cleft palate.

Alveolectomy is surgery to remove some of the bone of the alveolar ridge to improve the fit of a dental implant or denture to replace an extracted tooth. Alveoplasty is surgery to shape the edges of the socket after a tooth is extracted so as to prepare the site for a denture. Alveolar remodeling is a loss of the bone in the alveolar ridge. Alveolar ridge augmentation is reconstructive surgery, using a BONE GRAFT or artificial bone to build up the alveolar ridge so that it can hold a denture.

See also CLEFT LIP AND/OR PALATE; DENTURE; IMPLANTOLOGY.

amalgam Also known as dental amalgam and silver fillings; a mixture of two or more metals such as powdered silver, copper, tin, or zinc, held together with mercury, a metal that may account for up to 50 percent of the mixture.

Amalgam, invented in France ca. 1820, has been used for close to 200 years to fill dental cavities. The material is durable, strong enough to stand up to the pressure exerted when the teeth come together to chew food, and it is relatively inexpensive. It is easy to put in place because the mouth does not have to be completely dry when the amalgam is inserted. As a result, in 2005 the AMERICAN DENTAL ASSOCIATION (ADA) estimated that as many as 100 million Americans have amalgam fillings, with dentists adding approximately 53 million new amalgam fillings that year.

Common Problems with Amalgam Fillings

Amalgam fillings are potentially allergenic. They also react to heat and cold, and they are unattractive.

Allergic Reactions to Amalgam Some patients experience an allergic reaction to amalgam fillings characterized by symptoms similar to other contact ALLERGIES: redness, rash, itching. Allergic reactions to amalgam are most likely to occur among people who are sensitive to other metals, including nickel. If a reaction occurs, the dentist will remove the amalgam filling and replace it with another type of restoration.

Physical Reactions to Amalgam Like all metals, the metal in amalgam fillings transmits heat and cold and may expand or contract whenever the metal is warmed or cooled by food, drink, or even a breath of very cold air. In extremely rare cases, the filling's expanding and contracting may be sufficiently pronounced to cause tiny cracks that weaken the tooth, requiring either a new filling or a more extensive restoration.

Cosmetic Drawbacks to Amalgam Fillings Amalgam fillings present two cosmetic problems: the metal's color and the possibility of metal fragments staining the tissue near the tooth.

Because the silver-colored filling does not match the color of the tooth, an amalgam filling is clearly visible. As for staining, when the dentist smooths or removes amalgam with a high-speed tool, fragmentary particles of silver from the amalgam may be forced into the gum, or tongue, or inside the cheek next to the tooth. The fragments produce one or more gray or blue spots, a mark called an amalgam tattoo. The mark is permanent but benign; no treatment is required. However, if the tattoo is unsightly and clearly visible—for example, on the gum in the front of the mouth—the dentist may be able to significantly and safely lighten or eradicate the stain by exposing the tissue to a Q-switch alexandrite LASER. The removal process usually requires three sessions.

Exposure to Mercury in Amalgam Fillings

Mercury is a metallic element that releases vapors known to be hazardous in high concentrations. The signs of mercury poisoning are: memory loss, irritability, sleeplessness, loss of appetite, nerve damage, loss of physical coordination, kidney failure, and death. They were first noted in the 19th century among London hatmakers who commonly used a mercury solution to wash the furs from which they made their hats. (The effects of mercury on these early workers inspired Lewis Carroll's "Mad Hatter" and his tea party in *Alice in Wonderland*.)

Concerns about Patient Exposure to Mercury in Amalgam Fillings By the 1970s, the introduction of tests sensitive enough to identify the presence of extremely small amounts of mercury vapors revealed that amalgam fillings release mercury vapors into the mouth and that these vapors are then absorbed into the body. However, the amount of mercury released by the fillings is so small, and the hardened mercury used so much less absorbable than the mercury in fish, that well-designed studies from the Environmental Protection Agency (1993), the U.S. Public Health Service (1997), and in 2009, the American Dental Association, once again concluded that amalgam fillings were safe. For example:

- In April 2006, the National Institute of Dental and Craniofacial Research, a division of the U.S. National Institutes of Health, released the results of two studies of more than 1,000 children who were randomly assigned to have their cavities filled with either amalgam or a COMPOSITE (resin, a tooth-colored plastic material). The studies—one in the Boston area with 534 children aged 6 to 10, the other in Portugal with 507 children aged 8 to 10—ran for seven years. In the end, children given amalgam fillings did excrete slightly higher than usual but nontoxic amounts of mercury in their urine. But the amount of excreted mercury was within normal usual ranges, and standardized intelligence tests sensitive enough to measure a three-point drop in IQ and several physical tests showed that none of the children in either group exhibited any symptoms of mercury poisoning. They

SUMMARY TABLE OF STATE MERCURY DENTAL WASTE PROGRAMS

State Name	Laws and Regulations Regarding Mercury Amalgam Use	Guidance on Mercury Waste in Dental Practices
Alabama	Y	
Arizona	Y	
California	Y	Y
Colorado	Y	
Connecticut	Y	Y
District of Columbia	Y	
Florida	Y	
Georgia	Y	
Illinois	Y	
Indiana	Y	
Kentucky	Y	
Maine	Y	Y
Massachusetts	Y	
Michigan	Y	
Minnesota	Y	Y
Montana		
New Hampshire	Y	
New York	Y	Y
Ohio		
Oregon	Y	Y
Vermont		
Virginia	Y	Y
Washington	Y	Y
Wisconsin	Y	

Source: U.S. Environmental Protection Department, State Mercury Medical/Dental Waste Programs. Updated December 5, 2007. Available online. URL: www.epa.gov/epawaste/hazard/tsd/mercury/medical.htm. Accessed December 17, 2009.

showed no loss of intelligence or memory, no problems with coordination or nerve function, and no reduction in kidney function.

- Six months later, in September 2006, a panel of experts at the Food and Drug Administration voted to reject an agency statement that amalgam fillings were safe because the panel wanted more research on amalgam safety for specific population groups such as the developing fetus. At the same time, the panel said that amalgam fillings do not pose a risk to patients who have them and that there is no need for anyone to have an amalgam filling removed. In Europe, several countries have either limited the use of amalgam fillings for pregnant women and small children or banned them completely.

However, in June 2008, as part of the settlement of a lawsuit filed by a group opposed to the use of any amalgam fillings, the FDA issued a new statement warning that the mercury in amalgam might pose a risk to the nervous systems of developing fetuses and young children. The statement advised pregnant women not to avoid seeking dental care but to discuss alternatives to amalgam fillings with their dental professionals.

Environmental Concerns about Amalgam Fillings Amalgam waste from dental products can be a significant source of environmental contamination if it is not treated as hazardous waste. The use of technologies such as *amalgam separators* to separate amalgam from dental waste water, and simple precautions in disposing of amalgam materials, can reduce or eliminate the problem. For example, the New York State Department of Environmental Conservation requires that dentists using or removing amalgam follow specific practices in handling and/or disposing of amalgam, directing that dental personnel:

- never put scrap amalgam in the sharps container.
- never put scrap amalgam in the red biohazard bag.
- never discard scrap amalgam in the trash.
- never rinse scrap amalgam down the drain.
- never remove excess amalgam from the amalgam well with the high-speed suction vacuum line.

- never clean up a mercury spill using a vacuum cleaner.
- never place extracted teeth with amalgam restorations in the red biohazard bag. They should be placed in a container that is acceptable to their recycler. Precautions, such as glasses, gloves, and mask, should be used when handling extracted teeth.
- always collect and store all contact and noncontact scrap amalgam, capsule waste, and extracted teeth with amalgam restorations in separate, appropriately labeled, tightly closed containers.
- always recycle scrap amalgam through an amalgam recycler.

As of 2007, several other states had also introduced rules to govern the use and disposal of dental amalgam material. The table on page 8 lists the 23 states (plus the District of Columbia) that have such rules in place as of December 2009 and shows whether the rules are laws or guidelines or both.

See also CAVITY; COMPOSITE, DENTAL; RESTORATION.

amelogenesis imperfecta (AI) Rare, inherited birth defect characterized by thin or soft dental enamel covering on both primary and adult teeth. The National Organization for Rare Disorders lists four types of AI:

- *Type I: Hypoplastic amelogenesis imperfecta:* In this form of AI, there is not enough enamel on the tooth; the surface is usually pitted.
- *Type II: Hypomaturation amelogenesis imperfecta:* In this form of AI, there is sufficient enamel but the crystals of enamel do not develop normally. The enamel is brittle and cracks easily.
- *Type III: Hypocalcified amelogenesis imperfecta:* In this form of AI, there is sufficient amount of enamel but the enamel does not contain enough minerals. The enamel is soft and will

wear away within a few years after the teeth erupt from the gum.

- *Type IV: Hypomaturation-hypoplasia with taurodontism:* With this condition the molar's roots are very near the bottom of the tooth, producing a long chamber inside the tooth and very short root canals. This form of AI includes the characteristics of Types I and II plus smaller than normal teeth.

Symptoms and Diagnostic Path

The diagnosis of amelogenesis imperfecta usually follows a dental examination that identifies the signs of the disorder: teeth that look yellow or darker than normal and enamel that breaks or chips easily. In addition, patients with AI often suffer from MALOCCLUSION (the failure of the teeth and jaws to meet correctly), and AI has been linked to other malformations such as weakened, poorly formed bones.

Treatment Options and Outlook

In treating AI, the dentist aims to restore the appearance of the teeth and/or make them stronger so as to protect them from future damage and enable the patient to chew food efficiently. To do this, the dentist uses a variety of restoration techniques; the exact choice depends on the type and severity of the condition.

Patients with Type I AI and minimal loss of enamel benefit from simple techniques such as use of a SEALANT to protect the surface of the teeth or BONDING to create a new, smooth surface. Patients with Type II, Type III, or Type IV AI who have badly malformed teeth or missing teeth often require more radical restoration such as CROWNS to cover existing teeth and DENTURES (partial or full) to replace missing teeth. Some patients require orthodontic treatment to correct malocclusion.

To achieve the best dental and psychological results, dentists usually advise beginning restoration very early in life. Before restoration begins, the patient often undergoes periodontal treatment to remove CALCULUS (hardened deposits) on and between misaligned teeth, as well as various rinses and/or antibiotics to reduce any related inflammation.

Risk Factors and Preventive Measures

Amelogenesis imperfecta is an inherited condition transmitted as a dominant trait, which means that if one parent has AI and passes the dominant gene to the child, the child will also have the condition. Other than the family history, there is no known risk factor for amelogenesis imperfecta and no known preventive measure.

See also CALCULUS, DENTAL; GENETICS.

American Association of Women Dentists   See WOMEN'S DENTAL ASSOCIATIONS.

American Dental Association (ADA)   The American Dental Association was founded in 1859 by 26 representatives of contemporary dental societies meeting at Niagara Falls, New York. Today, as the world's largest and oldest dental association, ADA represents more than 150,000 American dentists in 55 states and territories and more than 500 local dental societies/associations practicing one or more of the nine ADA-approved dental specialties: PUBLIC HEALTH DENTISTRY, ENDODONTICS, ORAL AND MAXILLOFACIAL PATHOLOGY, ORAL AND MAXILLOFACIAL RADIOLOGY, ORAL AND MAXILLOFACIAL SURGERY, ORTHODONTICS AND DENTOFACIAL ORTHOPEDICS, PEDIATRIC DENTISTRY, PERIODONTICS, and PROSTHODONTICS.

To serve the needs of its members and their patients, ADA:

- oversees the Commission on Dental Accreditation, the national accrediting group for dental schools and postgraduate studies programs.
- runs the Council of Dental Therapeutics to evaluate products for oral health and, where

appropriate, grant these products the ADA Seal of Acceptance.

- promotes a strict code of professional ethics (see ETHICS, DENTAL CODE OF).
- publishes the *Journal of the American Dental Association* and other educational and news publications.
- maintains a library of dental literature at its headquarters in Chicago.
- maintains a comprehensive Web site (www.ADA.org) for patients and dental professionals.
- provides grants for dental research, education, and scholarship through the ADA Foundation.
- advocates for public health dental issues such as water fluoridation and issue-oriented events such as "Give a Kid a Smile Week."

American Dental Association Seal of Acceptance
The ADA Seal of Acceptance, first awarded in 1931, identifies for consumers dental products such as toothpaste, dental floss, toothbrushes, and mouth rinses that meet the association's standards of quality and effectiveness.

The seal is awarded for a five-year period, after which it must be renewed. When the seal is displayed on a product, the product must also carry a statement explaining why ADA approved the product. For example, the statement for a fluoridated toothpaste with the ADA Seal of Acceptance reads: "The ADA Council on Scientific Affairs' Acceptance of [product name] is based on its finding that the product is effective in helping to prevent and reduce tooth decay, when used as directed." The ADA Seal appears only on consumer products; professional products are evaluated in an ADA newsletter for dental professionals.

For more information on the ADA Seal of Acceptance, see "ADA Seal of Acceptance: Frequently Asked Questions (FAQ)" at www.ada.org/ada/seal/faq.asp.

See DENTISTRY; WOMEN'S DENTAL ASSOCIATIONS.

analgesic Any substance that produces analgesia, the relief of pain without a loss of consciousness, as opposed to anesthesia, the relief of pain with loss of consciousness. Analgesics are commonly used to reduce pain after surgery, including dental surgery.

Analgesics are classified as opioids or non-opioids. Opioids are natural derivatives or synthetic compounds that imitate opium, drugs that interrupt the transmission of pain impulses to and from the brain to other parts of the body. Opioids may be addictive; they are available only on prescription. Non-opioids such as acetaminophen (Tylenol and similar products) and the nonsteroidal anti-inflammatories (NSAIDs) such as aspirin, ibuprofen, and naproxen, are not addictive. These drugs alleviate pain by reducing the body's production of prostaglandins, natural chemicals that enable the body to perceive pain.

Although many analgesics are sold over the counter without a prescription, these drugs, like all medicines, have risks as well as benefits. For example, aspirin, the most common analgesic, is an anticoagulant (or blood thinner) that increases the time it takes for blood to clot; when taken by a person (most commonly a child) suffering from a viral infection such as the flu, aspirin may cause Reye's Syndrome, a potentially fatal reaction characterized by vomiting, irritability, confusion, convulsions, and loss of consciousness. Acetaminophen, considered a safe alternative to aspirin for children with viral infections, has its own drawbacks. Taken by a person who customarily has more than three alcohol drinks a day, it may cause liver failure and death.

See also ANESTHETIC/ANESTHETICS.

anchorage A base to support the bands or wires used in orthodontics to move teeth. There are two main classes of constructed anchorages: *intraoral* and *extraoral*.

Intraoral anchorages are anchorages situated inside the mouth; they are used in orthodontics or to wire a fractured jaw shut. The most basic anchorage, called a *simple anchorage,* is a tooth. An intermaxillary anchorage is an appliance linking a tooth on one jaw to an anchorage on the other—for example, a link from a band on a tooth on the upper to an anchorage on the lower jaw or vice versa. An intramaxillary anchorage is a link from a band on a tooth on one jaw to an anchorage on another tooth on the same jaw.

An intraoral anchorage may serve as a connection for headgear, a device such as a FACEBOW that circles the head and is connected to the intraoral anchorage, maintaining the pressure that moves the teeth.

Extraoral anchorages are appliances that sit outside the mouth, linked to bands on the teeth via small hooks or elastic bands. A cervical anchorage is an appliance resting at the back of the neck. A cranial anchorage is an appliance resting at the back of the head. A facial anchorage is an appliance resting on the chin or forehead.

The benefit of the intraoral as opposed to the extraoral anchorage is that the first is permanently in place and does not require the patient to put on and take off an appliance.

anemia   A condition characterized by a decrease in the number of red cells in the blood leading to a decrease in hemoglobin, the molecule in the blood that carries oxygen to every cell in the body. Some symptoms of anemia are present in the mouth and may be noticed by a dentist. Dentists must also consider the condition and take precautions when treating anemic patients.

Types of Anemia

The common causes of anemia are excessive blood loss, nutritional deficiency, an inherited disorder of the red blood cells, or injury to the bone marrow (the spongy material in bones where blood cells are made).

Anemias Related to Excessive Bleeding   Anemia may result from an obvious wound or heavy menstrual bleeding. "Hidden blood loss," such as gastric bleeding caused by an ulcer or medicines such as aspirin and other NSAIDs (nonsteroidal anti-inflammatory drugs), which irritate the lining of the stomach, may also be the cause. The treatment is to close the wound or change the medication.

Anemia Related to a Dietary Deficiency   When the diet lacks sufficient amounts of iron, folate, or vitamin B_{12}, anemia may occur. Adding supplements or food rich in these vitamins to the diet relieves or prevents the anemia.

Anemia Related to an Inherited Disorder   Inherited types of anemia include pernicious anemia (an inability to absorb vitamin B_{12}, most common among people of Scandinavian descent), sickle-cell anemia (a defect in the red blood cells most common among blacks, but found as well among people of Mediterranean or Middle Eastern descent), and thalassemia (a reduced ability to produce hemoglobin, most common among people of Mediterranean descent). Although genetic testing may reveal that a person carries the trait for these anemias, there are no preventive measures other than to forego having children. The most common treatment is transfusion.

Anemia Related to Damaged Bone Marrow (aplastic anemia)   Following an injury to the bone marrow anemia may develop. The spongy material inside bones produces red blood cells, white blood cells, and platelets, the particles that enable blood to clot. The trigger for anemia may be exposure to radiation (including radiation treatment for certain kinds of cancer) and/or chemotherapy; exposure to toxic chemicals; exposure to some medicines used to treat infections or rheumatoid arthritis; or a viral infection. Another possible cause is a previously dormant autoimmune disorder exacerbated by pregnancy. Prevention requires avoiding the triggers; again, the most common treatment is transfusion.

Dental Symptoms of Anemia

The symptoms common to all anemias are fatigue, weakness, shortness of breath, and dizziness. Some forms of anemia make the patient more susceptible to infection.

The dental/oral signs and symptoms of anemia include pale gums, cracks at the corner of mouth, and atrophic glossitis, which is a (flattening of the papillae (natural bumps on the tongue), making the tongue look smooth, slick, and redder than normal. X-rays of the jaw may show some changes in the bone structure. Patients with chronic anemias, such as sickle-cell anemia or thalassemia, may heal very slowly after any injury, including dental surgery. Those with very low red blood cell counts or whose blood clots abnormally fast or slowly are poor candidates for anesthesia or sedation because their blood carries reduced amounts of oxygen.

Dental Treatment for Anemic Patients

Dental treatment for patients with anemias is aimed a reducing infection and preventing bleeding. For example, to reduce the risk of infection, the dentist may prescribe oral antibiotics or an antibiotic rinse before any procedure. Prior to a major treatment such as extraction or periodontal surgery on an anemic patient whose blood clots slowly, the dentist, in consultation with the patient's doctor, may prescribe drugs to encourage blood clotting and reduce the risk of excessive bleeding. During the procedure, the dentist will tailor the anesthesia/analgesia to the patient, often avoiding injections that can cause bleeding.

See also INFECTION CONTROL.

anesthetic/anesthetics Any substance or technique that interrupts one or more of the chemical reactions by which the body transmits pain messages from the site of an injury to the brain, producing pain relief known as anesthesia.

The earliest anesthetics were natural substances such as alcohol and sedative plants such as cannabis, kef, hashish, hemp (active ingredient: tetrahydrocannabinol), coca (the source of cocaine), and poppies (the source of opium

and morphine). Each of these substances was effective in reducing pain; in large amounts some, such as alcohol, were able to render the patient unconscious. But it was difficult if not impossible to administer exact doses, and many had unpleasant side effects such as nausea or hallucination.

Although there is some dispute about who first introduced surgical anesthesia to the United States, there is no doubt that American dentists played an important role in the process. New England dentist William Thomas Green Morton (1819–68) is usually given the credit for bringing anesthesia into the operating room—or the dentist's office. In reality, it seems likely that another dentist, HORACE WELLS, treated a patient with ether gas before Morton did. But Morton, who had tried alcohol and opium before turning to ether gas, made his mark with the successful use of the inhaled anesthetic gas during a procedure to remove a tumor performed by John Collins Warren in October 1846 at Massachusetts General Hospital. After the surgery was complete, Warren turned to the audience in the operating theater and spoke the famous phrase, "Gentlemen, this is no humbug," thus cementing Morton's reputation as the man who enabled doctors to perform painless surgery.

Ether and nitrous oxide both had serious drawbacks. They have unpleasant side effects (nausea, vomiting, hallucinations, and a lingering "hangover" effect), and they are flammable. Modern inhaled or injected anesthetics produce a quick loss of consciousness and an equally quick return to consciousness with minimal adverse effects.

Types of Anesthetics

There are four basic types of anesthetics, characterized by the area of the body they affect and of the duration of the loss of consciousness they produce. A local anesthetic is a substance applied to skin or mucous membrane or injected under the surface to relieve pain in a small area of the body, such as a tooth. A regional anesthetic is a substance injected near or into a cluster of nerves to relieve pain in a larger area such as both the tongue and lower lip. A general anesthetic, which may be inhaled or injected intravenously, is a substance that causes loss of consciousness during major surgery. A short-acting anesthetic, which may be injected or inhaled, produces loss of consciousness that ends as soon as the administration of the anesthetic stops.

Dental Anesthesia

The most common dental anesthetics are local anesthetics such as lidocaine or bupivacaine (a longer-lasting drug), injected into the area in which the dentist is working. For surgery requiring longer periods of time or extending over a large area of the mouth, the dentist may perform a nerve block, the use of a regional anesthetic to block a large nerve and its branches. For example, a dentist might block the infraorbital nerve controlling sensation from the area below the eye to the top lip, or the mental nerve, which controls sensation from the lower lip down to the chin.

In dentistry, nerve blocks are commonly used to block sensation to one side of the mouth from the following nerves:

- *Anterior superior alveolar nerve:* Blocking this nerve numbs the pulp inside the incisors and canine teeth and the inside of the cheek on one side of the upper jaw.
- *Middle superior alveolar nerve:* Blocking this nerve numbs the pulp and soft tissue around the first and second premolars and the first molar on one side of the upper jaw.
- *Nasopalatine nerve:* Blocking this nerve numbs the gum surrounding the front teeth on one side of the upper jaw and the front of the hard palate (the roof of the mouth).
- *Greater palatine nerve:* Blocking this nerve numbs the tissue around the back teeth on the upper jaw and the back of the hard palate (the roof of the mouth).

- *Infraorbital nerve:* Blocking this nerve numbs the pulp and the soft tissue of the incisors and canine on one side of the upper jaw, as well as the adjoining upper lip and side of the nose.
- *V2 nerve:* Blocking this nerve numbs half of the upper jaw, the upper teeth, the lip, cheek, and under-eye area on one side of the face. (Also called the maxillary nerve.)
- *Inferior alveolar nerve:* Blocking this nerve numbs the lower lip on one side of the mouth.
- *Lingual nerve:* Blocking this nerve numbs the gum and the tongue on one side of the lower jaw.
- *Buccal nerve:* Blocking this nerve numbs the soft tissue inside the cheek next to the back teeth on one side of the lower jaw.
- *Mental nerve:* Blocking this nerve numbs the pulp and soft tissue of the incisors, canine teeth, first and second premolars, and lip on one side of the lower jaw.

Dental anesthesia is administered via a syringe fitted with a cartridge containing a measured dose of the drug, often combined with a vasoconstrictor (a drug that constricts blood vessels and reduces bleeding).

See also ANALGESIC; NERVES.

Angle, Edward Hartley (1855–1930)   Edward Hartley Angle is the American dentist credited with establishing orthodontics as a dental specialty. In this regard, Angle defined three classes of MALOCCLUSION in *Treatment of Malocclusions of Teeth* (Philadelphia: S.S. White Dental Manufacturing Co., 1887) and then went on to create and promote a wide variety of treatment regimens and appliances still used in straightening teeth.

In 1874, when he was 18, Angle served as an apprentice to a local dentist in his hometown of Herrick, Pennsylvania. At age 20, he applied to and was accepted at the Pennsylvania College of Dental Surgery in Philadelphia, where he earned his dental degree in 1897. Angle first practiced dentistry in Towanda, Pennsylvania, where his main interest was in what he called "regulating" the teeth (i.e., straightening them). He then began his career teaching orthodontics at the University of Minnesota, then at Northwestern University, and later at Washington University in Saint Louis.

His first exposure to the broader dental world occurred in 1887 when Angle delivered a speech to the Ninth International Medical Congress convened in Washington, D.C., entitled "Notes on Orthodontia with a New System of Regulation and Retention." This showed his classifications of malocclusion and the novel wire devices he proposed to correct defects in a patient's bite.

In 1900, while practicing in Saint Louis, he founded the Angle School of Orthodontia, the first postgraduate school in orthodontics. Seven years later he began publishing *The American Orthodontist,* the first professional journal for dentists specializing in orthodontia. Eventually, Angle and his school migrated from Saint Louis to New York City to New London, Connecticut, and finally to Pasadena, California, in 1916. In his lifetime, Angle taught nearly 200 students, among them eight women and 33 dentists from countries outside the United States, virtually all of whom went on to become leaders in orthodontic teaching, practice, and research.

Today, the Edward H. Angle Society and the E. H. Angle Education and Research Foundation remain vital forces in orthodontic teaching and research.

See also BROADBENT, B. HOLLY; SCHOOLS OF DENTISTRY; TWEED, CHARLES H.

anodontia Anodontia (from the Greek prefix *a-* meaning "not," and the word *dontus* or *donto-* meaning "tooth") is a congenital defect that occurs most frequently in persons with other genetic defects, commonly Down syndrome; one 2007 Brazilian study showed proven or sus-

pected anodontia in 30.9 percent of the subjects with Down syndrome. People with anodontia lack tooth buds, the tissue from which teeth develop, and thus fail to develop any teeth. The opposite of anodontia is hyperdontia, the development of extra teeth, most commonly in the front of the jaw. Like anodontia, hyperdontia is often associated with other genetic or developmental defects. For example, in 2003, when researchers in the Department of Pediatric Dentistry at the Oregon Health and Science University School of Dentistry examined the records of 120 cleft lip and/or palate patients at the Iowa Craniofacial Anomalies Research Center, they identified a positive association between a cleft and hyperdontia.

Symptoms and Diagnostic Path

Because all primary teeth usually appear by age three, anodontia and hyperdontia are visible when the dentist examines the child's mouth. All permanent teeth, except for the back molars (wisdom teeth) usually appear by age 14, so the absence is also visible on examination. Dental X-rays can confirm that the teeth are missing rather than that they have simply not erupted through the gum.

Treatment Options and Outlook

Anodontia is treated with DENTURES appropriate to the number of teeth that are missing. For example, if only one tooth is missing, an artificial tooth can be bonded/wired to the next tooth in line. If several teeth are missing, the patient may be fitted with partial dentures, crowns, implants, or a bridge. If all teeth are missing, the patient can be fitted with full denture attached to implants set into the jaw. Hyperdontia is treated by removing the extra teeth.

Risk Factors and Preventive Measures

The National Institutes of Health classifies anodontia as a rare disorder. In 2005, the National Center for Research Resources began recruiting volunteers with anodontia and hyperdontia for a study designed to identify the exact gene or genes responsible.

See also GENETICS; IMPLANTOLOGY.

antibiotic prophylaxis Antibiotics are medical drugs that destroy or inhibit the growth of disease-causing organisms. A broad-spectrum antibiotic is a drug considered effective against the two main classifications of bacteria, gram-negative bacteria and gram-positive bacteria. Antibiotics are used in dentistry to reduce the risk of infection after dental surgery and to reduce the incidence of periodontal infection leading to bone loss.

Beginning in the 1980s, the American Heart Association (AHA) and the AMERICAN DENTAL ASSOCIATION (ADA) recommended that patients with certain heart conditions take antibiotics (usually penicillin) before routine dental treatment such as tooth cleaning and extractions. This treatment, known as antibiotic prophylaxis or preventive antibiotic therapy, is believed to reduce the risk of infective endocarditis (IE). Infective endocarditis is a rare but potentially life-threatening infection of the heart lining or valves caused by bacteria normally found in the mouth and skin traveling through the bloodstream to the heart.

In 2007, AHA and ADA reversed this policy, issuing revised guidelines that recommend preventive antibiotics only for patients at high risk of serious damage from IE. This includes patients who:

- have previously had IE
- have certain congenital heart defects
- have recently gotten an artificial patch to repair a congenital heart defect
- have an artificial heart valve
- have cardiac valve problems following a heart transplant
- have had a joint replacement

The new guidelines, endorsed by the Infectious Diseases Society of America and by the Pediatric Infectious Diseases Society, recognize that even daily brushing and flossing may send oral bacteria into the bloodstream. In addition, for many patients the risk of adverse reactions, such as a potentially fatal allergic reaction, from preventive antibiotics outweighs the benefits. This includes patients with:

- rheumatic heart disease
- mitral valve prolapse (failure of the valve between the pumping chambers of the heart to close properly)
- bicuspid valve disease (failure of the valve between the heart and the aorta to close properly)
- calcified aortic stenosis (hardened plaque deposits in the aorta, the large artery leading out from the heart)
- some congenital heart valve defects
- hypertrophic cardiomyopathy (thickening of the heart muscle)

For these people, normal daily oral hygiene is more valuable than preventive antibiotics in protecting against IE.

Another consideration in limiting the use of preventive antibiotics is that widespread use of these drugs contributes to the development of drug-resistant bacteria, an ongoing problem.

aphthous ulcer Recurrent aphthous ulcer (RAU), from the Greek and Latin word *aphtha* meaning "eruption." It is more familiarly known as a canker sore, from the Latin and French words *cancre*.

An aphthous ulcer is a small, painful round ulcer on the soft tissue inside the mouth—that is, the inside lining of the lips and cheek, the tongue, and the soft palate. A pemphigoid aphthous ulcer is an aphthous ulcer triggered by a chronic disease of the immune system, for example HIV/AIDS or systemic lupus erythematosus (SLE).

Symptoms and Diagnostic Path

An aphthous ulcer is identified by its appearance and location, a small ulcer with a white or gray center and a red outer rim found on the soft tissue inside the mouth. Aphthous ulcers may occur singly or in clusters. Unlike a cold sore, which is a herpes infection that occurs most frequently on the outside of the lip, an aphthous ulcer is not contagious.

Treatment Options and Outlook

In most cases, treatment is unnecessary because the sore becomes less painful and begins to heal within several days, with complete healing occurring in two to three weeks.

Over-the-counter pain medicines (acetaminophen, aspirin, ibuprofen) are useful for relieving the discomfort of a canker sore. Other common ways to alleviate the discomfort include avoiding acidic or spicy foods or foods with sharp, irritating edges (i.e., chips, crisp crackers, crunchy raw vegetables); using a very soft toothbrush near the sore; rinsing with warm salt water or a solution prescribed by the dentist; and covering the sore with a small dab of a paste of baking soda and water. One may also apply a nonprescription local oral anesthetic cream, gel, or spray as directed by the dentist.

Risk Factors and Preventive Measures

Although some experts believe that aphthous ulcers are bacterial or viral infections, the actual cause of these small ulcers has never been conclusively identified. However, common stress factors such as fatigue, a seasonal or food allergy, the onset of the menstrual period, or emotional distress may increase the risk. So may an injury such as a bitten lip or cheek.

More serious triggers include a weakened immune system, as in a patient with HIV/AIDS. Nutritional deficiencies such as a lack of the B vitamins B_{12} and folic acid or the minerals iron and zinc have also been linked to aphthous ulcers. Finally, a tendency to aphthous ulcers appears to run in families. Although the sores may appear at any age, a first episode most frequently occurs between the ages of 10 and 40.

apicoectomy Also known as epicetomy or root-end resection, apicoectomy is endodontic surgery to remove all or part of the root of a tooth as a way to save a tooth in or around which inflammation or infection persist after a ROOT CANAL TREATMENT. The name of the procedure comes from the apex, or the end of the tooth's root; an infection around the root of the tooth is called an apical or periapical infection.

The process by which the root develops, or by which it closes after surgery when material such as calcium hydroxide is inserted to stimulate the growth of new tissue, is apexification. Apical curettage is surgery to remove damaged or disease tissue and bone around the root.

Procedure

After numbing the area with local ANESTHETIC, the endodontist loosens the gum tissue near the tooth root to examine the bottom of the tooth and the surrounding bone. She removes the apex (tip of the root) along with any infected surrounding tissue. Once the tip and tissue have been removed, the endodontist may place a small filling at the root to seal off the root canal. If required, she will suture the incision closed to help it heal neatly. Provided there are no complications, the sutures are usually removed within a week to 10 days.

Risks and Complications

Slight bleeding, swelling, and pain are common complications after this type of surgery. Severe or increasing pain or swelling may be signs of infection and should be reported to the endodontist.

Outlook and Lifestyle Modifications

Once the wound has healed and the sutures have been removed, the tooth should feel completely normal.

appliance, dental A device used to improve dental/oral health or function. Dental appliances include restorations such as DENTURES; more commonly the term is used to refer to devices used to move teeth during orthodontic treatment.

Some common orthodontic dental appliances include:

- The Andresen appliance, created by Norwegian orthodontist Viggo Andresen, is used to strengthen the muscles around the mouth as an aide to moving the teeth.
- The Begg appliance, developed by Australian orthodontist P. R. Begg, is fixed in the mouth using round wires to move the teeth.
- The Bimler appliance, named for German-born oral surgeon Hans Peter Bimler, is used to stabilize fractures of the jaw.
- The Crozat appliance, created by New Orleans orthodontist George Crozat, is a heavy, removable wire device that fits behind the teeth.
- The Frankel appliance, developed by German Rolf Frankel, is used to improve occlusion (the way the teeth meet) by moving the top teeth forward and strengthening the facial muscles.
- The Hawley appliance is a retainer.
- The Kloehn appliance, also known as the orthodontic facebow, is an extraoral (outside the mouth) device created by S. J. Kloehn and used to move teeth during orthodontic treatment.

See also ORTHODONTIC BRACES; ORTHODONTICS AND DENTOFACIAL ORTHOPEDICS; RESTORATION; RETAINER; WIRE.

arch A curved structure; the dental arch is the structure comprising the teeth and the bony ridge holding the sockets (alveoli) into which the teeth fit. The dental arch of the upper jaw is larger than that of the lower JAW, so that when the mouth is closed, the teeth in a normal upper jaw extend slightly out in front and at the sides over those in the lower jaw.

The shape of the dental arch may be described as ovoid, U-shaped, tapering, or trapezoidal. An ovoid dental arch is one that curves so smoothly that placing two pictures of the arch together at the open end (at the molars) forms an oval; a U-shaped dental arch is a smooth curve, but broader than the ovoid shape. A tapering dental arch has a more pointed front end; a trapezoidal dental arch is also pointed, but less so than the tapering arch.

The dental arch may also be characterized by the number of the teeth in the mouth. For example, a dentulous dental arch has all the natural teeth in place; an edentulous dental arch is missing all the natural teeth; a partially edentulous dental arch is one from which some natural teeth are missing.

See ALVEOLUS; EXPANDER.

Atkinson, William Henry (1815–1891) The first president of the AMERICAN DENTAL ASSOCIATION, Atkinson originally trained as a physician but later turned to dentistry. Atkinson, who was born in Pennsylvania, built a successful practice in Cleveland before moving to New York. As an innovator, he is credited with a number of important methods used in dentistry. For example, he reintroduced the hand mallet to condense gold fillings and designed new instruments to build contour fillings. He was a frequent contributor to dental journals and a student of the natural sciences. His wide range of professional interests include the diagnosis of dental conditions, the loss of tooth enamel, the replacement of lost teeth, and the development of medicines to be used in dentistry. Atkinson was also a pioneer in dental economics, the first dentist in Cleveland to bill higher fees for dental surgery than for plain dentistry, and the first to bill his patients based on the time he spent with them.

atrophy The word *atrophy,* from the Latin *atrophia* meaning "badly nourished," describes a decrease in body tissue due to illness, injury, or failure to use a body part. The last, known as disuse atrophy, occurs when a muscle is not exercised either because a person voluntarily refrains from exercise or because he is bedridden or because the muscle is paralyzed. Gravitational atrophy is a loss of muscle and bone tissue experienced by astronauts after even short periods in a gravity-free environment in space.

In dentistry, the most common form of atrophy is loss of bony tissue in the jaw due to repeated infections linked to PERIODONTAL DISEASE. In severe cases, the loss of bone in the jaw may be so extensive that ordinary implants are too short to be useful. However, the results of one pilot study reported in the *Journal of Prosthetic Dentistry* in 2008 suggest that extra-long implants placed outside the upper jaw and anchored in the cheekbones may provide a solution. In this study with 21 women and eight men, the patients were comfortable and able to function effectively with extra-long implants that appeared intact and stable after one year.

See HEMIFACIAL ATROPHY.

avulsed tooth See "KNOCKED-OUT TOOTH."

baby bottle tooth decay   See DECAY.

baby teeth   See TEETH.

bacteria, oral   See DECAY; HALITOSIS; INFECTION CONTROL; MOUTHWASH; PERIODONTAL DISEASE; SALIVA.

bad breath   See HALITOSIS.

base metal alloy   An alloy is a mixture of two or more metals. A base metal, also known as a non-noble metal, differs from the precious or noble metals such as gold because it is common, and it oxidizes (tarnishes) when exposed to air. Base metal alloys are used in dentistry as building material for some parts of dental restorations such as crowns, fixed bridges, and partial dentures.

Base metal alloys are tough and durable, but they have drawbacks. First, they expand when heated and contract when cold, which means that, as fillings, they may be uncomfortable (at least initially). Second, they are silver colored, which means that they would be cosmetically unattractive if used in a place where the repair is easily visible. Finally, the base metal nickel is a common allergen that may trigger a reaction in sensitive persons such as those who develop contact dermatitis when wearing jewelry that is not gold, silver, or platinum.

See CAVITY; GOLD (AU).

Bass, Charles Cassidy M.D. (1875–1975)   Bass was a medical doctor and microbiologist, not a dentist, on the faculty of Tulane University in New Orleans, where he specialized in research on the organisms responsible for tropical diseases, primarily malaria and hookworm. However, he soon became intrigued by the microorganisms naturally present in saliva, and this study led him to a theory linking these organisms to the development of dental PLAQUE and then to dental decay.

Having proven his theory, Bass went on to create an effective method of tooth brushing and oral hygiene known as the modified Bass technique (see TOOTHBRUSH), the most common technique of brushing currently taught in dental schools in the United States. Bass, whose work with dental bacteria earned him the honorary title, Father of Preventive Dentistry, eventually served as dean of the Tulane Medical School (1922–40), where bronze doors were hung in the library in his honor in 1981.

biofeedback   Behavior modification technique designed to increase the patient's ability to influence normally automatic body functions such as blood flow, blood pressure, body temperature, brain wave activity, breathing, gastrointestinal functions, heart rate, and muscle tension. For example, one stratagem used in biofeedback is to visualize an iceberg in an effort to lower body temperature so as to reduce tension, alleviate pain, and minimize the effects of a condition or situation such as anxiety during dental treatment or pain after a dental procedure.

Procedure

During a biofeedback training session, a therapist applies electrical sensors to different parts of the patient's body to monitor the body's physiological responses to stress and then feed the information back to the patient via auditory and visual "cues" such as a beeping sound or a flashing light.

With this feedback, the patient can begin to associate behavior such as clenching the jaw and/or grinding the teeth with stress and then to alter the behavior and reduce stress. In some cases, the patient is given a portable biofeedback device that enables him to practice the technique at home.

Repeated studies show that persons trained in biofeedback can use the technique to affect a number of otherwise involuntary body functions. For example, biofeedback has been used to help slow the heartbeat, control respiration, ease discomfort due to gastrointestinal muscle spasms, and relax blood vessels so as to lower blood pressure and relieve conditions such as migraine headaches and Raynaud's phenomenon ("cold hands") caused by swollen or constricted blood vessels. The technique also seems to be a valuable tool in alleviating chronic pain and sleep disorders.

Risks and Complications

There are no known health risks or complications associated with biofeedback.

Outlook and Lifestyle Modifications

A patient who is able to master the biofeedback technique is likely to experience a positive result in alleviating symptoms of various conditions such as those listed above.

biopsy Diagnostic examination of body tissue, such as the inside of the cheek, the gums, LIPS, and TONGUE, commonly but not exclusively to test for the presence of malignant cells.

Procedure

Most dental biopsies are done as outpatient procedures; all require at least a local anesthetic. Depending on the site and size of the sample to be removed, some biopsies may require stitches to close the wound. The types of biopsies used in dentistry include aspiration biopsy, bone biopsy, brush biopsy, excision biopsy, punch biopsy, and shave biopsy.

Aspiration Biopsy This procedure, also known as a needle biopsy or a fine needle biopsy, obtains a specimen by inserting a hollow needle through the skin or mucous membrane into the area to be examined, such as a tumor in the mouth.

Bone Biopsy This procedure, to examine a sample of bone tissue, most commonly to diagnose a bone tumor or to identify the cause of bone pain or the condition of bone, is performed with local anesthesia, allowing the dental surgeon to cut a small incision in the skin and insert a biopsy needle into the bone to extract tissue. A biopsy requiring a larger sample or one where a malignant tumor is suspected is performed under general anesthesia so that the tumor can be removed immediately if necessary. Occasionally, a dentist or plastic surgeon may perform a bone biopsy to ascertain the health of the bone before performing a reconstructive procedure.

Brush biopsy This procedure is performed by rotating a very small sterile brush against a suspicious area to remove cells for examination.

Excision Biopsy This procedure surgically removes an entire lesion, such as a white spot on the gum, lip, or tongue.

Punch Biopsy This procedure employs a sharp, round instrument to pierce the skin or mucous membrane to remove a cylindrical-shaped piece of tissue.

Shave Biopsy This procedure uses a sharp blade to remove a lesion sitting above the surface of the skin or mucous membrane.

Risks and Complications

Soreness and/or swelling at the site are common after a biopsy. Less frequent complications may include excessive bleeding and/or infection of the skin, mucous membrane, or bone. Fracture of the bone is a rare complication of bone biopsy.

Outlook and Lifestyle Modifications

Biopsy is an important diagnostic tool that enables the physician to determine the nature of the patient's lesion and thus choose an appropriate treatment.

birth defects   See ANODONTIA; CLEFT LIP AND/OR PALATE; DENTIN; ENAMEL; FUSED TEETH; JAW; TONGUE.

bisphosphonates   Medical drugs that interfere with the activity of osteoclasts, body cells that normally break down old bone tissue so that it can be absorbed and replaced with new bone tissue (see BONE). As a result, people taking bisphosphonates loose less bone tissue, which means that their bones stay denser and should theoretically be more resistant to fracture. Based on this assumption, doctors have prescribed bisphosphonates to treat conditions such as osteoporosis (age-related loss of bone density) and bone-destroying metastases in cancer patients. Examples of bisphosphonates, also called diphosphonates, are: alendronate (Fosamax), alendronic acid, cyclical etidronate (Didronel PMO), ibandronate (Boniva), pamidronate (Aredia), risedronate (Actonel), tiludronate (Skelid), and zoledronic acid (Reclast, Zometa).

In the early 2000s, soon after bisphosphonates were introduced, reports began to circulate linking the drugs to an increased risk of progressive, untreatable osteonecrosis (bone death) of the jaw, a disfiguring condition often accompanied by unremitting pain. At the start, the problem was blamed on the more potent intravenous bisphosphonates, but in May 2005 a report in the *Journal of Oral and Maxillofacial Surgery* described 63 patients with bone death in the jaw, seven of whom had taken the less potent oral form of the drug. Since then, warnings about the adverse effects of bisphosphonates have proliferated.

- In August 2007, a review of the articles regarding osteonecrosis of the jaw among patients with osteoporosis who have been treated with biphosphonates showed that the risk factors for adverse effects from these drugs include older women who have had invasive dental surgery such as extractions, dental implants, or ROOT CANAL TREATMENT, an alarming discovery given that older women are often treated with bone conservation and replacement therapies.

- In January 2008, the Food and Drug Administration issued an FDA Alert warning that taking oral bisphosphonates had been linked to an increased risk of muscle, bone, and joint pain that might appear within days, months, or years after the patient began taking the drug. Previously, bone pain, along with fever and chills, had been linked only to an acute reaction following the administration of intravenous bisphosphonates.

- February 2008, data from a study at the University of British Columbia and Vancouver Coastal Health Research Institute study showed that taking bisphosphonates may triple the risk of osteonecrosis of the jaw.

- In April 2008, researchers at the University of Southern California's School of Dentistry reported in the *Journal of Oral Maxillofacial Surgery* that they had found a direct link between taking bisphosphonates and increased presence of biofilm (a naturally occurring layer of bacterial debris) in the jawbone.

- Finally, in the same month, a report in the *Archives of Internal Medicine* warned that taking bisphosphonates might increase the risk of atrial fibrillation (an irregular heartbeat).

As of this writing, it remains unclear exactly how many patients have suffered osteonecrosis of the jaw after taking bisphosphonates. Also unknown is whether the risk is significantly higher with the intravenous form of the drugs, and exactly how the drug triggers the bone loss. One possible explanation, bolstered by the results of the April 2008 study at the University of Southern California, is that interrupting the body's natural cycle of bone loss and replacement leaves worn-out bone in place and that this old bone is more sensitive to bacterial invasion, infection, and destruction. But that remains to be proven.

bite   See MALOCCLUSION; OCCLUSION.

Black, Greene Vardiman (1836–1915) Self-taught and apprenticed early American dentist, author of *Operative Dentistry,* a two-volume work that remained a standard of dental teaching for nearly half a century. Black also developed a system for classifying dental caries, introduced various new techniques, created an AMALGAM for filling teeth, and produced standards for surgical procedures. He invented dental instruments and appliances such as the foot-powered drill engine and the gnathodynamometer (an instrument for measuring the force exerted by a person's teeth when biting), and was among the first in dentistry to use visual aids when teaching dentistry.

Black taught at the Missouri Dental College, which awarded him a D.D.S. degree in 1877, and eventually moved on to the Chicago College of Dental Surgery (later the Loyola University School of Dentistry). He received a medical degree from Chicago Medical School, and became dean of the Northwestern University Dental School (since closed). Today, the G. V. Black collection of 43 manuscripts, 55 letters, and several photographs covering the period between 1867 and 1915 is housed in the Galter Health Sciences Library at Northwestern University.

bleaching, tooth   See TOOTH; WHITENING.

blood circulation   See CIRCULATORY SYSTEM.

blood count   See COMPLETE BLOOD COUNT (CBC).

blood gases   Blood gases, shorthand for *blood gas test,* measures the levels of oxygen (O), carbon dioxide (CO_2), and bicarbonate (HCO_3) in the blood plasma, the clear liquid in blood.

CO_2 is a waste product eliminated through the lungs and kidneys. HCO_3, a compound that helps maintain a balance between acid and base, is regulated through the kidneys. Any imbalance between oxygen and carbon dioxide or any abnormal increase or decrease in bicarbonate upsets the body's pH (acid/base balance) and endangers the patient.

As a result, blood gases are a valuable tool for determining the status of patients anesthetized for surgery, including dental surgery, as well as those with respiratory disorders such as COPD (chronic obstructive pulmonary disease), kidney disease, or head or neck injuries that may interfere with breathing.

Examples of oxygen/CO_2 imbalances are:

- *Respiratory acidosis:* This condition, characterized by an excess of CO_2 and a lowered pH, may result when the lungs are unable to eliminate CO_2.
- *Respiratory alkalosis:* This condition, characterized by lower than normal levels of CO_2 and a heightened pH, may occur when the lungs eliminate too much CO_2.
- *Metabolic acidosis:* This condition, characterized by too little HCO_3^- and a lowered pH, may occur when the kidneys cannot effectively regulate HCO_3^-.

• *Metabolic alkalosis:* This condition, characterized by an excess amount of HCO_3^- and a heightened pH, may result from low blood levels of potassium, perhaps due to chronic vomiting or an overdose of sodium bicarbonate (baking soda).

Bolton Standards of Dentofacial Developmental Growth   A method for evaluating the differences in size between teeth in the upper and lower jaws. The system, created in 1958 by American orthodontist A. Wayne Bolton, provides two measurements of ideal OCCLUSION (how the teeth meet when the jaws are closed). The measurements are ratios derived from facial images and X-rays of subjects gathered between 1931 and 1959 by researchers at Case Western Reserve School of Dentistry in Cleveland, Ohio.

The first Bolton measurement is the overall ideal ratio of the length of the mandibular ARCH to the length of the maxillary arch. Bolton put the ideal ratio at 91.3 percent, meaning that the length of the lower dental arch should be about 10 percent shorter than the length of the upper dental arch.

The second Bolton measurement is the ideal ratio of the width of the distance across the mouth between the back teeth (premolar and molars) on the lower JAW to the distance across the mouth between the back teeth on the upper jaw. Bolton put this ideal ratio at 77.2 percent, meaning that the ideal distance between the back teeth on the upper jaw is 22.8 percent longer than that between the back teeth on the lower jaw.

Bolton's system is used today when planning a course of orthodontic treatment to ameliorate the effects of teeth that are too large or too small or crowded together or set in an overbite (the upper teeth sit too far in front of the lower teeth when the jaws are closed) or an underbite (the front teeth sit behind the lower teeth when the jaws are closed).

See BROADBENT, B. HOLLY; MALOCCLUSION; ORTHODONTIC BRACES.

bonding   Dental procedure to repair chipped or cracked teeth, to replace the surface on discolored teeth, to fill in gaps between teeth, or to reshape or lengthen teeth. Bonding is also done to protect a tooth root that has been exposed due to gum recession by covering the surface of the tooth with dental COMPOSITE, a plastic-based material commonly used to fill dental cavities.

Porcelain VENEERS are also bonded (i.e., pasted) to the surface of the tooth, but the term bonding commonly refers to repairs made with composite.

Procedure

First, the tooth is etched with a mild acid solution to roughen the surface, which is then painted with a conditioning liquid that helps the bonding material stick to the surface. Next, the dentist applies the clear plastic bonding agent, and then one or more layers of a durable, puttylike resin/plastic material colored to match the natural teeth. The surface is then exposed to high-intensity light that cures (hardens) the plastic. Finally, once the surface has hardened, it is polished to smooth away any irregularities.

Risks and Complications

The only risk associated with bonding is an allergic reaction to resin compound. Some stages of the preparation—grinding down an edge, for example—may be uncomfortable, but if necessary, the dentist can remedy that by administering a local ANESTHETIC.

Outlook and Lifestyle Modifications

Because the plastic surfacing adds some bulk to the tooth, some patients experience a short period of adjustment to the "new" teeth.

The plastic surface itself is breakable and can be damaged simply by biting down on hard food or by nervous habits such as BRUXISM (grinding the teeth) or chewing on hard objects such as a pencil.

The plastic stains, cracks, or chips more easily than porcelain veneers or CROWNS, but the simple bonding procedure can be done in one session in the dentist's office while porcelain veneers must be made in a dental laboratory and require additional visits.

Bonded surfaces typically last from three to 10 years; exactly how long the surface remains intact depends on:

- how smoothly the composite is applied
- how the patient's teeth come together when biting
- how carefully the plastic surface is maintained during regular dental checkups that enable the dentist to identify and repair small chips or cracks before they become large enough to dislodge the entire bonded surface

bone Hard, multilayer, calcified connective tissue and the major component of the skeleton, including the bones that shape the head and face, enclose and protect the brain and the organs of smell, sight, and taste, and, in tandem with the facial muscles, make it possible to eat, speak, breathe, and create facial expressions.

Starting at the top of the face and moving downward, the facial bones that affect the oral cavity are:

- *ethmoid bone,* the floor of the front part of the skull and the roof of the nose
- *temporal bone,* front of the skull, above the eyes
- *orbit,* socket around the eye
- *lacrimal bone,* irregular thin bone of the round socket
- *nasal bone,* bone forming the structure of the nose

- *palatine bone,* bone behind the upper jaw, forming part of the nasal cavity and the socket around the eye
- *omer,* triangular bone at the center of the nostrils
- *zygoma,* cheekbone
- *maxilla,* upper jaw
- *mandible,* lower jaw
- *hyoid bone,* U-shape bone between the lower jaw and larynx

The Life Cycle of Bones

Bone is active, living tissue. Cells called osteoclasts continually destroy old bone tissue. Cells called osteoblasts continually build new tissue via bone morphogenetic protein, a natural or engineered growth factor identified and named in 1965 by orthopedic surgeon and researcher Marshall Urist (1914–2001).

As the body ages, it continues to resorb old cells at the normal rate, but the production of new cells declines, thus leading to a loss of bone density that may result in the condition called osteoporosis (from the Latin *os* meaning "bone" and *porus* meaning "passage" or "gap").

According to *Oral Health in America: A Report of the Surgeon General* (2000), some studies of postmenopausal women suggest that bone loss in the lower jaw may precede the skeletal bone loss seen in osteoporosis.

Activities that put stress on bone stimulate bone growth. Thus, just as weight-bearing exercises such as walking or weight lifting help keep the arms, legs, and spine strong, chewing and talking provide healthful stress for jawbones. The major causes of jawbone loss is severe PERIODONTAL DISEASE.

When a tooth is lost to an injury or periodontal disease, an implant replacement appears to act as an artificial root, stimulating the alveolar bone (the bone sockets in which the tooth sat) more efficiently than either removable or permanent dentures, thus helping to retain bone tissue in the jaw.

Counting and Classifying Human Bones

A newborn human being has as many as 300 separate and distinct bones. Some, such as those in the skull, wrist, and ankle, will eventually fuse to produce an adult body with 206 bones.

The longest bone in the human body is the thighbone, which grows to a length approximately 25 percent of the adult body's height. The smallest bone in the body is the stirrup bone in the middle ear, which is about one-tenth of an inch long.

Bones may be grouped into three broad categories. The first category are essentially tubes, the larger (long bones of the arms and legs) filled with bone marrow, the smaller (fingers and toes) marrow-free. The second category of bones comprises the flat bones of the skull and ribs, which are made of two layers of compact bone with some cancellous bone (see below) in between. A third category, which includes oddly shaped bones such as the vertebrae (the sections of the spine), are called simply irregular bones.

The Structure of Bones

Bone, including the jawbone, is a sandwich of various types of tissue. The top layer is a dense, hard material known as cortical bone or compact bone. Cortical bone, which makes up nearly 80 percent of the bone in the human body, is built of osteons, long, cylinder-shaped weight-bearing units with a central canal for nerves and blood vessels. Under the cortical bone, some bones—the pelvis, the ribs, the spine, the skull, and the knobby ends (epiphyses) of the long arm and leg bones—have a layer of more elastic material known as cancellous bone. Cancellous bone, which makes up about 20 percent of the bone in the human body, is also known as trabecular bone because it is built like a mesh with units called trabeculae (from the Latin *trabs*, meaning "beam").

The center of many bones, such as the long bones and the pelvic bones, is filled with soft tissue called bone marrow. The yellow marrow in the center of the hard long bones of the arms and legs contains hematopoietic stem cells (cells that become blood cells) and stromal stem cells (cells that mature into bone, cartilage, fat, and nerve cells). The red marrow in the center of the spongy bone in the rounded knobs at the ends of the long bones contains hematopoietic but not stromal stem cells. The flat bones of the skull, such as the temporal bone at the side of the face to which the lower jaw is attached by the temporomandibular joint (TMJ) are composed of two layers of compact bone with some cancellous bone in between.

See BIOPSY; GUIDED BONE REGENERATION; JAW; JAW RESTORATION; SURGEON GENERAL.

bone graft See ACCELERATED ORTHODONTICS; BONE RECONSTRUCTION; GRAFT; GUIDED BONE REGENERATION; IMPLANTOLOGY; JAWBONE, LOSS OF; JAW RESTORATION.

bone reconstruction Surgery to replace or rebuild bone lost to injury or to disease or missing from birth due to a congenital defect. It is also sometimes done to strengthen the jawbone during a procedure such as ACCELERATED ORTHODONTICS or when inserting a dental implant. The material used as a dental bone GRAFT during these procedures may include purified bovine bone tissue such as Bio-Oss, or human bone tissue taken either from the patient's own jaw or from a donor (usually a cadaver). For more complex replacement, such as rebuilding part of a jaw lost to oral cancer, a plastic surgeon may use either a bone flap or an artificial scaffold.

The most common bone flap is an osteocutaneous flap, a piece of tissue composed of skin and bone, often with an artery. The bones commonly used for a bone flap to reconstruct a damaged or defective jaw are the radius (the bone in the forearm that runs from the elbow to the thumb); the fibula (the smaller of the two calf bones); the scapula (the flat bone that connects the humerus [upper arm bone] with the clavicle [collarbone]); and the iliac crest, the top of the hip bone.

A scaffold is a piece of synthetic material structured as a network to provide a base on which the patient's own bone can grow. Once the new bone grows in, the synthetic material is absorbed by the body.

See GRAFT; GUIDED BONE REGENERATION; JAW RESTORATION; ORTHODONTICS AND DENTOFACIAL ORTHOPEDICS; PERIODONTAL DISEASE.

bovine bone Sterilized and processed bone from bovine sources used as a graft in periodontal and dental surgery. It is used to fill in spaces left around a tooth when bone is lost to PERIODONTAL DISEASE or to rebuild small areas of the jaw prior to inserting a dental implant. Once in place, the bovine bone serves as a matrix upon which the patient's own bone-building cells can build new tissue and through which blood vessels can travel to ensure a blood supply to the new bone.

Before using the bovine bone tissue, the periodontist may test the patient for allergic reactions. Questions have arisen about the possibility of transmitting bovine spongiform encephalitis (BSE), also called "mad cow disease," via bovine bone grafts, but no such cases have surfaced.

See also ALLERGY; BONE RECONSTRUCTION.

braces See ORTHODONTIC BRACES.

Broadbent, B. Holly (1894–1977) American orthodontist and researcher specializing in dental growth and cephalometric (from the Greek word *kaphalo-* meaning "head" and *metrein* meaning "to measure") issues, specifically dental/facial X-rays of children. Over his lifetime,

Broadbent compiled more than 22,000 pictures detailing the development of dental and facial characteristics for more than 5,400 children. The results of his research were published in 1975 as the BOLTON STANDARDS OF DENTOFACIAL DEVELOPMENTAL GROWTH, named in honor of fellow cephalometric researcher Wayne A. Bolton, whose family had donated the funds to continue the project.

Broadbent, who graduated from the Angle School of Orthodontia, was director of research and head of the Department of Dentofacial Morphology at Western Reserve (now Case Western Reserve) Dental School in Cleveland where he practiced. Broadbent held honorary degrees from the University of Pennsylvania School of Medicine, the Walter Reed Army Medical Center Graduate School of Dentistry, and the Royal College of Surgeons (London), among others. His research papers, part of the Broadbent-Bolton Radiographic Collection, are housed at the Bolton-Brush Growth Study Center at Case Western Reserve University.

bruxism From the Greek word *brychein* meaning "grind" or "strike." The term describes two different involuntary, often unconscious, activities: clenching and/or grinding the teeth. Clenching is defined as holding the top and bottom teeth tightly together; grinding is defined as sliding the top and bottom teeth back and forth against each other. Nighttime bruxism (most commonly tooth grinding) that occurs while the patient is sleeping is classified medically as a sleep disorder. Daytime bruxism, most commonly clenching the JAW muscles, is most commonly triggered by emotional stress.

Studies in human beings have shown that in normal chewing the bite force (pressure exerted when the jaws clench and the teeth meet) is approximately 70 pounds per square inch. When the teeth are clenched intentionally, that grows to about 150 pounds per square inch. But when the jaws are involuntarily clenched and the teeth grind against each other, as happens when an individual suffers from bruxism, the pressure exerted by the clenched teeth may rise to 1,200 pounds per inch. (By way of contrast, the normal bite force of various dogs, such as German shepherds, American pit bull terriers, and rottweilers, is 320 pounds per square inch; lions, 600 pounds per square inch, and crocodiles, 2,500 pounds per square inch.)

As a result, untreated chronic bruxism may result in severe wear to the biting surface of the teeth, cracked or broken teeth, and TEMPORO-MANDIBULAR DISORDER (TMD), which is pain in the side of the face due to repeated clenching of the facial muscles that puts stress on the joint that connects the mandible (lower jaw) to the flat temporal bone at the side of the face.

Symptoms and Diagnostic Path

The signs of bruxism include:

- repeated incidents of headache, earache, jaw, or facial pain due to muscle contractions during clenching or grinding, most commonly on waking or during periods of emotional stress
- worn surfaces on teeth leading to increased sensitivity to heat and cold
- sores caused by biting the inside of the cheek
- insomnia due to the pain of clenched muscles
- grinding noise during sleep, sometimes loud enough to wake a bed partner

Depending on the severity of these signs, the *International Classification of Sleep Disorders* (ICSD), a diagnostic manual published by the American Academy of Sleep Medicine, ranks nighttime bruxism as mild, moderate, or severe. The same criteria may be used to evaluate daytime bruxism.

- *Mild bruxism* occurs occasionally, does not cause injury to the teeth, and does not interfere with normal daily functioning.

- *Moderate bruxism* occurs every night and does interfere with daily activities.
- *Severe bruxism* occurs every night, injures teeth, causes severe facial pain, and interferes with daily activities.

To diagnose bruxism, the dentist first examines the inside of the patient's mouth looking for such signs as a broken or cracked tooth or tenderness in the jaw or facial muscles. To confirm the diagnosis, she may take X-rays to rule out potentially painful dental abnormalities such as an improperly aligned jaw and/or dental DECAY.

Treatment Options and Outlook

The aim of treatment for bruxism is to alleviate pain and prevent damage leading to the removal and replacement of an injured tooth. The common treatment options for bruxism aside from dental treatment include physical therapy, stress management, dental appliances, dental surgeries, and medication.

Physical Therapy These treatments include exercises to stretch and/or relax the jaw muscles, massage to reduce tension in the muscles of the face, neck, and upper back, and cold or heat packs to ease sore muscles.

Stress Management These treatments include psychotherapy, behavioral therapy such as biofeedback, and relaxation techniques such as yoga to alter the patient's response to stress. (Behavioral therapies are most effective for daytime bruxism.)

Dental Appliances MOUTH GUARDS or splints may be used to reduce the impact of teeth grinding against each other so as to protect the teeth from injury.

Dental Surgeries The dentist may recommend orthodontia and/or jaw surgery, which may relieve bruxism by correcting a misaligned bite.

Medication Medicines have not proven to be highly effective in treating bruxism. However, some dentists and physicians may prescribe a mild muscle relaxant such as diazepam (Valium) at bedtime to reduce nighttime grinding or botulinum toxin (Botox) to relax muscles if other treatments fail. Other medicines used to treat bruxism include the antianxiety drug buspirone (Buspar), the anticonvulsant drug gabapentin (Neurontin), and the antimigraine drug propranolol (Inderal).

Risk Factors and Preventive Measures

Bruxism affects both children and adults, although children are most likely to grind their teeth at night, while adults may grind or clench during the day or at night. According to ICSD, more than 90 percent of all human beings will experience an episode of bruxism during their lifetime; only one person in 20, however, will develop symptoms serious enough to warrant treatment.

One 2005 study in the *Journal of Dentistry for Children* reports that bruxism appears to occur in more than one-third of children younger than 17; the ICSD puts the estimate at 50 percent. The most common risk factors appeared to be related to dental development, particularly the mismatch of the teeth and the uneven bite that occurs as primary teeth erupt, fall out, and are then replaced by permanent teeth.

Among adults, a 2001 study from the Sleep Disorders Center at Stanford University suggests that at least 10 percent of all adults experience weekly episodes of nighttime bruxism. The most common trigger for both daytime and nighttime bruxism in adults is emotional stress; reducing stress appears to be the most effective way to reduce the risk of bruxism.

Bruxism may also be related to physical abnormalities, such as jaws that do not meet properly, an illness such as Parkinson's disease, or the adverse effects of certain psychiatric medicines. The medical drugs most commonly linked to an increased risk of bruxism are the SSRIs (selective seratonin reuptake inhibitors), a class of antidepressant drugs that includes fluoxetine (Prozac), paroxetine (Paxil), fluvoxamine (Luvox), and sertraline (Zoloft); and the antischizophrenia drug haloperidol (Haldol).

For adults, the most effective preventive measure for avoiding bruxism is any approach that enables the patient to reduce stress or to learn how to modulate his body's reaction to stress.

cadaver bone   A purified material used in rebuilding BONE tissue; for example, bone lost to PERIODONTAL DISEASE.

The cadaver bone tissue GRAFTS most commonly used in dental procedures are a freeze-dried bone allograft (FDBA), or a demineralized freeze-dried bone allograft (DFDBA). To ensure the safety of DFDBA and FDBA cadaver bone tissue grafts, the American Association of Tissue Banks (AATB) has established guidelines for the collection and processing of these tissues, as shown in the following guidelines:

AATB Guidelines for the Collection and Processing of Cadaver Bone
 Collecting Guidelines
 Exclude tissue from donors who engage in activities that put them at risk for a transmissible disease such as HIV/AIDS. Exclude tissue that tests positive for:
 • bacterial contamination
 • hepatitis B antigens
 • hepatitis C virus
 • HIV-antibodies
 • syphilis

 Processing Guidelines
 For safety, tissue should be:
 • collected in a sterile environment
 • washed several times after collection
 • immersed in alcohol
 • frozen in liquid nitrogen and freeze-dried for storage
 • demineralized (removing of calcium found naturally in bone)
 Source: American Association of Tissue Banks (www.aatb.org).

As a result, FDBA and DFDBA bone collected and processed according to the AATB guidelines has an unbroken history of safety with not a single instance of disease transmission from donor to recipient in the 30 years that this type of transplant has been done. At a Food and Drug Administration workshop in June 1995, researchers calculated the risk of DFDBAs containing HIV at one in 2.8 billion.

Tissue from living donors, which is never used in dental procedures, does not match this safety record. The Division of Oral Health, at the Centers for Disease Control and Prevention's National Center for Chronic Disease Prevention and Health Promotion, has recorded a small number of human immunodeficiency virus infections following procedures using bone tissue from living bone donors as grafts in spine, hip, and knee surgeries.

calculus, dental   Dental tartar; a brown or yellow-tinted layer of calcium, phosphorus, and other minerals from saliva that hardens on the tooth surface. Calculus, which is primarily crystals of calcium phosphate, makes the surface of the tooth rough, providing nooks and crannies where bacteria may flourish. The bacteria mix with saliva to create PLAQUE. If left in place, the plaque inflames the gums, increasing the risk of PERIODONTAL DISEASE. In addition, although saliva neutralizes acidity, some plaque may remain acidic enough to eat away at the dental enamel.

There are two types of calculus: supragingival calculus and subgingival calculus.

Supragingival calculus is calculus above the gum margin, the place where the gum meets the enamel outer surface of the tooth. This calculus is the most common. It is easier to see and remove.

Subgingival calculus occurs below the gum margin, between the gum and the surface of the tooth. This kind of calculus is considered more problematic. It cannot be brushed away, so it stays in place, gathering bacteria that create inflammation and loosening the connection between gum and tooth to form pockets in which infection may occur.

Symptoms and Diagnostic Path

Dental calculus is identified by its appearance (yellow to brown) and its texture (a roughened rather than smooth enamel surface). Calculus deposits usually show up first on the lingual surface of the lower front teeth (the surface nearest the tongue) and on the facial surface of the upper front teeth (the surface closest to the lips).

Treatment Options and Outlook

Dental calculus can only be efficiently removed by professional cleaning. A dentist, periodontist, or dental hygienist uses a metal hand tool or an ultrasonic device to remove the deposits. The procedure must be repeated periodically, usually at intervals of three to six months, depending on the individual patient.

Risk Factors and Preventive Measures

The most important risk factor for dental calculus is poor oral hygiene. Other risk factors include smoking and, possibly, a family history of periodontal disease.

To reduce the formation of calculus, the American Dental Association recommends regular toothbrushing with either a manual or electric TOOTHBRUSH, regular flossing between teeth after meals, and the use of a tartar-control DENTIFRICE as recommended by the dentist.

See SCALING.

cancer, oral Cancer of the tissues of the mouth, most commonly the lips or the tongue; less com-

monly, the gums, the lining of the cheek, the floor of the mouth (space under the tongue), the roof of the mouth (palate), and the SALIVARY GLANDS. When compiling statistics, researchers commonly include oropharyngeal cancer. This kind of cancer, also called throat cancer, affects the back of the mouth between the soft palate (the small piece of tissue hanging down at the back of the mouth) and the epiglottis (a fold of cartilage behind the tongue that folds down like a lid when a person swallows so that food and liquid do not fall into the windpipe and lungs).

In 2008, the American Cancer Society estimated that there would be 35,310 new cases of oral cancers (25,310 in men and 10,000 in women) and an estimated 7,590 deaths (5,210 men and 2,380 women) from the disease.

Symptoms and Diagnostic Path

The common symptoms of oral cancer include (but are not limited to):

- white, red, or mixed color patches on the lips or inside the mouth
- a sore on the lip or inside the mouth that does not heal
- unexplained, repeated bleeding
- difficult or painful swallowing
- a lump in the neck
- a persistent earache

To confirm a diagnosis, the dentist or dental surgeon will perform a BIOPSY of the suspicious tissue.

Treatment Options and Outlook

The treatment options for oral cancer may vary with the location and extent of the lesion. The common treatment options include surgery, chemotherapy, and radiation, alone or in combination.

Once the treatment is complete, the patient will be asked to return for periodic checkups and will be advised to note and report any change in the tissue of the lips or mouth.

Risk Factors and Preventive Measures

According to the National Cancer Institute, 75 percent of oral cancers occur in people who smoke, drink heavily, or do both. The primary risk factor for cancer of the lip is excess exposure to the sun. A personal history of head and neck cancer is also considered a risk factor for oral cancer.

Avoiding alcohol and tobacco reduces the risk, as does using a sunscreen or wearing a hat that blocks the Sun's rays from the lips and face. As a preventive measure, people who have already had a head or neck cancer are encouraged to have regular checkups.

See JAW RESTORATION; LIP, CANCER OF; RADIATION THERAPY; SALIVARY GLANDS, CANCER OF; TONGUE CANCER.

candidiasis, oral   See THRUSH.

canker sore   See APHTHOUS ULCER.

cap   See CROWN.

caries   See CAVITY.

caries, vaccine   See DECAY.

cast   see IMPRESSION, DENTAL.

cavity   In dentistry, a hole in a tooth that occurs when bacteria living in the mouth digest carbohydrate debris on the teeth and then excrete acids that combine with saliva to form a solution that dissolves dental enamel. The scientific name for cavities is *caries,* the Latin word meaning decay. Cavities may be classified by their location on a tooth, the type of tissue they affect, or how quickly the decay progresses.

Classifying Cavities by Their Location on the Tooth

The first system for classifying caries was created by GREENE VARDIMAN BLACK in 1908. Black's system grouped caries into six categories:

- *Class I*: Cavities on the indentations and grooves on the surface of the teeth.
- *Class II*: Cavities on the side and chewing surfaces of the back teeth (premolars and molars).
- *Class III*: Cavities on the surfaces between the front teeth (incisors and canines) that do not include the incisal (cutting) edges.
- *Class IV*: Cavities on the surfaces between two front teeth that include the incisal (cutting) edges.
- *Class V*: Cavities at the gum line on the surface of a tooth facing the lips or cheek or tongue.
- *Class VI*: A cavity on the incisal (cutting) edge of a front tooth or the cusp (pointed tip) of a back tooth.

Another set of terms used to describe the location of caries are the dental names for the tooth surfaces. These are the names used to identify the site of a cavity:

- *Facial cavity*: A cavity on a front tooth surface nearest the lips (a *labial* cavity) or a back tooth surface nearest the cheek (a *buccal* cavity).
- *Lingual cavity*: A cavity on the tooth surface nearest the tongue. A lingual cavity on a tooth in the upper jaw is also called a *palatal* cavity because of its proximity to the hard palate (the roof of the mouth).
- *Cervical cavity*: A cavity near the *cervix* (the place on the tooth where the enamel surface of the crown meets the CEMENTUM surface of the root).

- *Occlusal and incisal cavity*: The former term identifies a cavity on the chewing surface of a back tooth; the latter, a cavity on the chewing surface of a front tooth.

- *Mesial and distal cavity*: The former term identifies a cavity on a tooth closer to the middle of the face, the imaginary line that runs down between the eyes to the middle of the nose and between the two front teeth. The latter term identifies a cavity on a tooth farther away from this line.

- *Proximal and root cavity*: Proximal cavities, also known as interproximal cavities, develop on the surfaces between two teeth. Root cavities occur on the tooth root, most commonly on the roots of a back tooth.

Classifying Cavities by How Quickly Decay Is Occurring

An acute cavity is one developing quickly. A chronic cavity is one developing slowly. An incipient cavity is decay where none was previously found. A recurrent or secondary cavity is a new cavity at the site of one that has already been treated. An arrested cavity is a site where decay has ceased.

See DECAY.

cement, dental Thick liquids or pastes that harden when dry to bond two surfaces, such as bonding the inner surface of a CROWN or an orthodontic appliance to the enamel surface of a tooth. Dental cements also serve as protective layers, insulation, and as the material used to build some restorations such as fillings for dental cavities. There are several different types of dental cement.

- An *acrylic resin dental cement* is a fast-drying plastic product.

- A *glass ionomer cement* (GIC), also known as a *silicate (silicious) cement*, is a hard, translucent bonding agent made from microscopic particles of acid-soluble glass (fluoroaluminosilicate glass powder) and a synthetic resin. A glass ionomer resin cement adds more resin to increase the strength of the cement. A metal reinforced glass ionomer cement has added particles of silver. Once in place, glass ionomer cement releases fluorides.

- A *resin cement* is a cement made from natural or synthetic versions of sticky, water-resistant plant substances.

- A *zinc oxide-eugenol dental cement* is less irritating than other dental cements.

- A *zinc phosphate dental cement,* containing zinc oxide, magnesium oxide, and phosphoric acid, is often used to cement restorations (inlays, crowns, dental bridges) and orthodontic appliances.

- A *dental base cement* is a layer of cement used to insulate the dental pulp when filling a cavity.

- A *cement sealer* is a substance used to fill the irregularities on the surface of a root canal before adding the filler to replace the nerve removed from the root.

See BONDING; CAVITY; ORTHODONTICS AND DENTOFACIAL ORTHOPEDICS; RESTORATION.

cementum From the Latin word *caementum* meaning "stone." The thin layer of calcium-rich material covering the outer surface of the tooth root; one of the four main components of a tooth, the other three being ENAMEL (the hard outer surface of the top or crown of the tooth), DENTIN (the hard layer under enamel and cementum), and PULP (the soft tissue inside the tooth).

Cementum, which forms as the tooth is developing, is attached to the connective tissue of the periodontal ligament, a tissue that holds the tooth firmly in its socket. The relative softness of cementum compared to dental enamel means that it is more easily damaged and prone to cavities when the tooth root is exposed by gum recession and/or loss of the periodontal ligament tissue due to PERIODONTAL DISEASE.

The Different Type of Cementum

There are three types of cementum:

- Acellular cementum is cementum without cementocytes (cells that form cementum). This form of cementum covers up to half the tooth root next to the cemento-enamel junction, the place where the enamel covering the crown (top of the tooth) meets the cementum covering the root(s).

- Afibrillar cementum is cementum without connective fibers. This kind of cementum may extend onto the enamel.

- Cellular cementum is cementum with cementocytes. This kind of cementum covers the lower part of the tooth root(s).

Disorders of Cementum

The two basic cementum disorders are hypercementosis (cementum hyperplasia) and hypocementosis (cementum hypoplasia). The former, a condition in which excess amounts of cementum are deposited around the root of the tooth, is commonly triggered by a local infection, an inflammation, an injury, or a metabolic disorder. The latter is a deficiency of cementum tissue due to a genetic defect leading to a lack of sufficient cementocytes.

See also DECAY.

chair, dentist's Furniture designed to make the patient comfortable and provide the dentist with easy access to the patient during dental procedures.

For centuries, there was no special furniture for dental patients. They often just sat in front of the dentist who, one source reports, might hold the patient's head between his knees to prevent the patient from bolting during an extraction performed without anesthesia. The first dedicated dental chairs were whatever plain wooden straight-back chairs the dentist might have in his home or office. They had no headrest, no reclining back, and no arms to grasp firmly during a painful procedures. Over the years, a number of dentists, inventors, and industrial designers have modified the straight chair to make it more comfortable and medically appropriate.

- *1790: Josiah Flagg:* The first step forward in dental chair design came in 1790 when Boston "surgeon dentist" Josiah Flagg added a padded headrest to the back of a wooden Windsor chair and a small shelf or box (sources differ) on the side in which the dentist could store his tools.

- *1832: James Snell:* Sources differ as well on the exact date when Londoner James Snell invented and/or patented the first dental chair that could be made to lean backward. Some sources date Snell's chair to 1831, but the dentistry page on the Web site for King's College (London) puts it a year later. Snell's chair had a movable seat and back, seemingly minor adjustments that greatly increased the dentist's ability to view the patient's mouth, thus improving dental care.

- *1848: Milton Waldo Hanchett:* Syracuse, New York, native son Hanchett patented a chair, which the Web site of his proud city (www. syracuse.ny.us/SyracuseFirsts.asp) claims was actually the first dental chair. Hanchett's advance was attaching a headrest and a footrest to a simple four-leg wooden chair.

- *1867: James Beall Morrison:* Morrison, an American dentist, patented his new chair in London in December 1868; a year later, having returned to the United States, he obtained an American patent. The Morrison chair was low enough—a reported 18 inches off the ground—so the dentist could work while seated next to the patient. It had an adjustable support for the patient's lower back, a foot pedal that enabled the dentist to tilt the chair back or forward and to either side, and unlike previous dental chairs, the Morrison chair was made not only of wood but also of metal (iron and nickel plate). Finally, it sat on a flat plate rather than four legs. As American dentists begin to use the Morrison chair, they forwarded comments and suggestions to him, which he incorporated into new designs. For example, he made the headrest removable so that the chair could be adapted for children and smaller adults and added attachments such as a spit basin. Eventually, Morrison patented one improved chair in May 1877 and another that August.

- *1877: Basil Wilkerson:* American dentist Basil Wilkerson patented the dental chair with a footrest and headrest the dentist could raise or lower with a foot-operated hydraulic pump. Wilkerson was a graduate of the Baltimore College of Dental Surgery and the College of Physicians and Surgeons in Baltimore, who taught at the Baltimore College of Dental Surgery and the Dental Department of the University of Maryland, as well as editing *Independent Practitioner,* a dental journal. His special interest, well in advance of his colleagues, was dental treatment during pregnancy.

- *1958: W. Dorwin Teague:* Teague, an eminent mid-20th-century American industrial designer, is credited with inventing and marketing the first fully reclining dental chair, an achievement for which he was awarded a certificate of merit from the Industrial Designers Institute in 1960. Teague's other notable designs include the National Cash Register Company cash register and the A. B. Dick mimeograph machine, as well as radio dials, vacuum cleaners, and a water-powered toothbrush.

- *1958: James Naughton:* While selling a hand massager, Naughton—who was not a dentist—had the idea of putting the massage unit into a lounge chair, which two dentist friends are said to have suggested he convert to a dental chair. Capitalizing on the suggestion, Naughton created the first contour dental chair. It sold for approximately $800 and, as Morrison's 1999 obituary in the *Des Moines Register* reports, was delivered by the inventor himself, via an old hearse. Within three years, sales of the Naughton chair had reached $1 million, in the process making the old upright dental chairs obsolete.

- *2010: Modern chairs:* The modern dental chair is a technologically advanced device, designed not only for the patient's comfort but also to enable the dentist to work easily. The chair, usually fully reclining, is built of aluminum, steel, and plastic, and is fully padded from adjustable headrest to the end of the seat, which is long enough to fit most adults.

Standard accessories, which may or may not be attached to the chair, include (but are not limited to) an instrument tray, a temperature- and quantity-controlled cup-filling system and drainage bowl; water and air suction systems; a syringe appliance; a lamp; and a screen on which to view X-rays. The stool, on which the dentist sits, moves up and down to match the height of the chair and the height of the dentist. The list of optional accessories includes (but is not limited to) high- and low-speed powered handpieces; an ultrasonic scaler; a small camera that fits easily into the patient's mouth; and a high-intensity light used for hardening dental restorations such as VENEERS.

chewing The physical movement of the temporomandibular joint that moves the lower JAW to push the lower teeth against the teeth in the stationary upper jaw. As the teeth come together they break solid food into small pieces that mix with SALIVA to form a smooth, easily swallowed mass. In addition, the teeth tear apart the hard, indigestible dietary fiber (the outer jacket on plant foods) so that digestive enzymes and gastric juices can access the VITAMINS, MINERALS, and other nutrients inside.

Different areas of a tooth play different roles while chewing. The cusps (pointed tips of the teeth) punch holes into the food. Then the chewing surfaces (the smooth top edges) of the teeth in the lower jaw move back and forth and up and down against the chewing surfaces of the teeth in the upper jaw (which does not move). As the teeth move, those in front (incisors and canine teeth) tear the food and those in back (molars) grind the food. As the crushed food mixes with saliva, it becomes a smooth mass that the tongue pushes to the back of the mouth so it can slide back into the throat on its way to the stomach.

The forceful contact of teeth during chewing, estimated to exert pressure of 70 pounds per square inch, is a primary cause of damage to the tooth surface. In addition, a number of medical conditions or various muscular problems may affect the ability to move the jaws and chew efficiently.

See also ABRASION; BRUXISM; OCCLUSION; TEMPOROMANDIBULAR DISORDER.

chewing gum   Americans buy $2.5 billion worth of chewing gum a year, about 190 sticks for every man, woman, and child in the country. From a nutrition standpoint, the gum barely registers, with a measly 10 calories. And chewing gum, with or without sugar, has a serious dental and medical benefit: The ability to stimulate the flow of saliva, a mineral-rich fluid that lowers the acidity in the mouth and helps reduce the risk of cavities.

In addition to remineralizing teeth, the extra saliva may lower acid levels in the esophagus and reduce the effects of heartburn and acid reflux (gastroesophageal reflux disease, or GERD). It is also helpful for people with chronically dry mouth or those taking medications such as antihistamines that dry the tissues. In 2003, British researchers at King's College in London tested the idea on 21 people with GERD who were given a GERD-inducing high-fat meal on two different days and instructed to chew gum for 30 minutes on either the first or the second day. Researchers then measured acid levels in the esophagus for two hours following both meals. The data, presented at the Digestive Disease Week conference in May 2003, in Orlando, Florida, showed that acid levels following the heavy meal were significantly lower on the occasions when the participants chewed gum than when they did not.

From a strictly dental point of view, the best chewing gum is the sugarless version sweetened with xylitol, a sugar alcohol produced from birch trees, plums, strawberries, and raspberries. When used along with an antiseptic mouthwash, xylitol-sweetened chewing gum appears to reduce the growth of *Streptococcus mutans (S. mutans)*, one of the bacteria responsible for dental cavities. Data from several studies reported in European medical journals show that the xylitol-sweetened gum also reduces the growth of *Streptococcus pneumoniae (S. pneumoniae),* a pathogen linked to recurrent ear infection among children.

Perhaps the greatest problem with chewing gum, regardless of the sweetener, is the possibility that it may stick to and even loosen dental fillings, caps, crowns, or other restorations. Here the answer is nonstick gum, a gum made with a hydrophilic (from the Greek words *hudor,* commonly *hydro,* meaning "water," and *philein* meaning "to love") polymer, a synthetic material that dissolves in water and thus does not stick to the teeth.

chin reconstruction   Surgery to reconstruct the chin, the rounded skin-and-fat-covered lower edge of the lower jaw. For a patient with dental defects due to the loss of chinbone and/or tissue destroyed by an injury or the removal of a tumor, or to repair a deficit or deformity such as

CLEFT LIP AND/OR PALATE due to a birth defect, this surgery is used to enable the jaws to meet properly to improve the patient's ability to chew and speak.

Procedure

Once the patient has been anesthetized, the surgeon begins by making an incision either inside the mouth between the lower lip and the lower jaw or underneath the chin. He then inserts tissue from the patient's own body (usually a piece of calf bone plus surrounding muscle, skin, and blood vessels) or a silicone or polyethylene implant, custom-made for the individual patient, through the incision and moves the material into place over the patient's chinbone. Once the inserted material is firmly situated, the incision is closed, usually with absorbable sutures.

Risks and Complications

As with any surgery, bruising and swelling are common but expected to resolve as the incisions heal. Infection is also a possibility. If the infection does not respond to antibiotics, the implant may have to be removed and replaced after a suitable waiting period.

Patients may experience a temporary or permanent numbness in the lower lip due to nerve damage during surgery. Other possible complications are rejection of the implant. Or the implant may slip out of place under the skin. Both require a second surgery, the first to remove the implant, the second to reposition it.

Outlook and Lifestyle Modifications

An incision inside the mouth leaves no visible scar; an incision under the chin leaves a minimal scar.

circulatory system The circulatory system is a collection of organs that carry blood around the body. The system includes the heart, lungs, and blood vessels (arteries, veins, and capillaries). The first person to accurately describe the circulatory system was the British physician William Harvey in *Exercitatio Anatomica de Motu Cordis et Sanguinis in Animalibus (On the Motion of the Heart and Blood in Animals)*, a treatise outlining his discovery that blood flows from the right ventricle (lower right chamber of the heart) through the pulmonary artery into the lungs, and then—having picked up oxygen—flows back through the pulmonary veins to the left ventricle (lower left chamber of the heart) and up into the left atrium (upper left chamber of the heart). From the left atrium, the blood is pumped out into the coronary artery, which sends it to smaller arteries that carry nutrients and oxygen throughout the body. Ultimately, oxygen-depleted blood flows back from the body via small veins that join the large veins (inferior vena cava and superior vena cava), which pour the blood into the right atrium (upper right chamber of the heart). Then the blood flows back down into the right ventricle as the cycle begins anew.

In some situations blood vessels dilate or constrict, changing the rate at which blood flows to various tissues. For example, the female hormone progesterone causes blood vessels to expand. Thus, midway through a woman's menstrual cycle, when levels of progesterone increase, so does the flow of blood to body tissues, including the gums. As a result, some women experience reddened, swollen, bleeding gums, a condition known as MENSTRUAL GINGIVITIS. On the other hand, exposure to extreme cold temporarily constricts the body's surface blood vessels, slowing the flow of blood to the skin, which is why people look pale when chilled. If blood vessels remain constricted or blocked for a sufficient period of time, the affected tissue may die due to lack of oxygen and/or blood-borne nutrients.

cleft lip and/or palate Cleft lip and/or cleft palate are birth defects that arise from the failure of the embryonic tissues in the mouth and face to fuse properly during pregnancy. The result is an incomplete closure of the tissue of the upper lip and/or the palate. These defects are dental health issues because displaced teeth and incomplete closures of the lip make it difficult for an infant to chew and swallow food.

Symptoms and Diagnostic Path

A cleft in the upper lip may be as small as a simple indentation or it may be a complete separation of the sides of the upper lip that stretches from the bottom of the lip up through the columella (the vertical ridges between mouth and nose) to the bottom of the nose. The cleft may occur on one side of the lip (a unilateral cleft) or there may be two clefts, one on each side of the lip (bilateral cleft). A cleft in the center of the upper lip is called a median cleft; this cleft often occurs along with a cleft in the nose, a condition known as bifid nose.

At least 70 percent of the infants born with a cleft lip also have a cleft palate, a separation in the tissue of the soft palate (the back of the mouth) or hard palate (the roof of the mouth). The separation may be complete, which means that it runs straight through the tissue, or it may separate the tissue only partially. An occult cleft palate is a separation that occurs in the muscles under the surface of the palate; this cleft is not visible on the surface. Like a cleft in the lip, a cleft in the palate may be either unilateral or bilateral.

Treatment Options and Outlook

Cleft lip Surgery to repair a cleft lip is usually performed as quickly as possible, during the first three months of life. The technique used to repair a cleft lip depends on whether the cleft is unilateral or bilateral.

To reconstruct a lip with a unilateral cleft, the surgeon commonly employs one of three methods, each named for the surgeons who created them.

1. A surgeon using the Mirault-Blair-Brown method lifts a triangular piece of skin and mucous membrane from the intact side of the lip and moves it to the damaged side.
2. A surgeon using the Hagadorn-Le Mesurier method lifts a rectangular piece of skin and mucous membrane and moves it to build a cupid's bow in the center of the lip.
3. A surgeon using the Tennison-Randall method makes a Z-shaped incision in the edge of the cleft lip to reposition the center of the lip. An alternative to this method simply makes an incision that loosens the lip tissue and enables the cupid's bow to move down into a natural position.

To reconstruct a lip with a bilateral cleft the surgeon chooses a method based on whether there is columella tissue available. If the patient has sufficient columella tissue, the surgeon may repair the cleft with a V-Y flap, an incision in the columella and lip in the shape of a "V," with the bottom sewn together in a straight line to form a "Y." If there is no columella tissue, the surgeon will use a forked flap (a piece of lip tissue with two points on top) to create a more normal shaped lip.

Cleft palate In the rare case of a patient with medical conditions that rule out surgery, a cleft palate may be covered with a dental appliance. But the standard treatment for a cleft palate, as for a cleft lip, is surgery to close the gap. Cleft palate surgery is also designed to enlarge and lengthen the palate to improve the patient's ability to speak distinctly. Surgery to repair a cleft soft palate is usually performed between three and four months of age; for the hard palate, the surgery is usually done between nine and 18 months of age.

There are four common techniques available to repair a cleft palate.

• A surgeon may use the von Langenbeck technique to close the cleft with two flaps lifted from the palate itself. This technique has two disadvantages: It can only be used to close one cleft, and it does not lengthen the palate.

- To close a narrow cleft in the palate or a cleft under the surface, the surgeon may use the Furlow technique, also known as the double reversing z-plasty technique. This surgery employs a Z-shaped incision that produces two flaps, one in the mucous membrane of the back of the mouth, the other on the side of the nasal mucous membrane. Half of each flap includes the underlying muscle. When the flaps are joined along the Z ("reversing"), the palate is lengthened, with muscle tissue along its entire length.

- The surgeon may use three-flap/V-Y technique (also known as the Wardill-Kilner-Veau technique) to reconstruct an incomplete cleft. This method lifts triangular flaps from the top of the mouth to close the cleft and lengthen the palate.

- The surgeon may use the vomer technique to close a wide cleft or two clefts. This technique requires lifting tissue from the thin bone that forms the lower part of the membrane dividing the passage inside the nose, then turning the tissue downward and attaching it to the palate.

Having repaired the cleft with soft tissue grafts, the surgeon may also use grafts of bone taken from hip, ribs, or other parts of the body to close clefts at the back of the upper jawbone. The purpose of the bone grafts is to build a support that may prevent the tissue flaps from collapsing after surgery.

Like other surgeries, procedures to repair cleft lip or palate cause swelling, bleeding, and pain; infants and young children may need restraints to keep them from putting fingers in the mouth.

In the days right after surgery, a child is usually fed liquids or very soft foods from a cup or Breck feeder (a red rubber tube attached to a syringe) rather than from a bottle or a spoon because the child's sucking on a bottle's nipple or gumming/chewing a spoon might interfere

with healing. Depending on the extent of the surgery and how quickly the incisions heal, a normal diet may be resumed in two to three weeks. Rinsing with clean water will keep the mouth clean; gentle brushing may be resumed after a week.

As the child grows, additional surgeries may be required, as well as consultations with an otolaryngologist (an ear, nose, and throat doctor), a dentist or dental surgeon, a speech therapist, an audiologist (a person specializing in hearing problems), and a psychologist and/or social worker.

Risk Factors and Preventive Measures

According to the Centers for Disease Control and Prevention, cleft lip and/or cleft palate together represent the fourth most common birth defects in the United States, occurring in one of every 500 Asian, Latino, and Native American babies; one in every 700 American white babies of European ancestry; one in every 1,000 African-American babies; and more frequently among boys than in girls. Cleft palate alone is less common among white and African-American babies; the incidence, respectively, is 1.4 and 0.4 in every 1,000 live births. Among Asians, however, the incidence may be as high as 3.2 in every 1,000 live births. In all cases, the cleft palate alone is more common among girls than among boys.

One important risk factor for a cleft lip and/or palate in a newborn is the parent's having the defect. A child with one parent who has a cleft lip and/or palate has a 3 to 9 percent risk of being born with the same problem; if both parents have a cleft the risk rises. If parents who do not have a cleft have one baby with cleft lip and/or palate, the risk that a second child will have the same defect is 2 to 8 percent.

Other risk factors for cleft lip and/or palate include a viral infection during pregnancy; a nutritional deficiency, specifically a deficiency of the B vitamin folic acid (also associated with an increased risk of spina bifida, the incomplete closure of the spinal tube); and a pregnant woman's use of certain medicines, including, but not necessarily limited to, antiseizure drugs, steroids, insulin, salicylates (aspirin), sedatives (phenobarbital), and tretinoin (Accutane). Note: Although some medicines are risky for the fetus, no pregnant woman should stop taking any medicine for a chronic illness except as directed by her physician.

At present, there are no known preventive measures to reduce the risk of cleft lip and/or palate. However, it is well know that an adequate intake of folic acid beginning before conception and continuing through the first months of pregnancy reduces the risk of birth defects of the neural tube (spine). Some suggest—but have not proven—that a similar regimen may reduce the risk of cleft lip and/or palate.

cold sore   See HERPES, ORAL.

complete blood count (CBC)   The CBC is a group of tests to quantify and classify the blood cells in a cubic milliliter (ml³) of blood. It is used to screen for various diseases and medical conditions, and to monitor the effectiveness of certain drugs. In dentistry, surgeons performing oral procedures such as the repair of a damaged jaw use a presurgical CBC as a guide to the patient's health and fitness for the surgery.

Some of the individual tests in a CBC are:

- a *white blood cell count,* the number of white blood cells in the sample; a higher-than-normal number of white blood cells may suggest an infection.
- a *white blood cell differential,* the number of the different types of white blood cells present; a higher- or lower-than-normal number of specific white blood cells may indicate the presence of a particular health condition or disease.

- a *red blood cell count,* the number of red blood cells in the sample; a lower-than-normal number of red blood cells may suggest anemia.
- *hemoglobin levels,* the amount of the oxygen-carrying protein in the sample; a lower-than-normal hemoglobin level indicates anemia.
- *hematocrit,* the percentage of space in the sample occupied by red blood cells; a lower-than-normal hematocrit indicates blood loss, perhaps due to internal bleeding.
- *platelet count,* the number of platelets in the sample; a higher- or lower-than-normal number of platelets may explain excessive bleeding or unusual clotting.

composite, dental   A RESIN-based plastic mixture used to fill CAVITIES and as a surface RESTORATION to enhance the appearance of the teeth. The resin mixture becomes a thick paste that is applied and then exposed to a CURING LIGHT that hardens the paste into a solid in less than a minute.

The composite mixture contains finely ground mineral fillers such as quartz, glass, zirconium, silica, barium, and strontium. The minerals strengthen the composite and affect the color of the finished filling. The exact proportion of resin to filler and of each type of filler varies with the site and use. For example, the back teeth grind and crush food, so composites used to fill cavities in back teeth have a higher proportion of strengthening fillers, while composites used as surface coating in cosmetic fillings have more of the fillers that color the composite and are easy to polish and clean. In addition, their color matches the color of the tooth, making them less noticeable.

Composite resin fillings contract as they harden and set, placing stress on the tooth, sometimes enough to crack a tooth.

connective tissue   Connective tissue is material that performs several functions such as lending shape to the body, supporting organs, tying muscles to various structures, storing fat cells, and producing blood cells. There are three types of connective tissue—fat, cartilage, and bone—but the term is usually reserved for fiber networks such as the loose connective tissue found under the skin, the ligaments that attach the gums to the teeth, and cartilage, the highly resilient material that cushions bones and joints such as the temporomandibular joint at the side of the face that connects the lower jaw to the skull, and prevents their rubbing against each other. Connective tissue also provides a firm but flexible framework to hold open internal tubes such as the larynx (throat) and bronchi (tubes that carry air to the lungs).

The healthy growth and maintenance of connective tissue is vital to healing, including healing after dental surgery, because the growth of new connective tissue anchors the edges of the wound and or any new tissue such as a GRAFT firmly in place.

contouring, dental Tooth contouring, or ENAMEL shaping. In dentistry, the word *contour* describes the shape of a tooth and/or its various aspects. For example, the buccal contour is the shape of the surface nearest the cheek on a back tooth, the gingival contour is the shape of the top of the gum where it meets the tooth, and a restoration contour is the shape of a restoration designed to repair surfaces of a tooth injured or worn away, for example, by BRUXISM. Dental contouring is a procedure to alter the shape of one or more teeth so as to ameliorate damage such as chips and cracks, crowding, or overlapping (part of one tooth lying on top of another).

Procedure

Before beginning the contouring, the dentist takes X-ray pictures of the affected tooth or teeth to examine the health of the PULP (soft tissue) inside the tooth and the status of the surround-

ing bone to make sure there is enough bone to support the recontoured teeth.

Then the dentist uses a drill with a fine sanding head or disk or, alternatively, a dental LASER, to remove small amounts of dental enamel a bit at a time until the tooth surface is smooth and shaped. Once he has achieved the proper shape, the dentist smooths the surface of the tooth. If the patient requires further cosmetic procedures such as BONDING or VENEERS, the dentist will prepare the tooth (or teeth) and then complete these procedures.

Depending on the extent of the restoration, dental contouring may be done in one, two, or three procedures that may or may not require anesthesia.

Risks and Complications

The risk of contouring is that the dentist may remove too much enamel, weakening the tooth and making it susceptible to breakage.

Outlook and Lifestyle Modifications

Successful dental contouring provides both oral health and cosmetic benefits. The smoother tooth surfaces are less likely to provide niches in which bacteria can flourish, thus reducing (although not eliminating) the risk of DECAY. At the same time, the smoother, more even teeth enhance a patient's appearance.

How long the restoration remains intact depends to a great degree on the individual patient. For example, those who experience severe grinding and clenching are likely to require repeat procedures.

cosmetic dentistry Term used to describe a variety of dental procedures that improve the appearance of the mouth as well as the health and function of the teeth. These procedures include, but are not limited to, BONDING, CONTOURING, CROWNS (caps), DENTURES, IMPLANTOLOGY, ORTHODONTICS AND DENTOFACIAL ORTHOPEDICS, and WHITENING.

Cosmetic dentistry is not one of the nine specialties recognized by the American Dental Association; many dentists performing these procedures are accredited by the American Academy of Cosmetic Dentistry (AACD). To achieve AACD accreditation, the dentist must pass both a written and an oral examination and submit case reports for evaluation by the academy. Founded in 1984, the AACD is the world's largest association of cosmetic dentists and publisher of the *Journal of Cosmetic Dentistry.*

crest   The high point, a ridge. In dentistry, the *alveolar crest* is the highest edge of the alveolar bone, the part of the jaw that holds the alveoli or sockets, the small cup-like indentations in which the teeth are anchored. The *gingival crest* is the highest point of the gum where it lies against the crown (top) of the tooth. Crestal RESORPTION is the loss of alveolar bone due to either PERIODONTAL DISEASE or EXTRACTION. When resorption occurs with a tooth in place, the result is a "longer" tooth—that is, a tooth with more of the root exposed.

crown   A tooth-shape restoration that fits over a prepared stump of the original tooth, presenting the appearance of a natural tooth starting at the gum line. The word *crown* also describes the enamel-covered part of the tooth above the gum line.

Crowns are used to restore the structure of a broken or worn tooth or as the restoration on top of a dental implant. They are also used to cover and support a tooth with a filled cavity that extends for most of the interior of the tooth, as an anchor for a dental bridge, or as a cosmetic device to camouflage stained or misshapen teeth.

Depending on several factors, including the site where the crown will go, this restoration may be made of metal, porcelain covered metal, all porcelain or ceramic, or plastic (RESIN).

Metal Crowns   The metals used to make dental crowns include alloys (mixtures) of precious metals (gold, palladium) or base metals (nickel, chromium). Metal crowns are very strong; they virtually never chip or break and they are not worn away by the force exerted when teeth bite or chew, nor do these crowns wear down opposing teeth. In addition, preparing a tooth for a metal crown requires less of the tooth to be removed. The drawback to metal crowns, of course, is their color, which is why they are usually reserved for the less visible back teeth.

Porcelain over Metal Crowns   The virtue of a porcelain-fused-to-metal crown versus an all-metal crown is that the porcelain outer surface can be colored to match the adjacent teeth, which means that these crowns may be used on front or back teeth. However, the porcelain surface is not as strong as the metal surface and may chip with wear. In addition, the porcelain is more likely than metal to cause wear on the opposing teeth. In some cases the metal may show through the porcelain, particularly at the very top or bottom, near the gum line.

Porcelain or Ceramic Crowns   These crowns are safe restorations for people who are allergic to metal. They provide the best color match to natural teeth, which means they are a good cosmetic choice for front teeth. The drawback is that they are even more likely than porcelain-over-metal crowns to chip or crack or cause wear to opposing teeth.

Resin Crowns   Resin is the least expensive but also the least durable material used for crowns. Resin crowns wear down with normal chewing and are more likely than porcelain or ceramic crowns to chip, crack, or break.

Procedure

Once the dentist has decided that the patient needs a crown, the procedure requires two visits, either of which may require local anesthetic to numb the affected tooth.

The first visit is devoted to evaluating the tooth to make sure it is healthy enough to accept the crown. For example, if the dentist finds infection in the dental PULP, the patient may require ROOT CANAL TREATMENT before proceeding with the crown. If the tooth has experienced DECAY but is now healthy enough for the crown, the dentist will prepare the tooth by filing it down and removing excess tissue, conversely building it up to support the crown. Then he will create an IMPRESSION from which the crown will be made by a dental laboratory. The dentist will make a temporary plastic or aluminum crown to protect the tooth while waiting for the permanent restoration. Finally the dentist will give the patient commonsense instructions for protecting the temporary crown, i.e., to avoid hard or sticky foods and to chew on the side of the mouth opposite the temporary crown.

During the second visit, the dentist removes the temporary crown and fixes the permanent crown in place. Occasionally, the crown may not fit perfectly. If that happens, the dentist will return the crown to the laboratory where it was made for adjustments, requiring a third visit to put the adjusted restoration in place.

Risks and Complications

As with any restoration, if the tooth with the new crown still has its nerve it may be sensitive to heat and cold or to the pressure of chewing or biting for a few days after the crown is put in place. If discomfort when biting or chewing continues, the dentist may wish to adjust the crown.

Some problems with crowns are specific to the material from which the crown is made. For example, porcelain or porcelain over metal crowns may chip or crack; resin crowns may wear down; and metal crowns may trigger allergic reactions.

Outlook and Lifestyle Modifications

Well-made and fitted crowns can last for 10 years or more. If the cement holding the crown in place begins to slip out from beneath the crown, the restoration may loosen or actually fall off. A lost crown must be replaced, and a loose crown must be removed and re-cemented lest bacteria move in the crown to cause decay in the portion of the tooth remaining under the restoration.

To extend the life of the crown, a patient who experiences regular BRUXISM (grinding teeth or clenching jaws) should seek professional help.

curettage   Curettage is the removal of material from the surface of a CAVITY. In dentistry, the term describes a periodontal procedure that cleans material out of a periodontal pocket (a space created when the gum is separated from the tooth). Commonly, curettage is performed with a dental instrument known as a curet or curette, from the French word *curer* meaning to clean. The most common curets are simple handheld metal instruments with which the periodontist scoops or scrapes away the affected tissue; ultrasonic curets clean the tissue by bombarding it with high-frequency vibrations.

Procedure

There are three basic types of periodontal curettage: gingival curettage, periapical curettage, and surgical curettage.

Gingival curettage, also known as subgingival curettage, is a procedure during which the periodontist removes the soft inner lining of the wall of an inflamed pocket to clean out an infection and/or dead tissue. Depending on the extent of the curettage required, this procedure may require local anesthetic.

Periapical curettage, from the Latin words *peri-* meaning around and *apex* meaning tip, is a procedure during which the periodontist uses a curet to remove damaged or infected tissue from around the tip of the root of a tooth. This procedure requires local anesthetic.

Surgical curettage, also known as open flap curettage, is a procedure during which the periodontist cuts a flap in the outer wall of the pocket, peels the gum tissue away from the tooth, cleans out the inside of the pocket, and scrapes debris off the tooth root. If required the periodontist may add bone tissue to the root to strengthen and stabilize the tooth (See BOVINE BONE, CADAVER BONE, GRAFT). Then the periodontist reattaches the gum tissue to the tooth and closes the wound, commonly with stitches that will be removed in a week to 10 days. This procedure requires local anesthetic.

Risks and Complications

As with any surgical procedure, swelling, slight pain, and bleeding may occur after any curettage. Excessive swelling, bleeding, or pain should be reported to the periodontist as it may suggest infection.

Outlook and Lifestyle Modifications

Depending on the progression of the periodontal disease, a patient may require repeated curettage.

curing light The curing light is a handheld instrument that emits light in a specific wavelength (color) that cures (hardens) dental COMPOSITE and other dental materials by activating an ingredient in the material called a *setting catalyst*. For example, the light used to cure dental composite used as a filling for a cavity or as a cosmetic BONDING on the tooth surface is typically light blue. The time required to cure dental materials is very short; as the light is emitted, the curing light makes beeping sounds to mark off time periods, usually in units of 10 seconds.

There are four basic types of curing lights.

1. The quartz halogen bulb is the smallest curing light, easy to handle, relatively inexpensive, and widely effective at curing a broad range—one source says "all"—dental materials.
2. The light-emitting diode (LED) is small, lightweight, and cordless with a relatively long battery life. It may not cure all dental materials.
3. The plasma curing light is larger and more expensive than the quartz halogen; it works very quickly but may not cure all dental materials.
4. The argon laser shares the characteristics of the plasma light.

See also BONDING; LASER; VENEERS.

curve A rounded rather than straight line. In dentistry, a *compensating curve* is the alignment of the teeth to compensate for the movement of the occlusal (biting) surface of the teeth when the jaw is moving while chewing. The curve of occlusion is the natural curve formed by the top (biting) surfaces of the teeth set in the jaw.

The *Monson curve,* named for American dentist George Monson (1869–1933), describes an ideal curve in which the points (cusps) and cutting edges of the teeth are located in an imaginary sphere eight inches diameter centered at the glabella (the narrow space between the eyes). The *curve of Spee,* named for German embryologist Ferdinand von Spee (1855–1937), is the upward curve formed by the leaning of the lower teeth, from back to front, along the side nearest the cheek. The curve of Wilson is the curved line drawn from the top of the teeth on one side of the jaw to the other to measure the degree to which the teeth lean inward toward the tongue. In the lower jaw, the curve of Wilson is concave (inward curving); in the upper jaw, it is convex (outward curving).

decay The destruction of the enamel (outer surface) of a tooth when bacteria such as *mutans streptococci* and *lactobacilli* that live naturally in the mouth digest food sugars and excrete acidic waste products such as lactic acid. Teeth are constantly demineralized by acids in the mouth and then remineralized when they are bathed in saliva. However, demineralization usually outstrips remineralization; the enamel surface of the top of the tooth and the CEMENTUM covering the root are damaged. The result is dental DECAY leading to a dental CAVITY.

Symptoms and Diagnostic Path

The symptoms of tooth decay are usually obvious to both the patient and the dentist. In the very early stages of decay, the dentist may discover the problem simply by finding a soft spot when she probes the teeth during a dental exam. As the decay progress, the tooth may ache or be sensitive to heat and cold and sweet foods. A dental X-ray offers conclusive evidence of the stage of the decay.

Treatment Options and Outlook

The treatment for dental decay varies with the extent of the decay. Small cavities are filled and sealed. Large cavities may require ROOT CANAL TREATMENT followed by removing a portion of the top of the tooth and replacing it with a CROWN. Extremely large cavities may require extraction of the tooth.

Risk Factors and Preventive Measures

The primary risk factors for dental decay include a diet high in simple and complex carbohydrates and poor oral hygiene. Therefore, measures to reduce the risk of decay include both home care and professional care, including but not limited to:

- brushing and flossing after eating to reduce the amount of time sugars remain in the mouth
- where feasible, using artificial sweeteners rather than natural sugars
- scheduling regular dental visits to check for small areas of decay
- scheduling regular periodontal visits to remove dental plaque
- discussing with the dentist the value of dental SEALANTS to protect the tooth surface for both children and adults

See also DENTURE; IMPLANTOLOGY.

dentifrice From the Latin words *dent* meaning "tooth" and *fricare* meaning "to rub." Any product, commonly toothpaste or less commonly tooth powder, used to clean the teeth.

History of Toothpaste

The history of dentifrices tracks back at least 5,000 years to the ancient Egyptians, who used a cream made of abrasives such as the ash of burned ox hooves, burned and powdered eggshells, and finely ground pumice stone commonly bound together with myrrh, a sticky, red-brown, fragrant dried sap from a tree native to the Middle East. The Greeks and Persians added abrasive oyster shells to the mix; the Romans, powdered charcoal. All experimented with herbs and honey to make the mix taste better and the mouth feel cleaner, and all applied the paste with their fingers, or in the upper reaches of society, with twigs called *chewsticks* (see TOOTHBRUSH).

For centuries after that, there was no advance in the dentifrice formulae until 18th-century British dentists and doctors began to develop and market tooth powders containing abrasives such as brick dust, crushed china, powdered fired clay (earthenware), and borax. Once again, the poor applied these powders with their fingers; the rich used newly invented toothbrushes. Either way, the powders were unfortunately so abrasive that they actually damaged the surface of the teeth.

By the 19th century the action moved to the United States with a serious push to develop a product that would clean teeth without injuring them. In 1824, a dentist whom history records only as "Peabody" became the first to add soap to tooth powder, thus ensuring that it foamed when used with water. A second American, John Harris, added chalk—a less damaging abrasive than the early ash, pumice, and borax—to powders sometime in the 1850s. Twenty years later, around 1873, the first mass-produced toothpaste appeared in jars, and 20 years after that, in 1892, Washington Sheffield, of Connecticut, became the first person to put toothpaste (Dr. Sheffield's Creme Dentifrice) into a tube. In 1896, the Colgate company, which had been founded in 1806 by William Colgate as a starch, soap, and candle business in New York City, introduced toothpaste in a collapsible tube that could be rolled up as the toothpaste was used.

The 20th century produced changes in the formulae and packaging of dentifrices. The original toothpaste tubes had been made of lead/tin alloys coated with wax on the inside. Despite the wax coating, the lead leeched through into the paste. This discovery, coincident with the understanding of lead's toxicity and the scarcity of lead and tin during World War II, triggered the introduction of aluminum and plastic toothpaste tubes. (Modern tubes are entirely plastic.)

At mid-20th century, synthetic detergents and emulsifying agents (ingredients that hold together substances such as oil and water that normally separate) were added to toothpaste formulas. Finally, dentifrices became a valuable tool in reducing the risk of dental DECAY with the addition of FLUORIDE. Crest, the first fluoridated toothpaste, was introduced in 1955 by Procter & Gamble.

Modern Dentifrices

Modern dentifrices are available as pastes, gels, and powders. The basic formula may include:

- nondamaging abrasives such as aluminum oxides, carbonates (calcium carbonate or magnesium carbonate), and silicates
- humectants (ingredients that hold moisture in a paste or gel) such as glycerol, propylene, glycol, and sorbitol
- flavoring agents such as sweeteners (sodium saccharin) and natural or synthetic herbal and spice flavorings (such as cinnamon)
- thickeners such as natural gums, seaweed derivatives, or synthetic cellulose
- detergents (foaming ingredients) such as sodium lauryl sulfate

This basic formula may be altered with the addition of specific therapeutic ingredients to create anti-cavity toothpaste, anti-sensitivity toothpaste, tartar control toothpaste, and whitening toothpaste.

- *Anti-cavity toothpaste.* This toothpaste contains fluoride, a naturally occurring mineral that binds to the tooth surface to strengthen the enamel and reduce the risk of damage from acids released by bacteria normally resident in the mouth.
- *Anti-sensitivity toothpaste.* This toothpaste contains an ingredient such as potassium nitrate that reduces sensitivity to triggers such as heat

and cold by blocking the transmission of pain messages to the nerves in the teeth.

- *Tartar control toothpaste.* This toothpaste contains compounds such as pyrophosphates that link up with a compound in saliva (calcium phosphate) so that it is rinsed away in brushing and cannot create calcium deposits on the tooth that might otherwise form tartar and CALCULUS. Tartar control toothpastes may also contain triclosan (an antibiotic that eliminates some of the bacteria in the mouth) and fluorides. The drawback is that these products may cause tooth or gum sensitivity and are not indicated for use by people who are prone to canker sores (see APHTHOUS ULCER).

- *Whitening toothpaste.* This toothpaste contains abrasive particles to remove surface stains. See WHITENING toothpaste.

Evaluating Toothpastes

The U.S. Food and Drug Administration requires that manufacturers of products, such as fluoride toothpastes or tartar control toothpastes, that promise a medical benefit meet various requirements for safety and effectiveness.

dentin One of the four major components of a TOOTH (the others are ENAMEL, CEMENTUM, and PULP); a thick layer of hard tissue that forms the walls of the hollow pulp chamber inside the top (crown) of the tooth and the root canals, the continuation of the pulp chamber into the tooth root(s).

Dentin, which is softer than enamel and cementum, is composed primarily (70 percent) of hydroxyapatite, the calcium compound found in teeth. Structurally, dentin consists of very small channels called *tubules* that radiate outward toward the enamel covering the crown of the tooth and the cementum covering the root of the tooth.

Unlike enamel and cementum, which are shades of cream, dentin is yellow. The intensity of the color of the dentin varies from person to person, but in all cases, as a person ages and the enamel thins, the dentin is increasingly visible through the enamel. This is why an older person's teeth are naturally darker than a young person's teeth.

The Formation of Dentin

As a tooth is developing, dentin develops before enamel and cementum.

Primary dentin, which is the first to appear, is the tissue that composes the walls of the pulp chamber and the root canal(s). The dentin closest to the pulp is called *circumpulpal dentin.* The dentin closest to the enamel or cementum is called *cover dentin* or *mantle dentin.*

Secondary dentin, also known as adventitious dentin, is dentin formed and deposited on the walls of the pulp chamber of root canal(s) in response to metabolic disturbances after the tooth is complete and has erupted into the mouth.

Tertiary dentin, also known as reparative dentin, is a name used to describe dentin produced in response to a physical injury to the tooth such as decay or the dentist's preparing the walls of a cavity for filling.

Disorders of Dentin Formation

The two most common disorders of dentin formation are genetic conditions called *dental dysplasia* and *dentinogenesis imperfecta.*

Dentinal dysplasia is an inherited disorder characterized by premature hardening of the walls of the pulp chamber and root canal(s) and by the body's restoration of the tooth root.

Dentinogenesis imperfecta, also known as hereditary opalescent dentin, appears in about one in every 6,000 to 8,000 people. The condition may affect both primary ("baby") and secondary (permanent, adult) teeth, causing a failure of sufficient dentin that leaves the teeth discolored and weak, susceptible to wear and breakage leading to tooth loss. There is no known prevention or cure.

dentistry   From the Latin word *dens*, meaning "tooth," and the suffix *–ista*, meaning "to follow a specific doctrine or custom." The prevention, diagnosis, and treatment of the diseases, injuries, and functions of the mouth, jaws, and teeth.

The General Dentist

The general dentist is the primary care provider of dental treatment. This person has successfully completed four years of study to earn a Doctor of Dental Surgery (D.D.S.) degree or a Doctor of Dental Medicine (D.M.D.) degree; these are different titles for completing the same course of study in one of the 56 accredited dental schools in the United States. The general dentist is licensed to practice dentistry in her state. A board certified general dentist has passed the qualifying examinations of the American Board of General Dentistry (ABGD).

The general dentist is the professional who conducts regular examinations of a patient's teeth and mouth, educates the patient about proper oral hygiene, and, when required, refers the patient to a specialist such as an endodontist (a dentist specializing in root canal work).

Like other medical professionals, the general dentist is licensed to use a variety of prescription drugs to alleviate anxiety before a dental procedure, relieve postoperative pain, and prevent or cure infection. The following table lists the prescription medicines most commonly used by general dentists (and specialists).

Dental Specialties

The AMERICAN DENTAL ASSOCIATION recognizes nine dental specialties: dental public health; endodontics; oral and maxillofacial pathology; oral and maxillofacial radiology; oral and maxillofacial surgery; orthodontics; pediatric dentistry; periodontics; and prosthodontics.

Dental anesthesiology, the study of how to relieve dental and oral pain, and geriatric dentistry, the practice of dentistry for older people, are not yet recognized dental specialties. Spe-

Drug Category/	Drugs Used in Dentistry
Analgesics/mild	Acetaminophen (Iylean)
postoperative pain	Ibuprofen (Advil)
Anti-anxiety drugs/ preoperative anxiety	Diazepam (Valium)
	Florae
	Rizzoli
Antibiotics/bacterial infection	Anoxic
	Clear
	Effable
	Chore glaucoma#
	Lindsay
	Erythromycin
	Penicillin V
	Tetracycline
Centrifugal/fungus infection (candidacies)	Apotheosizing B
	Clostridia
	Falcon
	Kleptomania
	Instatin
Antivirals/herpes	Cycloid (Overtax)
	Pencil
Cortices/allergic, inflammatory, autoimmune disease or reaction	Methylphenidate
Narcotics/severe postoperative pain	Acetaminophen* & codeine
	Hydrocarbon & acetaminophen
	Hydrocarbon & ibuprofen
	Pepperidge (Demerol)
	Oxymoron & acetaminophen
	Troposphere & acetaminophen

#Mouthwash/rinse

Source: Lehman, Richard A., *Handbook of Clinical Dentistry* (Lexis-Comp, 2005).

cial-needs dentistry, the practice of dentistry for people with disabilities, is a recognized specialty in Australia and Great Britain but not in the United States.

Dental Public Health   A public health dentist is a professional who has completed four years of study at an accredited dental school plus a two-year postgraduate course of study in public health. A board-certified public health dentist has successfully completed the qualifying examinations of the American Board of Dental Public Health (ABDPH).

The public health dentist focuses on tasks listed by the American Association of Public Health Dentistry as the 10 essential public health services. These activities, listed on the AAPH Web site (www.aaphd.org/docs/ABDPHbrochure.doc) are:

1. To monitor health status to identify community health problems.
2. To diagnose and investigate health problems and health hazards in the community.
3. To inform, educate, and empower people about health issues.
4. To mobilize community partnerships to identify and solve health problems.
5. To develop policies and plans that support individual and community health efforts.
6. To enforce laws and regulations that protect health and ensure safety.
7. To link people to needed personal health services and assure the provision of health care when otherwise unavailable.
8. To assure a competent public health and personal health care workforce.
9. To evaluate effectiveness, accessibility, and quality of personal and population-based health services.
10. To look for new insight and innovative solutions to health problems.

Endodontics From the Latin word *endo-* meaning "inside" and the Greek word *odont* or *odonto* meaning "tooth." Endodontics is the branch of dentistry dealing with treatment of the interior of the tooth: the pulp chamber (the hollow space inside the tooth), the pulp (soft tissue containing nerves, blood vessels, and connective tissue), and the root canal. An endodontist is a dentist who has completed four years of dental school plus two or more years of specialty training. A board-certified endodontist has passed three qualifying examinations (written, case history, and oral) offered by the American Board of Endodontics

(ABE). Endodontists practice three basic types of treatment: *nonsurgical endodontic treatment, endodontic retreatment,* and *endodontic surgery.*

- *Nonsurgical endodontic treatment:* This procedure, more commonly known simply as a root canal, treats an infection in the pulp by removing the infected pulp entirely, smoothing and shaping the pulp chamber and root canal, and then filling and sealing the tooth. A successful root canal produces a stable, healthy tooth that should last as long as a patient's other natural teeth.

- *Endodontic retreatment:* This procedure involves removing the original filling, again cleaning out the interior of the tooth, and again filling and sealing the tooth. Retreatment is most commonly required when the interior of the tooth has become infected.

- *Endodontic surgery:* Endodontic surgery comprises a group of procedures used for both diagnosis and treatment of problems at the tooth root. For example, the dentist may cut an incision into the gum and peel the tissue back to identify a small fracture that causes pain but does not show up on an X-ray, or he may perform an APICOECTOMY, surgery to trim and smooth the tip of the root or clean away infected tissue around the tip.

Most teeth can be treated with one or more of these three endodontic procedures. The exceptions are:

- teeth whose root canals are inaccessible due to a structural anomaly such as extremely narrow channels or abnormally twisted roots

- teeth with severely fractured roots that cannot be repaired

- teeth that are extremely loose due to a severe loss of the surrounding bone

In these cases, the only practical solution is to extract and replace the tooth.

Oral and Maxillofacial Pathology   The oral and maxillofacial pathologist is a dentist who has completed a postgraduate, in-hospital course in pathology (the study of the nature and causes of disease). Dentists practicing this specialty diagnose and treat health conditions of the mouth, upper jaw, and face including birth defects such as CLEFT LIP AND/OR PALATE. They also work with other medical and dental specialists such as plastic surgeons and pediatric dentists to identify links between oral conditions and systemic disease. A board-certified oral and maxillofacial pathologist has met the requirements of the American Board of Oral and Maxillofacial Pathologists. These requirements include qualifying examinations in surgical oral and maxillofacial pathology (diagnosis via microscopic slides); clinical and radiographic oral and maxillofacial pathology (diagnosis via clinical and radiological images); oral and maxillofacial pathology; and general, systemic, and clinical pathology (written exam on pathology, tissue chemistry, cell biology, and basic science).

Oral and Maxillofacial Radiology   The oral and maxillofacial radiologist is a dentist who has completed a postgraduate, in-hospital residency in radiology. These specialists use the entire panoply of imaging techniques including conventional X-rays, digital imaging, CT scans, MRI (magnetic resonance imaging), and radiation therapy to diagnose and treat illnesses of the mouth, head, and neck. A board-certified oral and maxillofacial radiologist, who is most likely to practice in a recognized medical center or hospital, has passed the examination administered by the American Board of Oral and Maxillofacial Radiology.

Oral and Maxillofacial Surgery   An oral and maxillofacial surgeon is a graduate of a four-year dental school who has completed (at a minimum) a four-year, in-hospital, postgraduate surgical residency. These specialists are trained to diagnose and perform reconstructive surgery to repair soft tissue and bone defects caused by injury, tumors, or birth defects. They are also trained in pain control and treating facial pain, and may perform dental procedures such as the extraction of impacted WISDOM TEETH. A board-certified oral and maxillofacial surgeon has successfully completed written and oral examinations administered by the American Board of Oral and Maxillofacial Surgery.

Orthodontics   Orthodontics and dentofacial orthopedics is the branch of dentistry that repairs defects in the alignment of the teeth and jaws as well as the development of the facial structure. An orthodontist is a dentist who has completed graduate studies in a program accredited by the American Dental Association. A board-certified orthodontist has successfully completed the voluntary written and oral examination of the American Board of Orthodontics (ABO) and continued to renew certification periodically as required by ABO.

Pediatric Dentistry   A pediatric dentist is a professional specializing in the dental care and treatment of children from infancy through adolescence, as well as patients with special health care needs. He has completed four years of dental school and a two-year residency in pediatric dentistry at an accredited dental school whose courses include oral pathology; advanced diagnostic and surgical procedures, including the management of oral and facial injuries and defects; radiology; sedation and anesthesia; child psychology and development; the use and effects of medicines in children; management of oral/facial trauma; and care for patients with special needs. A board-certified pediatric dentist has successfully completed this training and passed the American Board of Pediatric Dentistry's voluntary examination in the field.

Periodontics   Periodontology, from the Greek prefix *peri*-meaning "around" and the word *odonto* meaning "tooth," is a branch of dentistry specializing in the treatment of PERIODONTAL DISEASE, conditions affecting the tissues (gums, bone) that support and nourish the teeth. A periodontist is a graduate of an accredited dental school who has completed an accredited postgraduate residency in periodontal dentistry. A board-certified periodontist has successfully completed the American Board of Periodontology's qualifying examinations.

Prosthodontics   From the Greek word *prosthesis* meaning "an addition." Prosthodontics is the dental specialty dealing with the restoration and/or replacement of teeth using devices such as bridges, caps, CROWNS, DENTURES, IMPLANTOLOGY, and VENEERS. A prosthodontist is a dentist who has graduated from dental school and completed a two-to-three-year program in prosthodontics accredited by the American Dental Association. A board-certified prosthodontist is a dentist who has successfully completed a postgraduate course in prosthodontics and passed the written and oral examinations of the American Board of Prosthodontics. To maintain his certification, the prosthodontist must retake the examinations every eight years.

See also AMERICAN DENTAL ASSOCIATION; ANALGESIC; ANESTHESTIC; ANGLE, EDWARD HARTLEY; CAVITY; CHAIR, DENTIST'S; DENTIFRICE; DENTURE; DRILL; FAUCHARD, PIERRE; FLUORIDE; RADIATION; RESTORATION; SCHOOLS OF DENTISTRY; TOOTH; TOOTHBRUSH.

denture   A dental prosthesis that takes the place of missing teeth. Dentures may also be used in plastic surgery to alter a person's facial shape and/or features.

Over the centuries, human beings have used many different materials to replace lost teeth, including animal teeth, ivory, pieces of bone, and teeth extracted from another person. The artificial teeth in modern dentures are usually made of either strong, wear-resistant acrylic resin or porcelain, a material used most commonly for upper front teeth because porcelain reflects light in a manner similar to natural teeth. Porcelain is more attractive than acrylic resin but not as strong; it is more easily damaged by biting and chewing.

The Types of Dentures

The three basic types of dentures are complete (full) dentures, partial dentures, and overdentures.

Complete (Full) Denture   A full denture is a removable prosthesis that takes the place of all the teeth in the upper or lower JAW. This type of denture is held in place by simple suction or with a thick denture paste/cream or pad or with clips that attach the denture to dental implants in the jaw.

A conventional full denture is one made approximately three months after any oral surgery, allowing time for the wounds to heal. An immediate full denture is made in advance from measurements taken by the dentist; this denture is put in place right after surgery so that the patient has a full set of teeth even as the surgery is healing. The disadvantage of the immediate denture is that as the tissues shrink from healing, the denture will have to be adjusted.

Partial Denture   A partial denture replaces one or more teeth, holding the teeth on either side of the gap in place and, of course, improving the patient's ability to chew and speak as well as his appearance.

A partial denture (also known as a bridge) may be either removable or fixed. A removable partial denture clips to teeth on either side of the missing teeth. A precision partial denture is a removable prosthesis with clips inside the teeth rather than on the side. A fixed partial denture has artificial teeth attached to a CROWN on either side of the false teeth. The crowns are cemented onto the teeth on either side of the missing teeth.

Overdenture   A removable denture that fits over the top of teeth or is attached to dental implants. Overdentures are often more comfortable than full dentures. They are also less likely than full dentures to cause problems with OCCLUSION (how the teeth meet), and they require fewer adjustments over a period of years.

Preparing and Placing a Denture

The first step in preparing a full denture may be oral surgery to remove the last few remaining teeth or to smooth out irregularities in the top of the jaw that might interfere with the fit of the new denture. Once the surgical wounds have healed or if the patient has already lost all the teeth on the jaw for which the denture is being made, the dentist or prosthodontist (a dentist specializing in dental prosthesis) makes models—wax forms or plastic patterns—as templates for the denture. The wax mold is then put in place on the jaw and adjusted to fit snugly. A mold of the jaw is cast from the wax impression and sent to a dental laboratory, which makes the denture. While waiting for the denture, the patient wears a temporary denture.

To prepare the patient's mouth for an overdenture, the dentist shapes the teeth on which the prosthesis will sit and covers them with metal caps to reduce the risk of decay; if required, he inserts implants to hold the overdenture. Then the dentist makes a mold of the area to be covered by the denture and sends the mold to the dental laboratory, which makes the overdenture.

Removable partial dentures are prepared and fit in essentially the same way as an overdenture. A fixed partial denture requires the dentist to prepare the anchoring teeth as for a crown.

Wearing a Denture

A well-made denture fits as comfortably and as securely as possible in the mouth even while the patient speaks and eats. Some patients use a denture adhesive or a denture pad to hold a full denture more securely in place.

Denture paste adhesive is applied to a wet or dry clean denture in amounts sufficient to hold the denture without oozing out over the edges. The denture paste is commonly applied in three series of small "dots," with one series on the left, one on the right, and one in the center.

Denture powder adhesive is shaken onto the denture in a thin, even layer and the excess shaken off. The virtue of a powder adhesive is that it is easier to clean off the denture and the gum tissue.

Denture pads are soft pads that may be impregnated with an adhesive. Like denture paste, denture pads are usually applied in three small strips, one on the right, one on the left, and one in the center.

Denture adhesives and pads should not be used in an attempt to make a poorly prepared or loose denture fit better. Even with a denture adhesive or pad in place, an ill-fitting denture may injure the soft tissue and bone on which it sits, sometimes to the point of triggering an inflammation of the gum tissue or the loss of supporting bone.

Caring for a Denture

In the first few days or weeks, a new denture may be irritating or annoying while chewing or eating, especially if one has not worn dentures before. As a rule, lower dentures seem to be more irritating or annoying than dentures on the upper jaw. Nonetheless, the patient is usually told to wear the new denture 24 hours a day at the beginning to reduce the swelling that occurs naturally after dental work.

Once the dentures feel comfortable and the patient can eat and speak with ease, the dentures should be worn during the day and removed at night. Removing the dentures for several hours allows SALIVA, a mineralized and naturally antimicrobial liquid, to bathe the oral tissues. When the dentures are removed at night, they should be cleaned with a denture cleaner, a product specifically designed to remove debris from the dentures.

In the first year, the patient's gums continue to shrink as they heal, and a complete denture may require refitting or relining to ensure a secure fit. With proper care, if the patient does not have bone loss that changes the shape of the jaw, a denture may last more than 20 years.

See CROWN; IMPLANTOLOGY; PROSTHODONTICS.

disclosing solution   See PLAQUE.

discoloration   See TOOTH DISCOLORATION.

drill   A dental tool used to remove DECAY from the tooth, creating a clean CAVITY to be filled and sealed so as to prevent further damage to the tooth.

From Stone Picks to the Electric Drill

The first dental drills were probably cosmetic devices, tube-shaped jade sticks used by the Mayans to dig a hole into a tooth to insert a decorative jewel. Early Greeks and Romans twirled sharp instruments against a tooth to drill a hole. It was not until the 18th century that the development of a true dental drill began with the introduction of cutting instruments, picks, and scissors-type tools to remove decay from a tooth.

The following chronology details the next series of developments:

- *1728:* French dentist PIERRE FAUCHARD describes a drilling tool turned by catgut twisted around a cylinder.
- *1790:* John Greenwood, best known for being George Washington's dentist, invents the first pedal-powered drill.
- *1829:* Scottish inventor James Naysmyth (alternately, Naysmith) introduces a rotary drill driven by a coiled wire spring.
- *1838:* American dentist John Lewis patents a hand-cranked dental drill bit.
- *1858:* Saint Louis dentist Charles Merry adds a flexible cable to Naysmyth's design for the rotary drill.
- *1864:* In England, George F. Harrington creates a handheld device powered by the spring of a clock movement.
- *1868:* American dentist George F. Green invents a dental drill run by air pumped through a bellows operated with a foot pedal.
- *1871:* James B. Morrison enhances the speed and power of the Naysmyth-Merry designs by adding a flexible arm with a handpiece to hold the drill and a foot treadle.
- *1875:* On January 26, George F. Green patents the first dental drill powered by electricity. Green's drill, a revolutionary but awkward device run by a stand-alone motor, was eventually replaced by "plug-in" drills at the start of the 20th century when office buildings, including those housing dental offices, were wired for electricity.

The Modern Dental Drill

By 1908, most American dental offices were equipped with electricity, and the plug-in electric drill was becoming standard dental equipment. Three years later, in 1911, Emile Huet of Belgium perfected the first high-speed electric engine, capable of running at 10,000 rpms. Because a faster dental drill makes less noise and vibrates less intensely, it is more comfortable for the patient. Huet tried to interest dental manufacturers in his new engine. But he was ahead of his time—contemporary handpieces could not adapt to the speed.

By the 1940s, standard electric dental drills were running at speeds up to 6,000 rpms; those with faster motors were pushing up to 25,000 rpms. In 1953, Robert Neilsen, a research associate of the AMERICAN DENTAL ASSOCIATION (ADA) at the National Bureau of Standards (NBS) in Washington, D.C., created a water-powered turbine drill that ran smoothly at 60,000 rpms. Four years later, an NBS coworker, John Borden, invented a miniature compressed air–powered turbine called the Airotor that fit into the head of a dental handpiece designed to emit a fine stream of water to prevent the bit and the tooth from overheating while the dentist drilled.

Borden's basic design remains the standard, although the inevitable advances in technology have made it possible to push the speed of the engine up to 600,000 rpms on a modern drill. Regardless of the speed, the drill itself has three basic components: a motor, a handpiece, and a drill bit.

The Motor High speed drills are driven by a turbine powered by pressurized air that rotates a drill bit at speeds of more than 300,000 rpms. Because slower speeds may be needed for tasks such as polishing, dental drills usually have a second, slower electric motor.

The Handpiece The drill handpiece is a tube-shaped, lightweight device made of strong plastic, metal alloys, or titanium. In addition to the connection for the bit, the handpiece has connections for cooling water and air the dentist uses to flush or blow away debris, leaving a clear field in which to work. Some handpieces also have a fiber-optic light source to illuminate the tooth.

The Drill Bit The bit, a.k.a. the bur, is a small, highly durable instrument made of tungsten carbide. Bits come in several different shapes to accommodate different situations such as cutting into a tooth or cleaning out a cavity.

Alternatives to the Dental Drill

In the future, dentists may be able to enter a tooth or clean out a cavity without a conventional drill.

One alternative to the motor-driven drill is AIR ABRASION. This technique, which aims small air-driven particles of aluminum at the surface of the tooth, can be used in periodontal treatment to clean away plaque and may be used when treating small cavities or cleaning debris from otherwise hard-to-reach surfaces inside a cavity or between teeth.

A second alternative is the LASER. The Food and Drug Administration (FDA) has approved the use of argon and carbon dioxide lasers to activate tooth-whitening solutions and to work on soft tissue; for example, to treat gum disease. The FDA has also approved two lasers, the erbium YAG laser and the erbium chromium YSGG laser, whose energy is absorbed by water and hydroxyapatite, the calcium compound in teeth, to shape the inside of a cavity for a filling, to repair a defective filling, or to shape a tooth for bonding.

drill-less dentistry See AIR ABRASION; ANESTHETIC/ANESTHETICS; METH MOUTH; PAIN.

dry mouth See XEROSTOMIA.

dry socket The condition that occurs when the blood clot at the site of an extraction, such as the removal of a wisdom tooth, is dislodged. The loss of the clot exposes nerves and bone, triggering pain not only at the site, but also along the NERVES that run to the ear and eye on the same side of the face.

Symptoms and Diagnostic Path

The most common symptom of dry socket is pain that becomes increasingly severe in the days right after the extraction. There may be an unpleasant odor and taste in the mouth; the lymph nodes in the jaw and neck may be swollen. The loss of the clot is clearly visible on examination; the socket looks empty ("dry") and the bone may be seen at the bottom of the concavity.

Treatment Options and Outlook

Once the dentist has made certain that the cause of the postextraction discomfort is dry socket, she may prescribe one or more remedies for the pain. These treatments include (but are not limited to):

- medicated dressings packed into the socket
- rinsing out the socket to remove any irritating debris such as particles of food
- over-the-counter or prescription pain relievers
- home care, such as flushing the wound with salt water, mouthwash, or a prescription rinse; applying cold packs to the side of the face; and following all directions regarding medication

With treatment, the pain should be reduced and the wound begin to heal; complete healing usually occurs within two weeks.

Risk Factors and Preventive Measures

The risk factors for dry socket may include:

- *Tobacco*. The chemicals in tobacco and tobacco smoke, as well as the sucking action when drawing on a lit cigar, cigarette, or pipe, may irritate and/or contaminate the wound.
- *Infection*. Existing or previous infection around the site of the extraction, including incidents of periodontal disease.
- *Personal susceptibility*. A history of dry socket increases future risk.
- *Oral contraceptives*. The high levels of estrogen in oral contraceptives may dissolve the blood clot.

The best way to reduce the risk of dry socket is to follow the dentist's pre- and postextraction instructions to the letter.

E

eating disorder An eating disorder is a psychological illness characterized by eating too much or eating too little. The term covers a wide variety of medical conditions such as obesity and binge eating (eating very large amounts of food at one sitting). But it is most commonly used to describe anorexia nervosa (voluntary starvation) or bulimia (voluntary purging of food after eating, either through regurgitation or the use of laxatives and diuretics). Both these conditions produce visible changes in the teeth, gums, and JAWS. As a result, a dental professional rather than a primary care physician may be the first health care provider to identify the problem.

Symptoms and Diagnostic Path

The most obvious sign of anorexia nervosa or bulimia is a dramatic, unexplained weight loss and failure to gain back the lost weight even when food is freely available. The dental consequences of nutritional deficiencies due to anorexia nervosa or frequent vomiting among bulimics include:

- erosion of the dental ENAMEL due to repeated vomiting of acidic stomach contents (pregnant women who suffer from severe morning sickness with frequent episodes of vomiting may experience similar erosion of the enamel surface of the teeth)
- dry mouth; cracked and bleeding lips
- oral pain
- increased sensitivity to temperature changes
- frequent infection

- increased incidence of decay
- loosened teeth and loss of bone in the jaw due to nutritional deficiencies
- change in tooth shape, color, and strength
- enlarged salivary glands

Treatment Options and Outlook

Among psychiatric disorders, anorexia nervosa has the highest incidence of death—up to 15 percent. Chronic starvation produces serious medical problems, up to and including death by heart failure. And data from one study published in the *Archives of General Psychiatry* in 2003 suggests that women with anorexia were up to 57 times more likely than healthy women to commit suicide.

The first treatment option is to stabilize the patient's medical condition, if necessary. The second is to provide psychiatric therapy designed to address the patient's reasons for rejecting food. The conditions are difficult to cure; treatment is long-term and characterized by frequent relapses.

Risk Factors and Preventive Measures

Anorexia nervosa and bulimia are most common among young people in places where food is plentiful. They are at least nine times more common among young women than among young men. Many who treat eating disorders theorize that the illnesses represent a patient's attempt to exercise control over life decisions by controlling food intake. More information on eating disorders is available from the National Eating Disorders Association at www.nationaleatingdisorders.org.

embrasure From the French word *embraser*, meaning to "widen the opening in a door or window"; in dentistry, it refers to the space ("opening") between two teeth.

The embrasure has a serious dental function, providing an opening through which food can escape when a person is chewing so that it (the food) does not form a solid block of material that might interfere with either chewing or swallowing.

According to one 2008 study published in the *Journal of Prosthetic Dentistry,* as a general but not invariable rule, naturally occurring embrasures are larger and thus provide a more effective spillway than the embrasures in dental RESTORATIONS such as fixed or removable DENTURES. When creating restorations, the prosthodontist must keep this in mind so as to provide an adequate escape route for food and liquids.

An interdental embrasure is the space from front to back and top to bottom between two teeth. A buccal embrasure is the space between the teeth looking at the surfaces nearest the cheek; a labial embrasure, the surfaces facing the lips; a lingual embrasure, the surfaces facing the tongue; an occlusal embrasure, the surfaces on top where the teeth meet when chewing. An embrasure clasp is a device inserted between two teeth to hold them together. An embrasure hook holds a removable denture in place between two teeth.

emergencies, dental In the United States, dental emergencies such as a fractured tooth, fractured jaw, "KNOCKED-OUT TOOTH," and TOOTHACHE are an underreported but real problem for both adults and children. According to the National Center for Health Statistics of the Centers for Disease Control and Prevention's 1999 National Hospital Ambulatory Medical Care Survey, more than one out of 10 persons who go to an emergency room are seeking treatment for a facial injury or dental problem. These problems have real consequences: The National Institute for Dental and Craniofacial Research's Oral Health Survey 2002 reports that American students missed more than 1.5 million school days in 1996 due to dental or facial pain.

As a rule, dental emergencies fall into one of two broad categories: problems due to infection arising from decay or PERIODONTAL DISEASE and problems related to an injury. Early treatment for dental DECAY and periodontal disease plus good oral hygiene obviously lowers the incidence of complications due to advanced disease, while the use of protective dental appliances such as MOUTH GUARDS lowers the risk of facial injury in both adults and children engaged in contact sports.

However, in dentistry as in medicine, the American emergency room appears to function as an introduction to basic health care. According to the NIH/CDC 2002 survey, 80 percent of children under 3.5 years old first saw a dentist when they went to an emergency room for a dental/facial injury, and 69 percent of all dental emergency patients did not see a dentist on a regular basis.

When a person with a dental emergency goes to an emergency room, his problem is likely to be treated first by a physician rather than a dentist. In many cases, this is appropriate because the injury, such as a fractured jaw or bleeding in the mouth that does not stop, is a medical problem with dental effects. In other cases, such as a knocked-out tooth, a dentist or dental surgeon is the more appropriate choice. To meet this need, a few medical centers, such as Children's Hospital in Boston, maintain an emergency number for dental assistance so that an injured person who calls ahead may be met by a dentist in the emergency room.

See also JAW, FRACTURE.

enamel, dental The hard smooth outer covering of the crown (top) of the tooth; one of the four main components of a tooth, the other three being CEMENTUM (the outer surface of the tooth root), DENTIN (the layer of hard tissue under the enamel and cementum), and PULP (the soft tissue inside the tooth).

The Formation of Enamel

The enamel begins to form in the tooth bud, the embryonic structure inside the JAW that gives rise to a tooth. At this stage, the enamel is a soft mixture of mineral crystals called calcium hydroxyapatite embedded in a matrix (network) made of fibers of a protein called *amelogenin*. As a tooth bud develops into a tooth, the protein and fat matrix disappears, and the tooth emerges from the gum with a shiny mineral enamel surface over the crown (and a layer of cementum over the root) designed to resist damage from acidic foods or the acidic liquids excreted by the bacteria responsible for dental DECAY, the single most common cause of injury to the dental enamel.

Damaging Dental Enamel

Dental enamel is rightly characterized as the hardest substance in the human body. But it is formed from cells that disappear as the tooth matures so it cannot reconstitute itself, which means that it is not impervious to decay—the most common cause of damage to the enamel—or to physical injury, or to the destructive effects of certain medical conditions and environmental exposures. The list of situations in which the dental enamel is damaged includes but is not limited to the following:

- *Antibiotic exposure during tooth development:* A child who is given a tetracycline antibiotic while his teeth are developing or a child whose mother took a tetracycline antibiotic while she was pregnant may develop teeth with a mottled brownish color.
- *Birth defects:* One example of a birth defect affecting the dental enamel is AMELOGENESIS IMPERFECTA, a rare inherited disorder characterized by thin, soft enamel.
- *Tooth grinding and clenching:* The pressure of tooth-against-tooth exerted when a person

involuntarily clenches or grinds his teeth, a condition known as BRUXISM, may chip or wear away the biting surfaces of the teeth (the edges that meet during chewing). Occasionally the pressure is strong enough to crack the tooth.
- *Digestive disorder:* Celiac disease, a condition that prevents the body from absorbing nutrients in certain types of food, is sometimes accompanied by stained dental enamel.
- *Excess exposure to fluorides:* In areas such as the southwestern United States, the groundwater supply is naturally high in fluorides. Long-term exposure to these high levels of fluorides may stain the enamel. Moderate exposure, as with fluoridated water supplies, is beneficial; it strengthens teeth without producing these adverse effects.
- *Excess exposure to chlorine:* This situation, rarely encountered by anyone other than an athlete who spends long periods of time in highly chlorinated swimming pools, may result in erosion of the dental enamel.
- *Gastric reflux:* The repeated regurgitation of acidic stomach contents experienced by a person with gastroesophageal reflux disease (GERD) can erode the enamel surface of the teeth.
- *Nutritional deficiency:* A child with the vitamin D deficiency disease rickets may develop a rough band on the dental enamel. (Note: In adults, a vitamin D deficiency is called osteomalacia.)

Repairing Dental Enamel

Currently, dentists ameliorate damage to the dental enamel by bleaching away stains, filling cavities, and restoring the tooth surface with a variety of prostheses such as INLAYS, ONLAYS, and CROWNS to rebuild the parts of the tooth lost to decay or injury. Dental researchers, however, are working to discover means to repair the tooth surface by creating an artificial substance that mimics the hardness and durability of natural enamel and can be implanted or transplanted to the human tooth.

To do this they must be able to replicate the process by which minerals are deposited in an amelogenin matrix and then harden, replacing the soft matrix/mineral complex with a hard and durable enamel surface. While not yet completely successful, these projects have yielded intriguing first steps.

For example, in March 2005, a team of researchers at the University of Southern California, in Los Angeles, published a report in the journal *Science* explaining that they had been able to organize amelogenin crystals into long strands ("ribbons") that could be dipped into a mineral solution to form a structure resembling the natural matrix from which teeth emerge.

In March 2007 at the 85th general session of the International Association for Dental Research, a team of dental researchers from the Institute of Medical Science at the University of Tokyo, in Japan, reported finding a way to grow cells from the developing teeth of young pigs that showed promise as a way to create artificial enamel. However, this promise and that of similar research remains a work in progress.

See also ABRASION; EATING DISORDER; EROSION; FLUORIDE; RESTORATION; SEALANT; TOOTH.

endodontics From the Latin word *endo-* meaning "inside" and the Greek word *odont* or *odonto* meaning "tooth." Endodontics is one of the nine dental specialties approved by the AMERICAN DENTAL ASSOCIATION (ADA) Council on Dental Education and Licensure. Endodontics is the branch of dentistry dealing with treatment of the interior of the tooth: the pulp chamber (the hollow space inside the tooth), the pulp (soft tissue containing nerves, blood vessels, and connective tissue), and the root canal (the narrowing of the pulp canal inside the tooth root or roots). An endodontist is a dentist who has completed four years of dental school plus two or more years of specialty training. A board-certified endodontist has passed three qualifying examinations (written, case history, oral) offered by the American Board of Endodontics.

Endodontics includes three basic types of treatment: Nonsurgical endodontic treatment, endodontic retreatment, and endodontic surgery.

Nonsurgical endodontic treatment is a procedure more commonly known as a ROOT CANAL. It treats an infection in the pulp by removing the infected pulp entirely, smoothing and shaping the pulp chamber and root canal[s], and then filling and sealing the tooth. A successful root canal produces a stable, healthy tooth that should last as long as a patient's other natural teeth.

Endodontic retreatment is used to correct any deficits in the original root canal treatment or to resolve a new problem with the tooth such as decay, a broken filling, or an injury to the tooth that leads to infection. To treat this, the endodontist removes the original filling, again cleans out the interior of the tooth, and again fills and seals the tooth. If the endodontist discovers a problem with the structure of the root or the root canals that would lead to failure of the retreatment he is likely to recommend a third type of endodontic treatment, endodontic surgery.

Endodontic surgery is a group of procedures used for both diagnosis and treatment of problems at the tooth root(s). The treatment may be inside or outside the root. As an example of the former, the endodontist may go into the root canal to remove calcium deposits that narrow the canals and interfere with endodontic treatment. As examples of the latter, he may cut an incision into the gum and peel the tissue back to locate a small fracture that causes pain but does not show up on an X-ray, or he may perform an APICOECTOMY, surgery to trim and smooth the tip of the root or clean away infected tissue around the tip.

Most teeth can be treated with one of more of these three endodontic procedures. The exceptions are:

- teeth whose root canals are inaccessible due to a structural anomaly such as extremely narrow channels or abnormally twisted roots

- teeth with severely fractured roots that cannot be repaired
- teeth that are extremely loose due to a severe loss of the surrounding bone

In these cases, the only practical solution is to extract and replace the tooth.

See also DENTISTRY; IMPLANTOLOGY; ORAL AND MAXILLOFACIAL PATHOLOGY; ORAL AND MAXILLOFACIAL RADIOLOGY; ORAL AND MAXILLOFACIAL SURGERY; ORTHODONTICS AND DENTOFACIAL ORTHOPEDICS; PERIODONTICS; PROSTHODONTICS; PUBLIC HEALTH DENTISTRY; ROOT CANAL TREATMENT.

epidemiology Epidemiology is the study of how frequently an illness or condition such as dental DECAY or PERIODONTAL DISEASE occurs among human beings and how many people it affects. This information is derived from epidemiological studies, which show the incidence (the number of new cases of a specific problem) and the prevalence (the proportion of the population affected) of the condition.

Epidemiological studies may be prospective or retrospective. A prospective study begins with a group of people such as several nine-year-old children, and follows them forward in time to see how a factor such as what they eat or what medicines they take affects their risk of a certain condition such as developing dental cavities. A retrospective study looks at a group of people such as a sample of 50-year-old adults with periodontal disease and examines their medical and dental history to evaluate how their past behavior, such as poor dental hygiene, affected their current dental health.

The accuracy of an epidemiological study is influenced by a number of variables. One is whether the study included human beings. This is important because while a study on animals may indicate an effect on human beings, it cannot be regarded as conclusive because different species react differently to various chemicals and diseases. A second variable is the number, gender, race, and age of the people in the study. Unless the aim of the study is to seek results specific to one group—for example, the incidence of sickle-cell anemia among persons of African descent—the study must include several hundred or more men and women of all ages and races. Finally, a retrospective study is often considered less accurate than a prospective study because people inevitably have memory lapses about past behavior.

See also EVIDENCE-BASED DENTISTRY.

erosion, dental From the Latin word *erodere,* meaning "to eat away." Dental erosion is the term used to describe damage to the ENAMEL or DENTIN surface of a tooth due to a chemical reaction. This may occur due to the consumption of acidic liquids, for example, or when a person suffering from heartburn experiences gastroesophageal reflux, meaning the flow of acidic stomach contents rises back into the esophagus, up into the mouth, and against the teeth.

Symptoms and Diagnostic Path

Common signs of dental erosion include, but are not limited to:

- widespread sensitivity to changes in temperature and sweet foods
- fillings that look as though they are raised above the surface of the tooth
- worn spots and "scooped out" grooves on the sides of the teeth
- chipping of the edges of the teeth that meet when the teeth are closed
- increased translucency of the teeth

Treatment Options and Outlook

The treatment for dental erosion is tailored to the specific damage. As a rule, the longer the erosion had continued, the deeper the damage and the more complex the remedy.

If the erosion is superficial and its most troublesome problem is sensitivity to heat, cold, and sweets, the dentist may simply recommend the use of fluoride gels, rinses, or DENTIFRICES to strengthen the tooth surface, or toothpastes that contain ingredients that desensitize the tooth.

Once the erosion has progressed to minor but visible damage such as a depression in the surface of the tooth, the dentist may recommend coating the surface of the tooth with a tooth-colored plastic COMPOSITE material that hardens to form a protective and cosmetically appealing shield.

Severe erosion that has penetrated the enamel and exposed the dentin (the softer layer underneath the enamel) or reached into the center (pulp chamber) of the tooth requires a fuller restoration such as a CROWN or, depending on the damage, even a full replacement tooth.

Risk Factors and Preventive Measures

Dental erosion is an underreported but growing problem. In 2008, a team of researchers from the University of Texas Health Science Center, in San Antonio, Indiana University, and the University of California, San Francisco, interviewed 900 students age 10 to 14 and found that nearly one-third of the students already had measurable erosion of the dental enamel. The researchers attributed this to excess ingestion of highly acidic foods such as soft drinks, some fruit juices, herbal teas, and "energy" drinks.

Other known causes of dental erosion include (but are not limited to) excessive use of acidic medical drugs such as aspirin, excessive exposure to acidic chemicals such as the chlorine in a swimming pool, or occupational exposure to toxic fumes from substances such as battery acid. To reduce the risk and/or severity of dental erosion, patients are usually advised to:

- cut back on ingestion of acidic foods
- check with the doctor regarding use of acidic medical drugs such as aspirin
- wear protective equipment at work or during athletic activities involving exposure to acidic chemicals

- schedule regular dental checkups to evaluate the health of the dental enamel
- use FLUORIDE products as directed to strengthen the dental enamel

See also ABRASION; BRUXISM; DECAY; EATING DISORDER.

erythroplakia, erythroplasia See ORAL CANCER.

esthetic (aesthetic) dentistry See COSMETIC DENTISTRY.

etching Dental etching is a technique used to prepare a tooth to accept a restoration such as a composite VENEER by roughening the surface of the tooth so that the adhesive used to hold the restoration in place will attach more firmly. The dentist may choose one of three basic roughening techniques: An acid such a phosphoric acid; a LASER; or AIR ABRASION, a procedure that bombards the tooth surface with small particles of sand to create small indentations that facilitate bonding.

Dental etching is considered a safe procedure. The only risks are sensitivity to heat and cold for a short time after the etching is done and, if the etching is too vigorous, demineralization of the surface of the tooth.

See also ABRASIVE.

ethics, dental code of The American Dental Association (ADA) Principles of Ethics and Code of Professional Conduct is a guide to ethical interactions between the dentist, his patient, and his community. The report is organized into five sections, each addressing one of the following topics:

Patient Autonomy The dentist's duty to respect the patient's rights and confidentiality. To this end, ADA urges dentists to fully inform patients about the good and bad points in any treatment plan and enlist the patient's co-operation in choosing a treatment while keeping all details of the patient's health and treatment confidential.

Nonmaleficence The dentist's duty not to harm the patient. In service to this principle, ADA expects dentists to keep their knowledge and their staff's understanding of treatments current and, when required, to refer a patient to a specialist.

Beneficence The dentist's duty to promote the welfare of the patient. To do this, ADA encourages dentists to put the patient's needs first and, when possible, to engage in community service that benefits the larger community.

Justice The dentist's obligation to treat people fairly. This principle means that the dentist may not discriminate against patients based on individual characteristics such as race or religion and must, where feasible, offer care in an emergency.

Veracity The dentist's duty to speak truthfully. Quite simply, this means that the dentist should be truthful in all his dealings with patients, other professionals, and the community at large.

The entire *ADA Principles of Ethics and Code of Professional Conduct* is available online beginning at http://www.ada.org/194.aspx.

Eustachio, Bartolomeo (1520–1574) Italian physician who devoted himself to the study of the structures of the human body. Eustachio served as professor of anatomy at the Roman University and as physician to various officials at the Vatican.

In 1563, he authored the first published book on dentistry, *Libellus de dentibus* (A little treatise on the teeth). As an investigative dental anatomist, he detailed the muscles of the face, mouth, and neck. He also established the tissue composition of the tongue and identified the internal structure of the tooth, and he was renowned for his exploration of the structure of the inner ear. In addition to producing the first descriptions of the stirrup bone, also called the stapes, one of the three bones of the middle ear, he discovered the small but vital tube that connects the ear to the mouth, a small passage that was named in his honor: the eustachian tube.

Eustachio's greatest work, however, remained unpublished during his lifetime. The *explicatio tabularum anatomicarum* (Anatomical engravings), completed in 1552, could not be published during Eustachio's lifetime due to religious bans on dissection. But when the drawings were finally published for the first time in 1714, nearly a century and a half after his death, the book became a best-seller, firmly establishing Eustachio's preeminence in anatomical science.

evidence-based dentistry Like evidence-based medicine, evidence-based dentistry represents an attempt to use data obtained from various sources to:

- determine the accuracy of tests used to diagnose a disease or condition
- predict the course of the disease or condition
- evaluate the effectiveness of treatment options in light of a particular patient's dental and medical situation so as to determine the best course of treatment

Evidence-based data may support or discredit a theory or procedure. For example, there is clear evidence to support the idea that applying fluorides to the enamel surface of the teeth reduces the incidence of dental DECAY (see FLUORIDE). On the other hand, in 2008, information garnered from repeated studies was used to reverse the widespread practice of prescribing penicillin antibiotics to patients with certain forms of heart disease before any dental procedure. Studies showed no proof that the antibiotics were either effective or ineffective, but did show a clear risk of drug reactions and an unjustified increase in cost to the patient.

Evidence-based dentistry is a useful tool but not a perfect one. The primary objection is that this is really a one-size-fits-all option based on studies rather than the experience of a dental or medical professional with a specific patient. To counter this, proponents of evidence-based dentistry and evidence-based medicine say they are valuable tools so long as the possibility of benefit to many is balanced against the risk of harm to a specific patient, an evaluation to be performed by the patient's own physician.

For readers interested in the list of evidence-based dental assumptions, the AMERICAN DENTAL ASSOCIATION (ADA) maintains a page on its Web site offering access to the latest examples with data drawn from its own library plus the following sources:

- Medline, the National Library of Medicine's searchable database of over 12 million indexed citations from more than 4,600 medical, dental, health, and scientific journals
- The Cochrane Collaboration, an international nonprofit group that creates evidence-based health-care reports/reviews
- EMBASE, a database of more than 18 million biomedical and pharmacological entries
- SIGLE (System for Information on Grey Literature in Europe), a database comprising European "grey literature"—that is, technical and research reports, conference papers, doctoral dissertations, and other forms of scientific literature.

The Web address for the ADA page on evidence-based dentistry is www.ada.org/276.asp. For other patient-friendly dental Web sites, see Appendix V.

See also EPIDEMIOLOGY.

evulsed tooth See "KNOCKED-OUT TOOTH."

examination, dental The routine dental examination is designed to evaluate the state of a patient's dental and oral health. The examination is a multipart procedure that includes:

- collecting the patient's medical and dental history
- conducting a visual examination of the mouth
- performing a physical examination of the teeth and gums, including palpation of the tissue to check for ORAL CANCERS
- taking X-rays of the teeth (as required)
- consulting with and advising the patient

According to the University of Washington Dental Fears Research Clinic, in Seattle, as many as 8 percent of Americans are so badly frightened by the prospect of this basic examination and the prospect of dental treatment that they avoid seeing a dentist until absolutely necessary.

Perhaps the most frequently cited reason for avoiding dentistry is the fear of dental injections. For example, a 1995 survey by the Seattle researchers showed that more than one in four of the students and staff were wary of dental injections; one in 20 said they had avoided, cancelled, or failed to show up for a dental appointment due to fear of an injection. Most blamed the pain of the injections for their reactions. Others were afraid of being injured by the injection, or of contracting a contagious disease from the needle, or suffering a side effect, or not getting enough pain relief during a procedure.

Modern dental professionals have several ways to address the fear of dental treatment, beginning with an initial interview conducted with the patient in the dentist's office rather than in the dental chair. Other stratagems include explaining exactly what a dental procedure entails, agreeing on signals such as raising one's hand that enable the patient to stop the dentist's work, providing adequate pain control tailored to the patient's tolerance, and—if these are not sufficient—suggesting that the patient consider instruction in relaxation therapy and/or a referral for psychological counseling.

Procedure

The well-designed dental examination is designed to produce a full picture of the patient's dental health so as to enable the dentist to plan a successful course of treatment. It includes the following:

Medical and Dental History Before beginning the physical examination, the dentist or dental hygienist will ask a new patient to list any health problems as well as current medications. A returning patient will be asked to report any recent changes in her general health.

Visual Examination of the Mouth The dentist will inspect the TONGUE, gums, and inside of the LIPS and cheeks, looking specifically for any indication of oral cancer. This examination may also include an examination of the head and neck area. He will check the temporomandibular joint at the side of the head that connects the lower jaw to the skull for any discomfort that might indicate TEMPOROMANDIBULAR JOINT DISORDER. He will palpate (feel) the salivary glands under the tongue and chin and the lymph glands in the neck to check for any signs of infection or swelling that might indicate infection or disease, such as cancer.

Physical Examination Using specialized probes, the dentist will examine the teeth for signs of DECAY. He may, if required, evaluate the patient's bite (how the teeth meet when closed) to determine the need for orthodontic treatment. Finally, the dentist will use a probe to examine the spaces between the teeth and the gums for inflammation and bleeding or other signs of PERIODONTAL DISEASE.

Radiographic Examination Depending on the patient's history and current oral health, the dentist may recommend a series of X-rays to check for hidden decay and/or signs of bone loss consistent with periodontal disease.

Consultation The examination concludes with a consultation between dentist and patient during which the two discuss the patient's dental health and any proposed treatment.

Risks and Complications

The routine dental examination has no apparent risks or complications.

Outlook and Lifestyle Modifications

The dental examination affords the dentist and patient the opportunity to identify and solve dental problems. To this end, once the examination is complete, the dentist will offer the patient recommendations for continuing care, including proper home care methods and information about any further treatments for problems identified during the examination. If required, the dentist will refer the patient to a specialist such as a periodontist, endodontist, or orthodontist.

As a rule, the dentist will urge the patient to arrange his next appointment before leaving the office. Dental experts recommend that patients visit the dentist at least once or more properly twice a year for a checkup and cleaning. Patients with more severe dental problems may require more frequent visits. Setting the appointment while the patient is in the office helps to maintain a regular schedule.

See also DECAY; ENDODONTICS; EXAMINATION, PERIODONTAL; ORTHODONTICS AND DENTOFACIAL ORTHOPEDICS; PERIODONTAL DISEASE; X-RAY EXAMINATION.

examination, periodontal The routine periodontal examination is a specialized multipart procedure designed to evaluate the health of the patient's gums and underlying jawbone. The examination includes:

- collecting information to produce a dental and periodontal profile
- performing a visual examination of the patient's mouth

- examining the physical state of the teeth and gums
- evaluating the health of the supporting BONE

Procedure

Like the basic dental examination (see EXAMINATION, DENTAL), the successful periodontal examination proceeds in logical order starting with an interview between dentist and patient.

Dental and Periodontal History   Before beginning the physical examination, the periodontist or dental hygienist will ask a new patient to report any previous dental or periodontal problems and/or procedures. A returning patient will be asked to report any recent changes in her general health.

Visual and Physical Examination   Like all dental examinations, the periodontal examination begins with looking at the patient's mouth to assess the condition of the gums and identify any obvious inflammation, infection, or progression of disease since the patient's last visit. Following the visual examination, the periodontist or dental hygienist uses a dental probe to measure four common signs of periodontal disease:

- *Gum recession*: The movement of the gum up or down away from the cementoenamel junction (CEJ), the line where the enamel covering the top of the tooth meets the cementum covering the root
- *Pockets*: Spaces between the tooth and gum created when the attachment between the two is broken by PERIODONTAL DISEASE
- *Bone loss*: Erosion of the alveolar bone, the sockets in the jaw into which teeth fit
- *Tooth mobility*: The free movement of teeth that occurs when bone is lost

X-ray Study   While the physical examination provides clues to the extent of bone loss due to periodontal disease, an X-ray provides conclusive evidence of bone loss and/or disease

progression that enables the periodontist to plan future treatment.

Cleaning   Having completed the physical examination, the dentist or the dental hygienist will use a scaler, a specialized instrument designed to remove hardened tartar (CALCULUS) that has collected on the tooth surface beneath the gum line. When the teeth are clean, the dental hygienist will polish the teeth to remove stains and smooth out microscopic rough patches where food and bacteria might catch, a step that helps reduce the risk of decay and periodontal disease. If required, the cleaning may end with the application of a FLUORIDE solution to strengthen the dental ENAMEL.

Risks and Complications

After a routine periodontal examination, the patient may experience slight discomfort and bleeding at the gum line (the place where the top of the gum meets the tooth).

Outlook and Lifestyle Modifications

The routine periodontal examination offers the periodontist and patient an opportunity to assess the progression of existing periodontal disease, identify and treat new problems, and create or continue a treatment program. To this end, once the examination is complete, the periodontist (like the dentist after a standard dental examination) will offer the patient recommendations for continuing care, including proper home care methods and information about any further treatment for problems identified during the examination.

As a rule, the periodontist will urge the patient to arrange his next appointment before leaving the office so as to maintain a regular schedule of checkups.

exodontics   See EXTRACTION.

expander   An appliance used in orthodontics to increase the size of the dental ARCH. Examples of expanders include, but are not limited to, the following:

The biometric distalizing arch (BMDA/LA) is an appliance used on the upper JAW along with a lower lingual arch to push the six-year molars (molars that generally erupt from the jaw by age six) on the upper jaw back to make room for the rest of the permanent teeth. The BMDA/LA is attached to the lower lingual arch with rubber bands that the patient puts on and takes off himself.

The quad helix expander is a firm WIRE appliance that widens the upper jaw. It is cemented to the inner surface of the upper molars and remains in place for several months to move the jaw farther out to either side.

The rapid palatal expander (RPE) is an expander made of firm wires attached to a central plate that sits in the middle of the roof of the mouth. The wires are cemented to the molars on each side, and the plate contains screws that the patient can turn as directed to widen the jaw. Once the jaw has reached the desired width, the RPE is left in place for several months as the bone settles firmly into place.

The T-rex expander, an appliance used to widen the upper jaw and push back the upper six-year molars. This expander may be attached to a headgear, an external appliance that circles the head and holds an appliance inside the mouth in place.

See also ORTHODONTICS AND DENTOFACIAL ORTHOPEDICS.

extraction   Dental procedure to remove a tooth, usually recommended when a tooth is so badly damaged that it cannot be repaired. Removing even one tooth can allow shifting of adjoining teeth, leading to MALOCCLUSION, so dentists normally recommend extraction only for:

- a tooth so badly broken or decayed that it cannot be repaired
- a tooth whose nerve is damaged but which is not considered suitable for endodontic (root canal) surgery because the tooth structure itself is too fragile
- one or more teeth so loosened by PERIODONTAL DISEASE that they cannot be made stable
- an impacted wisdom tooth (a tooth set in the jaw in a position that makes it impossible for the tooth to erupt through the gum)
- a tooth on the top or lower jaw that has no opposing tooth and will eventually move out of the jaw
- a tooth or teeth that crowd the jaw, push other teeth out of line, and will interfere with orthodontic treatment (a dental procedure to straighten and realign the teeth)

Exodontics, from the Latin prefix *ex-*, meaning "out," and the Greek word *odonto*, meaning "tooth," is the branch of dentistry devoted to extracting teeth from the mouth.

Procedure

Once the dentist has numbed the tooth, gum, and jaw, he begins by moving the gum away from the tooth. Next, he starts to loosen the tooth from its socket (the indentation in the jaw in which a tooth sits) by inserting a small screwdriverlike instrument called an elevator between the tooth and the bone and moving the tooth back and forth. As the tooth moves, the bone around it is compressed. Once the dentist has enlarged the bony socket, he begins to turn the tooth from one side to the other so as to break its connection to the ligament (the tough band of connective tissue) that ties the tooth to the bone. When the ligament is loosened, the dentist uses a pliers-like tool called an extraction forceps to lift it from the jaw. Most commonly, the tooth is extracted whole. However, if its roots are curved rather than positioned straight down into the socket, the dentist may have to section the tooth—that is, to cut it into pieces to remove it.

Risks and Complications

The most common complications of an extraction are mild pain, bleeding, and swelling.

Ordinarily, the pain is controlled with a nonprescription analgesic. Postextraction heavy bleeding, bleeding that lasts longer than an hour or two, or swelling or pain that increases after the first day may be a sign of infection. If these occur, the patient should check with his dentist, who may recommend antibiotics.

The first sign of healing after an extraction is the formation of a blood clot at the site. The clot, which closes the wound and stops the bleeding, is composed of cells specifically designed to begin the healing process and the formation of new tissue. Dislodging the clot leads to DRY SOCKET and exposure of the bone under the extracted tooth, a complication that occurs in about 5 percent of all extractions. To avoid dislodging or dissolving the clot, patients are advised to avoid hot liquids, alcoholic beverages, hard foods, vigorous rinsing, or sucking actions such as smoking or drinking through a straw that might create a vacuum that pulls out the clot. However, it is important to keep the mouth clean as the wound heals by brushing the other teeth and gently rinsing the extraction area as directed by the dentist.

The long-term complication of extraction may be shifting of the teeth on either side of the extraction. If this occurs, it may affect the way the upper and lower teeth meet, and eventually interfere with the ability to chew. As the adjoining teeth shift, they may also loosen, becoming a more likely site for periodontal disease. A second consequence of extraction is extrusion, the movement of a tooth upward or downward and out of its place in the jaw. Extrusion may occur because the tooth above (or below) the extracted tooth no longer meets an opposing force when the teeth are closed. To forestall these problems, the dentist may recommend replacing the extracted tooth with an artificial one that is put in place either immediately after the surgery or once the area has healed.

Outlook and Lifestyle Modifications

Removing a damaged or decayed tooth and replacing it with an artificial tooth relieves pain and reduces the risk of infection, and thus protects the patient's dental health.

facebow A facebow is a form of orthodontic headgear, a device that encircles the head and hooks up to an ANCHORAGE on the back teeth to exert pressure on the molars so as to move them farther back in the dental arch in order to accommodate crowded front teeth.

A generic facebow is made of two curved metal components. The first goes around the outside of the face. The second component fits inside the mouth; its ends slip into tubes fastened to the buccal (cheek) side of the back teeth. An elastic band attached to the outer part of the appliance goes around the neck to hold the two components in place. Tightening the elastic band increases pressure on the back teeth, moving them farther back.

The facebow, which may be worn up to 14 hours a day, is considered annoying and unattractive but not actively uncomfortable. It is commonly removed at night so as to avoid injury should the ends of the inner structure accidentally come loose from the buccal tubes or the ends of the outer structure slip from the elastic bands while the patient is sleeping.

See ORTHODONTICS AND DENTOFACIAL ORTHOPEDICS.

facial bones See BONE.

facial cleft A birth defect; the failure of the bony plates in the fetal skull to fuse normally during pregnancy, leaving a visible separation in the bones and/or other tissues of the face. As might be expected, facial clefts often affect the positioning of the lips and teeth and thus the ability to eat, speak, or breathe properly.

Facial clefts usually occur where they appear on the skull or face. For example:

- A *lateral facial cleft* is a cleft that stretches up from the corner of the mouth toward the ear. The scientific name for this type of cleft is *prosoposchisis,* from the Greek words *prosopo,* meaning face, and *schisis,* meaning fissure.
- A *midline facial cleft* is a cleft in the center of the face that may produce various deformities, including a bifid nose (cleft nose) and eyes set abnormally wide apart.
- An *oblique facial cleft is* a cleft that extends up one side of the face from the outer corner of the mouth to the inner edge of the eye. The scientific name for this type of cleft is *macrostomia,* from the Greek words *macro,* meaning large, and *stoma,* meaning mouth.
- A *cleft cheek* is a congenital separation in the cheek due to the failure of the bones of the embryo's maxilla (upper jaw) to fuse properly with the forehead and nose bones.
- A *cleft palate* is the failure of the bones at the top of the mouth (palate) to meet.

Each of these deformities may be repaired or alleviated by appropriate plastic surgery procedures.

The failure of the bones in the fetal skull to fuse properly causes clefts. The premature fusing of the bones in the skull, a condition known as *craniosynostosis* (from the Greek words *kranion,* meaning skull, *osteon* meaning bone, and *osis,* meaning condition), leads to another set of problems such as the harlequin deformity, an upward tilt of the bone around the eye. This deformity, like facial clefts, may be repaired with craniofacial plastic surgery.

facial expression   See LIPS.

facial landmarks   Imaginary structural characteristics of the features of an ideal face (forehead, eyes, ears, nose, mouth, and chin). These perfect but unrealistic features are used by plastic surgeons solely as guidelines in planning cosmetic and reconstructive surgery. In dentistry, ideal standards for lips and teeth are used to plan dental restorations such as dentures and procedures such as orthodontic treatment.

The Ideal Lips

The ideal lips are full. At rest they are centered under the nose. The outer edges of the top lips are on an imaginary straight line down from the center of the iris (the dark circle in the middle of each eye). The lower lip is slightly fuller than the upper.

When seen from the side, in profile, the closed lips ideally line up with the chin. The columella (the strip of skin running from the tip of the nose to the upper lip) and the upper lip form a right angle (90°). If the angle is less than this ideal, the upper jaw is described as prominent and the profile as convex; if the angle is greater, the upper jaw is described as retruded and the profile as concave. Regarding the relationship between nose, lips, and chin, the Ricketts E-Plane (E = esthetic; see RICKETTS, ROBERT) is an imaginary line drawn down from the tip of the nose to the tip of the chin. Ideally, the upper lip should be 4 mm (millimeters) back from this line, and the lower lip 2 mm.

Finally, when the lips are open to reveal the teeth in a full smile, the ideal upper lip is neither high enough to show the gums nor should it extend down over the lower teeth, and the top of the ideal lower lip just touches the top of the lower teeth.

The Ideal Teeth

Ideally, the upper and lower teeth are both centered under the philtrum, the grooved space between the nose and the upper lip. An imaginary straight line runs down the center of the philtrum to pass between the upper center front teeth.

The ideal teeth are straight, with no crowding or overlap of one tooth over another. They are unstained, with an ivory tint, free of chips or uneven wear on the biting edges and firmly anchored in the jawbone. The gums are symmetrically situated at the midpoint on each tooth, clear pinkish in color, with no recession (reduction in height on the tooth) and no active PERIODONTAL DISEASE. Some formulas suggest that the ideal center teeth are 80 percent as wide as they are long. A similar formulation, the Golden (Divine) Proportion created by Robert Ricketts, says that the most pleasing esthetic relationship between two objects is when one is approximately 62 percent as large as the other. This "rule" is sometimes used by all dental professionals when creating dentures, so that the two center teeth are made 1.6 times as wide as the incisor next to each of the center teeth.

fatty tissue   See ADIPOSE TISSUE.

Fauchard, Pierre (1678–1761)   Fauchard, a self-styled *chirurgien dentiste* (surgeon dentist), is often called "the father of modern dentistry." His two-volume, 863-page work, *Le chirurgien dentiste* (The surgeon-dentist), was the first scientific text devoted entirely to teeth and the instruments used to treat dental problems. It was soon translated into several languages and regarded for years as the standard text on dentistry.

Fauchard's achievements in dentistry occurred at a time when the practice was emerging from the barbershop into an authentic medical specialty, helped along by Louis XIV's attention to appearance, including the appearance of the teeth. The situation was tailor-made for Fauchard. Not only was he an indefatigable researcher and teacher, he was also a dental innovator who advocated the excavation and filling of dental cavities so as to save a damaged tooth. He also built dentures with natural teeth connected by wire springs; described crowns and bridges to hide or replace missing teeth; and suggested ways to straighten teeth (making him the father of orthodontics as well as dentistry). Today his name lives on in a number of professional awards and in the International Pierre Fauchard Academy, which supports various aspects of dental research.

fibroma A common, benign tumor made primarily of CONNECTIVE TISSUE. Fibromas, which are the most common growths found in the mouth, are located on soft tissue such as the inside of the cheek, the gums, and the tongue.

An *ameloblastic fibroma* is composed of connective tissue plus epithelial tissue (cells on the top layer of skin or mucous membrane) and tissue usually found in fetal teeth/tooth buds. A *cementifying fibroma* is a growth between two teeth composed of fibrous tissue and hard material similar to CEMENTUM, the material on the surface of the tooth root. An *irritation fibroma* is, as its name implies, a growth caused by constant irritation, usually to the tissue of the cheek or gum. An *odontogenic fibroma* is a tumor in the jaw composed of connective and other kinds of dental tissue. A *periapical fibroma* is found at the end of the tooth root.

Symptoms and Diagnostic Path

The typical fibroma develops slowly and painlessly over a long period of time into a round, smooth, clearly defined growth, lighter pink than the tissue to which it is attached by a stalk.

Treatment Options and Outlook

The area to which the fibroma is attached is numbed with local anesthetics and the fibroma is cut off. After the fibroma is removed, the dentist or oral surgeon may close the incision with a stitch, which will be removed within a week to 10 days. The patient may experience some discomfort for a few days. The fibroma is unlikely to recur.

Risk Factors and Preventive Measures

For unknown reasons, fibromas are more common among women than among men, but there is no known way to predict or prevent their development.

fillings See RESTORATION.

fixation From the Latin word *figo* meaning "to fasten" or "to make stable." In dentistry, the word *fixation* may mean either a device that holds something securely in place (such as a fixation splint used to immobilize a fractured jaw) or the process of securely attaching the device, such as positioning a dental implant in the jawbone. The CEMENT, wire, or plate used to make the attachment is called a fixative.

Dental fixation devices are commonly named for where they sit in the mouth; dental fixation techniques, for the part of the mouth they affect or simply the material from which they are made.

For example, an *osseous fixation* is the generic term for a device or technique that holds pieces of bone together, while a *maxillomandibular fixation* is a wire used to keep the jaws together so as to enable a fractured upper (maxilla) or lower (mandible) jaw to heal. A *restorative fixation* secures (usually with cement) a permanent restoration such as an inlay or a fixed denture. Finally, an *elastic band fixation* uses elastic bands attached to splints to hold fractured jaws together.

flaps Piece of skin or mucous membrane partially lifted from one place on the body (the donor site) and turned or moved into place on an adjacent (recipient) site to repair or rebuild a deficit due to disease, injury, or a birth defect. The flap may include underlying tissue (fat, blood vessels, muscle, bone) lifted from the donor site and turned toward or transferred to the recipient site. In dentistry, the dental surgeon or periodontist may create a flap from lip tissue or from the mucous membrane inside of the mouth.

A flap differs from a GRAFT in that a flap is still partially attached to the donor site and maintains its own blood supply, thus increasing the chance for successful transfer. Once a flap is in place, the surgeon may prescribe anticoagulants (blood thinners) to reduce the risk of blood clots—the most likely complication after flap surgery—at the connection between the blood vessels in the flap and those in the recipient site.

The flaps used in dental and oral procedures may be named for their source (the donor site) or for the surgeons who created the technique.

Dental and Oral Flaps Named for the Donor Site

The lip-lip flap is a piece of tissue lifted from one side of the upper or lower lip and moved to repair the other side of the same lip.

The nasolabial flap is lifted from the side of the nose and turned down to repair the area between lip and nose.

The over-and-out cheek flap is lifted from the cheek and turned over and down so that the pink underside of the flap is used to match and repair a damaged lip.

The palatal flap is lifted from the roof of the mouth and turned to repair a defect of an adjacent gum.

The semi-lunar gum flap is a half-moon-shape piece of gum tissue lifted and moved to cover the root of a tooth left bare by recession due to periodontal disease.

Dental and Oral Flaps Named for Surgeons

The Abbe flap, also called the Abbe switch flap, is skin lifted from the side of an intact upper lip and part of the cheek to which it is attached and moved down to rebuild a lower lip or, less frequently, an upper lip. The flap is named for Robert Abbe (1851–1928); variations on the original flap include the Abbe-Estlander flap, used at the corner of the mouth, and the Abbe-Sabbatini flap, used to reconstruct the center of the upper lip.

The Estlander flap, named for Finnish surgeon Jakob August Estlander (1831–81), is tissue taken from one side of the patient's lip and used to repair an injury to the same place on the opposite side of the same (upper or lower) lip.

The Karapandzic flap is skin lifted from one part of the upper or lower lip, turned, and moved forward to cover a defect on another part of the lip. The flap was introduced in 1974 by Miodrag Karapandzic, one-time director of the Clinic for Burns, Plastic and Reconstructive Surgery of the Belgrade University Clinical Center.

The Widman flap, introduced in 1918 by Leonard Widman, among the first dental practitioners to use flaps to reduce a pocket (the gap between gum and bone left by periodontal disease), is the most common flap used in dental procedures. Also known as flap curettage, the Widman is created when the periodontist makes incisions in the gum to lift a flap of tissue away from the tooth in order to scrape away debris from the surface of the tooth underneath the gum. When the cleaning is finished, the flap is sutured back in place.

See also CLEFT LIP AND/OR PALATE; LIP RECONSTRUCTION.

floss, dental Threadlike dental aid used to remove bacteria and other debris from the surfaces between teeth.

The Types of Dental Floss

The first practical dental floss, introduced by American dentist Levi Spear Parmly early in the

1800s, was simple silk thread. By the mid-1890s, the pharmaceutical firm Johnson & Johnson had patented its own brand of silk dental floss. Within 50 years, when the supply of silk to the United States was interrupted by the Japanese during World War II, nylon thread replaced the silk. Modern dental floss comes in several versions, each with specific benefits and drawbacks.

Unwaxed or *plain floss* is a thread made of multiple strands of nylon twisted together. Waxed floss is plain floss with a thin coating of wax. The waxed floss is stronger than the unwaxed, but bulkier and thus more difficult to thread between the teeth. Braided floss is a stronger version of the basic thread.

Dental tape, which comes unwaxed or waxed, is similar to dental floss but flat and ribbonlike rather than round like a thread. Like waxed floss, dental tape such as Reach Dental Tape is larger and more difficult than plain floss to insert between teeth positioned closely together.

Expanded polytetrafluoroethylene (ePTEF) floss is a thread of Teflon, the synthetic material used for protective clothing such as Gore-Tex. ePTEF is very strong and smooth enough to slide easily back and forth between the teeth; Glide, the ePTEF dental floss, was introduced in 1992.

"Super" floss, sometimes known as bridge or denture floss, is a nylon length of floss with bulky nylon mesh in the middle to offer additional scrubbing power and stiffened needlelike ends that enable the patient to insert the floss more easily through tight spaces. Examples of super floss are Oral-B Super Floss and Thornton Bridge and Implant Interdental Cleaners.

Like other health products, dental floss is under continual review. Possible developments for new floss include:

- putting bumps or soft brushing extensions down the length of the floss to improve its ability to dislodge debris
- coating the floss with antibacterial substances to reduce DECAY and PERIODONTAL DISEASE

- coating the floss with fluoride to strengthen the teeth
- adding compounds that whiten the teeth
- impregnating the floss with chemicals that make the teeth less sensitive to pain stimuli such as heat and cold

Flossing Technique

To floss, the patient may simply thread the floss between teeth, move the floss back and forth and up and down to dislodge debris, and then withdraw the floss. Or the patient may use a floss threader, a needlelike device through which the floss is threaded and then inserted between the teeth in a manner similar to the super floss. A floss holder is a slingshot shape device that holds a piece of floss securely in place so that the patient can insert the floss between the teeth. A battery powered flosser is a device with a replaceable slim nylon tip that slides between the teeth to clean the interdental surfaces.

Evaluating the Effectiveness of Dental Floss

Several studies attest to the effectiveness of flossing along with a manual toothbrush at reducing bacteria and debris on the interdental (between the teeth) surfaces. For example, when a team of researchers from the University of Washington, Seattle, the University of the State of Rio de Janeiro, Brazil, the Schulich School of Medicine and Dentistry at the University of Western Ontario, Canada, and the School of Dentistry at the University of Michigan, Ann Arbor, reviewed six trials with more than 800 children aged 4 to 13, they found that having a dental professional floss the children's teeth on school days for nearly two years reduced the incidence of interproximal cavities (cavities between the teeth) by as much as 40 percent. Data from a small (25-person) 2008 study at the University of Texas Health Science Center at San Antonio Dental School, published in the *Journal of Periodontology,* showed that flossing after brushing with a manual (nonpowered) toothbrush significantly increased plaque removal. The study included three basic flosses (unwaxed, waxed, shred-resistant), which were equally effective, and a powered flosser that was slightly more so.

See also IRRIGATION; TOOTHBRUSH.

fluoride A fluoride is a compound containing the element fluorine and another element such as sodium (sodium fluoride—NaF) or calcium (calcium fluoride—CaF_2). Fluorides occur naturally in bones and in the enamel surface of the teeth.

The Dental Benefits of Fluorides

In the mouth, the fluorides consumed in drinking water and food release electrically charged fluoride particles called ions that combine with the hydroxyapatite (a calcium compound) in teeth to harden the dental enamel and reduce the natural loss of minerals from the tooth. This reaction occurs not only in teeth already in the mouth but also in teeth that have not yet erupted through the gum. While fluorides are often assumed to be most useful for protecting children whose teeth are developing, they are also important for adults. Data from an Indiana University School of Dentistry, Indiana University–Purdue University, in Indianapolis, and colleagues in a study published in the fall 2007 issue of the *Journal of Public Health Dentistry* demonstrate that while fluoridation of drinking water reduces cavities among people of all age groups (see below), those likely to experience the greatest reduction in the need for fillings are older adults. Perhaps this is because the fluorides reduce the natural loss of mineralization that occurs as people grow older.

Sources of Fluorides

Fluoride compounds occur naturally in groundwater and in some plant foods such as tea that absorb fluorine from the soil in which they are grown. The most common sources of fluorides, however, are fluoridated community water systems and bottled water, fluorides applied by the dentist, and fluoridated homecare products.

Fluoridated Community Water Systems On January 25, 1945, Grand Rapids, Michigan, became the first community to deliberately fluoridate its public water system to reduce the risk of tooth decay. Today, nearly 200 million Americans get their drinking water from public water systems treated to deliver a concentration of 0.7 to 1.2 parts fluoride ions to 1 million part water (0.7–1.2 ppm), the level considered ideal to protect dental health. Nonetheless, fluoridation of water systems has drawn and continues to draw criticism from individuals and groups that consider it detrimental to health. In fact, no such link has ever been proven. Fluoridation of public water systems has an unparalleled record of safety and effectiveness in reducing the incidence of dental decay.

The following table shows the extent of fluoridation of public water systems as of December 31, 2006.

Fluoridated Bottled Water In 2006, the Food and Drug Administration's Center for Food Safety and Applied Nutrition announced that

FLUORIDATION OF PUBLIC WATER SYSTEMS UNITED STATES, 2006	
Number	**Population/Systems**
299,398,484	Total population, United States
262,690,043	Total number or persons in the United States served by public water systems
184,028,038	Total number of persons in the United States served by fluoridated water systems
53,429	Total number of community water systems in the United States
16,413	Number of community water systems in the United States providing fluoridated water
3,339	Number of community water systems in the United States with naturally occurring fluoride at or above optimal levels

Source: Centers for Disease Control and Prevention, "Water Fluoridation Statistics for 2006" (www.cdc.gov/FLUORIDATION/statistics/2006stats.htm).

manufacturers had permission to print claims on their labels that drinking fluoridated water may reduce the risk of dental caries or tooth decay. To qualify for the label copy, the bottled water must contain 0.6–1.0 mg of fluoride for each liter of water.

Professionally Applied Fluoride Products These products, available only in dental offices, are gels, foams, and rinses with concentrated amounts of fluorides. Fluoride "varnish" is a solution of resins and gums used to coat the surface of teeth to protect the surface against some of the ingredients in fillings or other dental restorations. These products have a proven record of reducing the risk of decay and the incidence of cavities.

Fluoridated Topical Home Care Products This group of protective products includes toothpastes, tooth powders, and rinses with 0.05 percent fluoride as well as tooth gels with up to 0.4 percent fluoride. The pastes and powders effectively reach the top and outer surfaces of the tooth. Gels and rinses do a better job of reaching the surfaces between adjoining teeth.

When used as directed, all the fluoridated topical home care products safely strengthen teeth and help remove dental PLAQUE, thus also reducing the risk of PERIODONTAL DISEASE. In addition, some contain ingredients to make the teeth less sensitive, a particularly important point for patients whose gums have receded, exposing part of the CEMENTUM-covered root, which is more sensitive than the enamel-covered crown.

Fluoride Supplements These single ingredient products are prescription-strength drops, tablets, or chewable lozenges meant for children and young adults lacking access to a fluoridated public water system.

Potential Adverse Effects of Fluorides

Public health experts consider a concentration of 0.7 to 1.2 parts fluoride ions to 1 million parts water (0.7–1.2 ppm) to be the upper acceptable limit. Ingesting higher amounts, either at one time or over a period of time, has been linked to fluorosis and potential fluoride poisoning.

Fluorosis In some parts of the American Southwest, the groundwater is naturally fluoridated to levels as high as 10 ppm. A person who drinks water with fluoride levels higher than 2 ppm may develop fluorosis, a nonfatal condition characterized by stains on the teeth that begin as white patches but eventually turn brown, pits on the enamel surface of the teeth, and abnormal hardening of the bones.

Fluoride Poisoning Fluoride poisoning is a potentially lethal event that may occur following the consumption of excessive amounts of fluorides either from supplements or from fluoridated dentifrices and rinses. Like iron poisoning, which is most common among children younger than six, fluoride poisoning is frequently due to a child's accidental ingestion of fluoride supplements or failure to spit out fluoridated pastes or rinses after brushing or rinsing. For young children, 100–300 mg of fluorides may cause nausea and diarrhea; a dose of 400 mg at one time may be lethal. For adults, the single lethal dose is 5 gm (5,000 mg).

To reduce the risk of such incidents, the American Academy of Pediatrics and the American Academy of Pediatric Dentistry recommend keeping all fluoridated products out of the reach of young children and withholding fluoridated rinses (which may provide up to 2 mg fluoride per dose) from children younger than six.

The most recent report of the AMERICAN DENTAL ASSOCIATION on fluorides, "Fluoridation Facts," is available online at www.ada.org/public/topics/fluoride/facts/index.asp9.

foil See GOLD (AU).

fold A structure created by a piece of tissue, such as a mucous membrane folding back on itself. For example, in the mouth, the mucobuccal fold is the area between the outer side of the upper or lower jaw to the inner surface of the cheek. The mucolabial fold is the area between the center of the upper or lower jaw to the inner surface of the upper or lower lip. And the sublingual fold is the area on the floor of the mouth, under the tongue, that runs from the center of the inner edge of the lower jaw back toward the tongue.

forensic dentistry The use of dental information as a tool in identifying human remains.

The Forensic Dentist

Like a person's fingerprint or DNA, the size, shape, and arrangement of the teeth, as well as the presence of various RESTORATIONS, is both individual and unique. In addition, teeth are virtually impervious to destruction by fire and other elements, which makes them a valuable tool in identifying persons who have died in a disfiguring situation such as a car crash or a fire, or when the body has been immersed in water for a period of time or is discovered after other body tissue has decomposed.

The person charged with collecting, preserving, and evaluating dental evidence so as to identify a body is the forensic dentist, usually a professional certified by the American Board of Forensic Odontology (ABFO), an organization established in 1976 under the auspices of the National Institute of Justice, which is the research, development, and evaluation agency of the U.S. Department of Justice. To achieve ABFO certification, the dentist must:

- graduate from a dental institution accredited by ABFO
- participate in a forensic dental organization approved by the ABFO certification committee
- be affiliated with and active in a medical/legal agency such as a coroner's office

- perform a requisite number of autopsies and identifications
- pass the board's written and oral examinations

Collecting Dental Evidence after Death

When conducting a postmortem dental examination, customarily under the direction of a coroner or medical examiner, the forensic dentist has a number of tools available, including (but not limited to) physical examination of the teeth, jaws, and prostheses, DNA profiling, and, on the horizon, a national dental database.

The Teeth and Jaws To evaluate teeth and jaws, the forensic dentist does what amounts to a postmortem ("after death") dental examination. The number of teeth present in the mouth after death and the way they are arranged in the jaw are valuable for confirming the identity of a person whose antemortem ("before death") records are available.

In identifying an unknown body, the forensic dentist pays attention to the general condition of the teeth and the care they received, which may reflect social or economic status. The size of the jaw may offer a clue as to gender, with males generally having larger jaws than females do, but the size of the teeth is not gender-specific. Other factors, such as shape, size, and color may suggest age, race, and ethnicity, dietary habits, health, and behavior of the person to be identified.

Age The presence of primary teeth clearly suggests a younger body as compared to a mouth with a complete set of permanent teeth. Forensic dentists commonly use a guide such as the Ubelaker chart. The chart, created by forensic anthropologist Douglas Ubelaker, curator of anthropology at the Smithsonian Institute, shows the development of teeth from the fetal stage to the age of 35.

Race and Ethnicity The shape and size of the teeth offer some clues to the race and ethnicity of the body. For example, African Americans generally have a thicker layer of dental enamel than do Caucasians. "Shovel shape" teeth (front top teeth that curve out rather than in) are likely to occur in Asians and other non-Caucasians. A cusp of Carabelli—a fifth cusp (point) on the top of the first molars in the upper jaw—is usually a characteristic of Europeans.

Dietary Habits   Brown stains on the teeth may indicate excessive consumption of coffee or tea.

Health and Behavior   Serious erosion of the dental enamel may suggest frequent regurgitation of acidic stomach contents due to an eating disorder, frequent gastroesophageal reflux ("heartburn"), excessive consumption of alcohol, or drug abuse (see METH MOUTH). Staining of adult teeth may be due to smoking. Heavy wear or cracks on the biting surface of the teeth suggests BRUXISM (involuntary tooth/jaw clenching and grinding) or that the person was a pipe smoker who held a pipe tightly between his teeth.

Restorations and Appliances   Like the teeth, the pattern of dental restorations such as fillings, CROWNS, and permanent DENTURES is individual and unique. If antemortem records are available, these may provide conclusive identification. In rare cases, a restoration may be traced by the material from which it was made. Some prostheses, such as breast implants and pacemakers, are required by law to be labeled so that they are easily traceable, but there is no legal requirement that dental restorations be labeled. Nonetheless, some dental professionals do label their work, making it easy to trace these restorations back to the person in whose mouth they were placed.

DNA   Because teeth are hardy enough to survive intact in situations where other tissue is destroyed or decomposes, another reliable tool is DNA obtained from a tooth. In cases where the identity of a body is known or suspected, a person otherwise unrecognizable due to the nature of his demise may be conclusively identified by comparing DNA taken postmortem to a sample taken from a viable source available before death, such as hair remaining in a hairbrush.

Comparing Evidence to Identify a Body

If there is reason to know or suspect that the body belongs to a specific person and if antemortem dental records are available, the simplest tool in forensic dentistry is to compare the decedent's dental structures with the suspected person's dental records such as dental X-rays or a dental professional's written notes. In doing so, the dentist carefully notes similarities and discrepancies between the two sets of data. He may determine that explainable differences, such as a tooth present before death but not afterward, can be considered irrelevant. On the other hand, differences that cannot be explained, such as a tooth present after death but not before, may lead to the forensic dentist's ruling that the body is not that of the person it was once believed to be.

The sources for antemortem data include (but are not limited to) a person's own dentist or oral surgeon, a local hospital that may have X-rays of the person's skull that include the teeth and jaws, the person's insurance carrier, or friends and family members holding copies of his medical records. In special circumstances, the forensic dentist may consult law enforcement agencies such as the FBI National Crime Information Center (NCIC) and, for service veterans, the Military Records Depository.

In the future, forensic dentists may also be able to consult a national dental database. In 1997, the FBI's Criminal Justice Information Services (CJIS) established a Dental Task Force (DTF) charged with exploring the possibility of creating just such a tool, to be known as the Automated Dental Identification System (ADIS). Eight years later, in May 2005, CJIS management approved the creation of the National Dental Image/Information Repository (NDIR) to access and add to all dental records currently held in the national computerized database maintained by CJIS at the NCIC. It is hoped that eventually the dental database will be as useful as the current fingerprint databases in facilitating identification of bodies, as well as missing persons and those wanted by the justice system.

The ABFO Categories of Identification

As ABFO notes, the ability to identify a body via its dental characteristics depends wholly on the amount of evidence available. As a result, ABFO has set four categories of identification based on varying degrees of certainty, meaning that, as ABFO notes, because the forensic dentist cannot vouch for the absolute accuracy of data collected before death, these conclusions are considered valid but conditional.

The categories of identification are:

1. *Positive identification.* The term describes a situation in which the data collected after death and that available before death are sufficiently in agreement, with no unresolved differences, so that it is clear that they come from the same person. For example, the information from the person's dentist clearly matches what the forensic dentist finds in his postmortem examination.
2. *Possible identification.* This term describes a situation in which the data collected after death is clearly similar but cannot be positively matched, either because the circumstances of the death may have badly damaged the remains or because there are some unanswered questions about the data collected before the person died. For example, while the number of teeth in the mouth after death seem similar to what was in place while the person was alive, there is some question about the exact placement of a restoration such as a dental implant.
3. *Insufficient evidence.* This term describes a situation in which the forensic dentist simply does not have enough information to offer a firm conclusion as to the identity of the body. For example, there is no data available showing the number and arrangement of the teeth before death.
4. *Exclusion.* This term describes a situation in which the evidence before and after death definitely do not agree.

The complete ABFO Body Identification Guidelines are available online at www.abfo.org via the link to "ID and Bitemark Guidelines."

fracture   See JAW, FRACTURE.

fungal infections   See THRUSH.

furcation defect   In dentistry, furcation, from the Latin word *furca,* meaning "a fork, branch, or separation," is the place where a multiroot tooth, such as a molar, divides into branches. A furcation defect is a structural abnormality in the area of furcation; for example, an opening from the inside of the root out to the surface of the tooth. Furcation invasion is a loss of bone at the place where the roots divide; root furcation is a term used to describe loss of bone at the tooth root caused by PERIODONTAL DISEASE.

Symptoms and Diagnostic Path

The patient may experience pain due to an opening from the surface of the tooth to the interior or the tooth may be loose due to loss of bone.

Treatment Options and Outlook

The treatment of a furcation defect is designed to reduce the periodontal pocket and slow or halt the progress of the disease. To that end, the dentist or periodontist may scale (scrape) the surface of the tooth root, debride (remove) diseased tissue, and plane (trim) the root. Another possibility is a bone GRAFT to strengthen the remaining bone.

Risk Factors and Preventive Measures

The risk factors for furcation defect are the same as for all forms of periodontal disease: genetic susceptibility, emotional or physical stress, fluctuating hormone levels, and diabetes.

See also BONE.

fused teeth   Two teeth, almost invariably the front primary teeth, joined together so they look like one wider-than-normal tooth or one tooth with two CROWNS or two different roots.

Symptoms and Diagnostic Path

Fused teeth are clearly visible on physical examination. The two teeth may be joined at the crown (top of the tooth), at the outer surface of the root, or in both places. There is an increased risk of decay along the line where the teeth are fused.

Treatment Options and Outlook

The treatment of fused teeth depends on the health of the patient and the extent and nature of the fusion. For example, the dentist may prefer to separate and restore fused teeth if the patient is healthy, but not if the patient has another condition, such as severe mental retardation, that interferes with his ability to follow a complicated oral hygiene regimen necessary to recover from treatment.

There appears to be no correlation between fusing of primary teeth and the likelihood that fusing will occur in the permanent teeth. In cases of fused primary teeth, the dentist is likely to take X-rays as the permanent teeth begin to erupt to make certain that enough room exists in the jaw for the permanent teeth to emerge and for the fused teeth to fall out naturally.

Risk Factors and Preventive Measures

Some experts suggest that fused teeth are a birth defect influenced by genes; others note the fact that one member of a pair of identical twins may have fused teeth while the other does not, which makes this unlikely.

gag reflex Involuntary contraction of muscles at the back of the throat, a natural and involuntary reaction that protects the body by preventing unwelcome objects from passing into the throat.

Symptoms and Diagnostic Path

As the tongue pushes food back toward the throat, the gag reflex is normally suspended so that food can be swallowed. However, if the food does not move easily, the gag reflex can be activated to push the food back out of the mouth. The gag reflex may also be activated by reaching into the mouth and touching the back of the tongue or the soft palate, a stratagem used by some people with an EATING DISORDER to stimulate voluntary vomiting.

The gag reflex may also be activated by emotions—for example, when one is forced to eat a food one finds distasteful or when one visits the dentist. An uncontrolled gag reflex can interfere with oral health by making it difficult to get normal dental treatment or to wear dentures.

Treatment Options and Outlook

Numbing the back of the mouth with a local anesthetic spray may reduce the severity of the gag reflex in dental situations. Over the long term, patients may benefit from relaxation techniques such as BIOFEEDBACK or behavioral therapy.

Risk Factors and Preventive Measures

If the activation of the reflex is due to anxiety, any technique that lowers the fear level may prevent the reaction.

gender and oral health Men and women face different challenges regarding oral and dental health. Women are more likely than men to experience dental problems such as PERIODONTAL DISEASE related to hormonal fluctuations at different stages of life. Men are more likely than women to experience dental problems such as DECAY and lost teeth related to lifestyle choices such as oral hygiene, physical activity, and TOBACCO use.

Women and Oral Health

The female hormones estrogen and progesterone influence the flow of blood throughout the body, including to the gums. As a result, the environment in a woman's mouth changes dramatically as levels of these hormones rise and fall naturally at different stages of life such as:

- at puberty
- during the menstrual cycle
- when using oral contraceptives
- when undergoing fertility treatments
- during pregnancy
- at menopause

Hormonal Influences on Oral Health at Puberty and During the Menstrual Cycle The sudden increase in the secretion of estrogen and progesterone during puberty increases the flow of blood to gum tissue, making the gums more likely to swell and bleed.

A similar condition may occur midway through the menstrual cycle when a woman's body begins to secrete increased levels of progesterone to prepare the uterus for the implantation of a fertilized egg. At ovulation (the release of an egg from the ovary), when progesterone levels are at their highest and the blood flow to the gums increases, a woman may experience redness and swelling of the gums and slight bleeding at the gum line (the place where the top edge of the gum meets the tooth), a condition called MENSTRUAL GINGIVITIS. Once ovulation has occurred, if the egg is not fertilized, progesterone levels begin to drop, the gingivitis recedes, and the cycle begins anew. Note: The higher progesterone levels also increase the risk of canker sores and HERPES infections ("cold sores").

Hormonal Influences on Oral Health of Oral Contraceptives and Fertility Treatments   Like naturally secreted hormones, the hormones in birth control pills and fertility treatments may also trigger periodontal inflammation, even among women who practice good oral hygiene. In 2004, researchers at Cukurova University, in Turkey, published a report in the *Journal of Periodontology* showing that, among two groups of women with similar levels of dental PLAQUE, those taking fertility drugs with progesterone for more than three menstrual cycles in order to induce ovulation and increase their chances of conceiving experienced more inflammation and bleeding of the gums, as well as an increase in the production of crevicular fluid, an anti-inflammatory liquid released by epithelial cells in the mucous membrane lining of the mouth. (The level of crevicular fluid in the mouth may be a marker by which to estimate the progression of periodontal disease.)

Hormonal Influences on Oral Health During Pregnancy   The increase in progesterone levels during pregnancy may lead to PREGNANCY GINGIVITIS, a condition similar to menstrual gingivitis. More frequent dental cleanings during the second and third trimester of pregnancy help reduce the incidence of infection.

In addition, the American Academy of Periodontology notes that women with active gum disease characterized by infections may be more likely to give birth prematurely or to give birth to a low-birthweight infant because the bacteria associated with periodontal disease produce substances such as *prostaglandin E-2* that may stimulate labor contractions.

Hormonal Influences on Oral Health at Menopause   Throughout life, BONE tissue is constantly lost and replaced. Testosterone, the male hormone, is vital to building new bone, while estrogen is essential to the retention of existing bone. At menopause, when the natural secretion of estrogen declines, women experience a precipitous decline in bone density, including the density of the jawbone, which may lead to an increased risk of tooth loss. (Men also lose bone tissue as they grow older, but they begin with bones that are naturally denser, and they have lower natural levels of estrogen, so the age-related bone loss and decline in estrogen is slower and less dramatic.)

Men and Oral Health

Poor dental health habits, tobacco use, certain medications, and some kinds of physical activity are risk factors for oral health problems for both men and women. For reasons of personality, social norms, and physical characteristics, though, each appears to be a higher risk for men than for women.

Poor Dental Health Habits   It is a truism that men are less likely than women to attend to the nitty-gritty of personal health. In regard to oral health, this is confirmed by the American Dental Association's *2003 Public Opinion Survey: Oral Health of the U.S. Population,* which reports that men are:

- less likely than women to brush their teeth after every meal (20.5 percent men versus 28.7 percent women)

- less likely than women to brush twice a day (49 percent men versus 56.8 percent women)

- less likely than women to have a personal dentist (74.6 percent men versus 89.2 percent women) and to schedule regular dental appointments

- less likely than women to brush their teeth before a date
- less likely than women to brush their teeth at work or in a restaurant bathroom after eating or before an appointment
- less likely to floss their teeth on a regular basis

Although women's hormonal fluctuations put them at higher risk of periodontal disease than men, their attention to oral health, including regular dental visits, may explain the Centers for Disease Control and Prevention finding that men are more likely to have advanced gum disease.

Tobacco and Men's Oral Health According to the Centers for Disease Control and Prevention, an estimated 45.3 million American adults 18 or older (20.8 percent) were current smokers in 2006, 23.9 percent of all men and 18 percent of all women. Because smoking increases the risk of periodontal disease, while smoking and chewing tobacco raise the risk of ORAL CANCERS, men have a higher incidence of both.

Physical Activity and Men's Oral Health Men are more likely than women to participate in contact sports such as boxing, football, and hockey where facial trauma is common. Wearing a protective MOUTH GUARD reduces but does not eliminate the risk of tooth loss and other oral injury.

Oral Health Problems Common to Both Men and Women

Medication Many common medications, including allergy drugs, antidepressants, and drugs used to treat cardiovascular disease (heart disease and high blood pressure) reduce the natural secretion of SALIVA. Saliva contains substances that lower the number of decay-causing bacteria in the mouth. It also contains minerals that harden and protect the enamel surface of the teeth. As a result, people on these medications are at higher risk of dental decay and/or tooth loss. Men are more likely than women to be treated for heart disease, so their risk of problems with cardiovascular medicines is higher. Women are more likely than men to be treated for depression, so their risk of dental problems with antidepressants is higher.

Age-related Dental/Oral Changes An age-related decrease in salivary flow occurs in both sexes, presenting an equal risk of dental problems such as reddened, inflamed gums, changes in the sense of taste, and an increased risk of tooth decay for both men and women.

genetics Genetics is the branch of science dealing with heredity; that is, the passing of inherited characteristics from parent to child through chromosomes and genes. Several dental and oral health conditions such as tooth DECAY, susceptibility to PERIODONTAL DISEASE, and CLEFT LIP AND/OR PALATE, may be the result of a person's genetic inheritance or "family history" (a characteristic shared by closely related individuals).

How Genes Exert Their Effects

Genetic conditions are transmitted by a dominant gene, a recessive gene, or an X- or Y-linked gene. Only one dominant gene from either parent is required to produce a dominant trait such as dark hair. To inherit a recessive trait such as blond hair, an individual must receive two blond hair genes, one from each parent. Note: The terms X-linked and Y-linked describe a trait or an inherited medical condition associated either with a gene on the Y (male) or X (female) chromosome, or with a change in the structure of the X or Y chromosome, or with the presence of an extra X or Y chromosome.

One example of a genetic dental condition is ANODONTIA (missing teeth). This defect occurs in several forms ranging from a few missing teeth to the absence of all teeth. Some forms of anodontia are transmitted by a dominant gene; some by a recessive gene; and some by an X-linked gene.

Other dental conditions known to run in families are a susceptibility to dental decay and to periodontal disease; exactly how these conditions are transmitted remains to be explained.

Teaching Genetics to Dentists

Given the clear evidence of a genetic link to several dental and oral health conditions, genetics seems to be a valuable subject for dental students. But in 2001, when 53 of the 54 dental schools in the United States responded to a questionnaire about genetics education for dental students written by a team of genetics, dental, and craniofacial experts from the University of Pittsburgh and the National Institute of Dental and Craniofacial Research, the results were not reassuring. The data, published in the *Journal of Dental Education* in August 2004, showed that:

- 50 of the schools answering the questionnaire did not require a course in genetics for admission

- only two of the dental schools even recommended that candidates take a genetics course prior to entering dental school

- 32 of the dental schools thought that genetics should be part of the dental curriculum, but only eight schools offered a formal course in genetics taught either at the dental school or at a related medical school as a requirement for graduation

- six schools reported having a genetics course taught by dental school faculty; one reported a course taught primarily by medical school faculty

- 45 schools said that genetics information was incorporated into other courses; several of these schools said they were interested in adding more information about genetics to their existing courses, and one school said that genetics had no place in dental school

Noting that "Genetics concepts and principles will underlie many new diagnostic and treat-ment strategies in health care in the coming years," the researchers concluded that "if dental clinicians are to participate in development and clinical implementation of these new approaches, they will need to understand genetics. If dental students are to be prepared for lifelong learning, it is important for them to have a working knowledge of genomics to facilitate integration of this new information. This survey represents the most comprehensive evaluation of genetics education in U.S. dental schools. From the results, it is apparent that the presentation of genetics in U.S. dental schools is not standardized, and as such, the genetics content presented to students varies greatly. It is hoped that these data will form the basis for developing additional tools to further assess how to integrate genetics into the dental curriculum. Curriculum models, course designs, and competencies are all issues that must be evaluated. Educators may benefit from the experiences of other health fields, medicine, nursing, pharmacology, and expert organizations in these efforts. Given the shortage of dental faculty, it may be wise to leverage efforts to develop a core genetics curriculum that is available to all dental schools. In this way, common teaching experiences may also benefit from the continued reevaluation and development of such a course."

genioplasty See CHIN RECONSTRUCTION.

gingiva The mucous membrane that originally covers the top of teeth that have not yet erupted; then, after the teeth erupt from the JAW, circles each tooth. The gingiva is attached to the CEMENTUM (the outside of the lower part of each tooth) and to the alveolar bone, the part of the jawbone that supports the teeth. In people with light skin, the gingiva is lighter in color around the tooth than the membrane on the alveolar bone. In people with dark skin, the gum around the tooth contains pigment cells that make it darker than the alveolar mucous membrane.

Attached gingiva is the part of the gum tissue tightly bound to the bottom of the tooth. Alveolar gingiva is the part of the gum tightly attached to the alveolar process (the jawbone). Areolar gingiva is gum attached to the jawbone by areolar (loose) connective tissue, the most common connective tissue in the body. Free gingiva is the part of the gum around the tooth that is not directly attached to the surface of the tooth. The gingival margin is the top edge of the gum tissue circling the tooth. Interdental (or interproximal) gingiva is the gum tissue between teeth.

Gingival hyperplasia (*hyper* meaning "bigger," and *plasia* meaning "form") is an enlargement of the gum tissue due to poor oral hygiene, periodontal disease, gingivitis, or certain medical drugs including, but not limited to, cyclosporine (medication to prevent rejection after organ transplant), Dilantin (or phenytoin; antiseizure medicine), or calcium channel blockers (medicine for heart disease).

The medical term for an inflammation of the gums is gingivitis. Gingivitis is a symptom of various diseases or disorders. Simple gingivitis is an inflammation of the gingiva that does not destroy the tissue connecting the gum to the tooth or bone. Acute necrotizing ulcerative gingivitis is an inflammation of the gum characterized by rapid tissue destruction. Primary herpetic gingivostomatitis is an inflammation due to a herpes infection.

See also GUM RESHAPING; PERIODONTAL DISEASE.

gingivectomy   See GUM RESHAPING.

gingivoplasty   See GUM RESHAPING.

gold (Au)   *Aurum,* from the Latin word meaning "shining dawn." A soft, bright yellow chemical element found naturally as "grains" in rock. Gold, which is easily molded, nonallergenic, and durable, has reputedly be used in dentistry as far back at the seventh century B.C.E. when the ancient Etruscans and Phoenicians employed gold WIRE to hold fake teeth in place in the mouth.

Giovanni of Arcoli (Johanues Arculanus), a 15th-century professor of medicine and surgery at Bologna and Padua, is believed to be the first to suggest using gold as a dental filling. In 1563, the first printed book on dentistry—BARTOLOMEO EUSTACHIO'S; *Libellus de dentibus* (commonly translated as *A Little Treatise on the Teeth*)—mentions the use of gold leaf (gold pounded into very thin sheets) for dental fillings.

In modern dentistry, gold is occasionally used pure—for example, as gold leaf formed into pellets to fill small cavities. It is more commonly used as an alloy with other elements such as the nonreactive precious "noble" metals platinum and silver plus reactive nonprecious base metals such as copper and zinc, a mixture similar to that used in silver fillings.

The virtues of a gold alloy are its durability, its resistance to chemical reactions such as corrosion, and its biocompatibility. Gold alloys are nonallergenic and strong enough not to break under the pressure exerted by the teeth during chewing; when properly prepared and maintained they may last 20 years or more. As a result, gold alloy is used to make restorations that sit on the top of the tooth such as an INLAY (a restoration that sits inside the cusps, or tips, at the top of a tooth), an ONLAY (a restoration that covers one or more cusps of the tooth), or a CROWN (a restoration that covers the entire top of the tooth). The major drawback to gold alloys is that they do not match the color of the tooth and are thus often considered cosmetically unacceptable for visible restorations, as in front teeth. When used for bridges or connections between teeth, the gold is often covered with porcelain to match the teeth.

Golden (Divine) Proportion   See FACIAL LAND-
MARKS.

graft   A graft is a piece of healthy tissue lifted
from one site on the body and moved to cover
an area where skin, mucous membrane, or bone
is damaged or missing due to disease, an injury,
or a birth defect. For example, a dental surgeon
or periodontist may use a tissue or bone graft
to cover a deficit left when gum or bone tissue
is lost to recession due to PERIODONTAL DISEASE
or when rebuilding a damaged jawbone (see
BONE).

A graft differs from a FLAP. A flap has its own
blood supply; a graft does not. As a result, the
success of a graft depends on the blood vessels
in the graft being successfully joined to the blood
vessels at the transfer site to provide the graft
with an adequate blood supply, a process known
as vascularization. A successful dental gum or
bone graft is said to *take* (fix in place) when new
blood vessels and scar tissue form in the injured
area.

Grafts are categorized in three ways: By their
source, by their tissue structure, and by the
function they serve.

Categorizing grafts by their source   A graft
taken from a patient's own body—for example,
tissue lifted from the patient's palate and transferred to another place in his mouth—are called
autogenous grafts, from the Greek words *autos*
meaning "self" and *genein* meaning "to make."
Autogenous grafts are also known as autogenous
transplants, autografts, autologen, and autologus
grafts. The procedure using material from the
patient's own body is called *autoplasty*; the tissue
used in the procedure is called *autoplast.*

A graft taken from another person and transferred to a genetically similar patient is called
an *isogenic graft,* from the Greek word *iso-* meaning "equal or uniform." A homograft (from
the Greek word *homo-* meaning "same") is a
graft taken from a member of one species and
transferred to another member of the same

species. Cadaver skin is one important type of
homograft.

Tissue taken from a member of one species
and transferred to a member of another species is called a heterograft, from the Greek word
hetero- meaning "different." Another name for a
heterograft is *xenograft,* from the Greek word *xeno-*
meaning "stranger," or *zoograft,* from the Greek
word *zoion,* meaning "animal." The most common
zoograft is pig skin used as a temporary covering
for areas of a human body where the skin has
been destroyed by a burn.

Categorizing grafts by tissue and structure   A
mucosal graft is a piece of mucous membrane,
such as the lining of the mouth, transferred from
one site to another. Examples include tissue
from the inner side of the lip moved to the other
side or a piece of tissue from the palate used to
fill in a space left after gum surgery or surgery to
repair a damaged tongue.

Skin or mucous membrane grafts may be full
thickness, split thickness, or dermal. A full thickness graft is a piece of tissue that includes both
the epidermis (the top layers of skin or mucosa
cells) and the dermis (the two layers of skin cells
under the epidermis). A split thickness skin graft
is a piece of skin that includes the epidermis and
the top part of the dermis. A dermal graft is a
graft of tissue from the dermis, the second layer
of skin cells. A composite graft has two or more
types of body tissue such as skin and fat or skin
and connective tissue (cartilage).

See also ACCELERATED ORTHODONTICS; BONE
RECONSTRUCTION; CADAVER BONE; GUIDED BONE
REGENERATION; IMPLANTOLOGY; JAWBONE, LOSS OF;
JAW RESTORATION.

Gram's stain   One way to categorize bacteria is
to label them as gram-positive or gram-negative
depending on how they react to a laboratory
test, Gram's stain, created by Danish physician
Hans Christian Joachim Gram (1853–1938).

Because gram-positive and gram-negative
bacteria are treated with different antibiotics,

the test is valuable as it enables doctors and dentists to choose the most effective medicine when treating a bacterial infection before or after dental treatment.

How Gram's Stain Works

- *Step 1:* The laboratory technician places a bacteria specimen on a slide and floods the slide with a purple pigment called crystal violet. The pigment is left in place for one minute, then flushed away with water, leaving a bluish purple residue.
- *Step 2:* The technician covers the slide with an iodine solution, lets that remain in place for one minute, and once again rinses the slide with water, again leaving a blue/purple residue on the slide.
- *Step 3:* The technician adds ethanol (alcohol), one drop at a time, until the specimen is no longer bluish purple, and then rinses the slide with water.
- *Step 4:* The technician applies a red dye called safranine and again lets the slide stand for one minute. The stain on a slide containing gram-positive bacteria remains bluish violet; the stain on a slide containing gram-negative bacteria turns pink.

groove A narrow channel in a surface; in dentistry, a shallow horizontal or vertical channel on the jawbone or on the surface of a tooth or on the surface of the gum. Dental grooves may be naturally occurring or they may be cut into the tooth during a dental procedure.

The naturally occurring dental grooves include the following:

- The *dental groove* is an indentation in the surface of the embryonic jawbone along which the tooth buds (structures that become teeth) will eventually form.
- The *developmental groove* is a fine line that marks the place on the enamel of the tooth where the parts of the CROWN of the tooth come together.
- The *free gingiva groove* is a slight line on the gum (see GINGIVA) where the free gingiva and the attached gingiva meet.
- An *interdental groove* is an indentation on the surface of the gum between two teeth that allows food and liquids to spill out from between the teeth.
- The *linguogingival groove* (from the Latin word *lingua*, meaning "tongue") is a groove on the back of some of the teeth in the front of the mouth—the side nearest the tongue.

Grooves created during dental procedures include the following:

- An *abutment groove* is a channel cut into the jawbone so as to create a place in which to fix the framework that holds a dental implant.
- A *retention groove* is a vertical channel created on the surface of a tooth so as to provide a better grip for a RESTORATION.

guard See MOUTH GUARD.

guided bone regeneration In periodontal surgery, a type of guided tissue regeneration (GTR), a procedure for encouraging the growth of new body tissue. The procedure is labeled "guided" because the surgery involves the insertion of a piece of absorbable material (such as Gore-Tex) called a membrane that keeps gum tissue from invading the area and serves as a matrix upon which new bone cells fasten to create new bone tissue. In dentistry, guided bone regeneration is commonly used to repair a defect such as a long, narrow groove in the jawbone.

Procedure

Once the dental surgeon or periodontist has numbed the affected area with an injected local anesthetic, she loosens and peels back the gum, scrapes away all debris to smooth the surface of the tooth, inserts a bone GRAFT (commonly BOVINE BONE), and covers the graft with the membrane. Once the graft and membrane are firmly in place, the periodontist sutures the wound and covers the area with a dressing. The dressing and sutures are usually removed within a week to 10 days.

The membranes used in early GTR procedures were not absorbable; a second surgery was required several weeks later to remove the membrane.

Risks and Complications

Postsurgical pain and/or discomfort are common, as are mild swelling and bleeding. A less common but more serious complication is infection, which may destroy tissue and cause the replacement to fail. The signs of infection are increased swelling, pain, and oozing from the wound, along with swollen lymph glands in the jaw or neck.

Outlook and Lifestyle Modifications

Successful guided bone regeneration results in firmly anchored teeth.

gum reshaping Periodontal surgery to reposition and tighten gum tissue around the teeth. There are two broad categories of gum reshaping procedures: *gingivectomy* and *gingivoplasty.*

Gingivectomy (from the Latin words *gingiva* meaning "gum," *ect-* meaning "out," and *-tomy* meaning "cut") is most commonly performed as a cosmetic procedure to remove naturally occurring excess gum tissue caused by a GENETIC disorder, a disease, or an injury. This surgery not only improves the appearance of the mouth, it also makes it easier to keep the teeth clean and, in cases where the excess tissue has made natural speech difficult, improves speech.

Gingivoplasty (from the Latin word *gingiva* meaning "gum" and *plastos* meaning "mold or form") is periodontal surgery to remedy gum tissue loosened by the destruction of underlying bone in the jaw after repeated incidents of acute PERIODONTAL DISEASE. The loss of bone creates spaces called pockets around the teeth, providing an area in which bacteria thrive. Cutting away loose gum tissue, then tightening the remaining tissue to eliminate the pockets, reduces the risk of bacterial growth, infection, and further bone loss.

Procedure

Some periodontists perform a complete SCALING prior to gum reshaping to remove PLAQUE and provide a smooth surface on which to position the tightened gum tissue.

The gum reshaping itself is performed with a local anesthetic to numb the tissue. Once the anesthesia takes effect, the periodontist will peel back the gum and use a scalpel, electrosurgical instrument, or LASER to cut away the excess or loosened tissue. If the surgery removes a large amount of tissue, the periodontist will use SUTURES to close the wound. In extreme cases, the surgery may require a tissue FLAP or GRAFT to close the wound. Once the sutures, flap, or graft are in place, the surgeon covers the wound with periodontal dressing, which is left in place for up to 10 days to allow the wound to heal so that the sutures can be removed.

Risks and Complications

Bleeding, swelling, and mild pain are common immediately after either gingivectomy or gingivoplasty. To lessen discomfort, the patient usually avoids hard foods that are difficult to chew and spicy foods that might irritate or injure tissue. To reduce the risk of infection, the patient keeps the area clean with an antiseptic rinse. When the dressing is removed, there may be more but slight bleeding for a day or so once normal hygiene (i.e., brushing and flossing) are resumed.

Infection after gum reshaping is rare. Its symptoms include unusual swelling, increased pain or discharge in the area of the surgery, and/

or swelling of the lymph glands in the lower jaw or neck.

Outlook and Lifestyle Modifications

The gums will look better within a month, but it may take several months for complete healing and the final shape of the gum line to appear. Cosmetically, gum reshaping gives the patient a more natural and attractive appearance. Medically, it reduces but does not eliminate the risk of damage from periodontal disease.

gums   See GINGIVA.

gutta-percha   A rubberlike material, the coagulated latex (milky sap) from any one of a number of tropical hardwood trees belonging to the Palaquium and Payena families native to Southeast Asia, the Philippines, and India. Gutta-percha is used widely in commercial products. It is water-resistant and does not conduct electricity, which makes it a perfect insulator for electrical wiring. It is resilient, which makes it useful as a covering for golf balls. And it is sticky, which makes it a useful component for adhesives. In dentistry, gutta-percha's resistance to moisture, nonconductivity, and resilience make it useful as a root canal filling, the material that is packed into the interior of the tooth once the root is removed. For this purpose, the gutta-percha is formed into cones sized to match the size of the files the endodontist uses to clean and smooth the root canal.

See ENDODONTICS, ROOT CANAL TREATMENT.

habit *Stedman's Medical Dictionary* defines a habit as "an act, behavioral response, practice, or custom established in one's repertoire by frequent repetition." In other words, a habit is behavior that, if repeated frequently enough, becomes a virtually automatic response.

Habits may be either beneficial or detrimental. Examples of bad dental and oral habits include grinding or clenching the teeth, biting the inside of the lip or cheek, and sucking the thumb in response to stress. The first may damage the enamel surface of the tooth, or crack the tooth, or cause spasms in the muscles that control the jaws. The second may injure the mucous membrane lining of the mouth. The third may force the teeth out of their normal position, requiring braces and/or other orthodontic devices to move them back into proper alignment.

Bad dental habits may also include such non–stress related choices as failing to brush or floss after eating or failing to see the dentist on a regular basis, resulting in dental problems such as DECAY and tooth loss.

Good dental habits, on the other hand, promote dental health. Examples of good dental habits include brushing and flossing after meals or sugary snacks, or chewing sugarless gum to increase the flow of SALIVA, which washes away debris while helping to maintain the mineral surface of the teeth, and seeing the dentist on a regular schedule, a habit particularly important for people who are prone to CAVITIES or have PERIODONTAL DISEASE.

Stress-related behaviors, including those that affect the teeth and mouth, are particularly hard to break. To do so, the patient may require professional help, such as instruction in stress management techniques such as BIOFEEDBACK. On the other hand, good dental habits such as frequent brushing or flossing are simply adult decisions. Like any other good health habit, they can usually be accomplished by a patient who is willing to learn how to care for his teeth.

See BRUXISM; ORTHODONTIC BRACES; THUMB SUCKING.

halitosis From the Latin word *halitus* meaning "breath" and the suffix *–osis* meaning "condition," or in this case "disease of." It means bad breath; an unpleasant odor emanating from the mouth due to the patient's lifestyle or a medical condition. Causes of halitosis include:

- eating specific foods such as onions and garlic containing odiferous mustard oil compounds that are absorbed into the bloodstream and excreted, in part, in the air expelled from the lungs

- smoking or chewing tobacco, which also contains odiferous compounds that either remain in the mouth or are expelled in air from the lungs

- failing to practice good oral hygiene so that bacteria living naturally in the mouth rot (i.e., digest and excrete) food particles remaining on or between the teeth and under the gums

- suffering from a medical or psychological condition such as diabetes; an EATING DISORDER (the body's lack of food forces it to digest its own tissues, producing an unpleasant odor); a gastrointestinal illness such as reflux; liver or kidney disease; PERIODONTAL DISEASE, which may cause foul-smelling infections; respiratory problems such as postnasal drip or a sinus infection; or xerostomia ("dry mouth"), a condition in which the body does not produce enough saliva to wash away food from the mouth

Halitophobia, a continuing, unrealistic fear of having bad breath, is considered a form of mental illness.

Symptoms and Diagnostic Path

In the dentist's office, halitosis may be identified simply by its odor. However, because other factors such as diet, emotion, or a medical condition can affect the breath, dental researchers prefer to use more accurate tests such as gas chromatography, which identifies specific compounds in any substance, or a Halimeter, which identifies and quantifies sulfides (odorous compounds such as hydrogen sulfide and methyl mercaptan). A Halimeter reading showing a high level of sulfides in a person's breath is diagnostic of halitosis.

Treatment Options and Outlook

A brief incident of halitosis, such as that following a meal of odiferous foods, probably does not require treatment. Continuing halitosis may require identifying and treating the cause.

If the cause is eating odiferous food or using tobacco, the patient may be advised either to avoid the foods or to clean the mouth properly after eating or to stop smoking.

If the cause is a failure to keep the mouth clean, the patient is urged to brush and floss on a regular schedule so as to remove debris on the teeth.

If normal oral hygiene does not solve the problem, the patient may be advised to seek a medical explanation. If the bad breath is due to a specific medical condition, the patient is advised to seek treatment for the condition—i.e., to use antihistamines and/or decongestants to relieve a postnasal drip, to obtain antibiotics to cure a sinus infection, to control his diabetes, or to use a moistening agent to relieve dry mouth.

Risk Factors and Preventive Measures

Treatment of halitosis usually prevents its reoccurrence. Patients should avoid eating odiferous foods, smoking, and other activities that cause bad breath.

See also DECAY; DENTIFRICE; MOUTHWASH; SPE-CIAL-NEEDS PATIENTS.

health conditions, dental effects of See SPE-CIAL-NEEDS PATIENTS.

Healthy People 2010 The third in a series of reports from the U.S. Department of Health and Human Services identifying national public health priorities and goals for the United States. The reports are designed to be used by federal government agencies, state governments, and community/private organizations to develop health programs that increase quality and years of healthy life and eliminate disparities of health care among all Americans. The series includes the *1979 Surgeon General's Report, Healthy People; Healthy People 2000: National Health Promotion and Disease Prevention Objectives* (1990), *Healthy People 2010* (2000), and *Healthy People 2020* (2010).

Healthy People 2010 is of particular value to those dealing with issues of oral and dental health. The report, which has 28 chapters ranging alphabetically from "Access to Quality Health Services" through "Vision and Hearing," includes a chapter titled "Oral Health" coauthored by the Centers for Disease Control and Prevention Health Resources and Services Administration, the Indian Health Service, and the National Institutes of Health. The chapter lays out recommendations to "prevent and control oral and craniofacial disease, conditions and injuries, and improve access to related services" that serve as the basis for the Surgeon General's report, ORAL HEALTH IN AMERICA: A REPORT OF THE SURGEON GENERAL.

The oral health issues and objectives described in *Healthy People 2010* are listed below. The baseline (starting point) for each objective is either the number of persons affected or the programs in place in the year indicated in parentheses, i.e., (1999). The target for each objective is the percentage of persons the report expects to be covered or the programs to be in place by the year 2010. The source for the issues, objectives, baseline statistics, and targets is *Healthy People 2010,* which is available in its entirety online at www.healthypeople.gov.

Issue: The Incidence of Dental Decay
Objectives

Reduce the proportion of all children who have cavities in their primary and/or permanent teeth

Baseline: 18 percent of children aged 2–4 years had one or more cavities in their primary teeth (1988–94)

Target: 11 percent

Baseline: 52 percent of children aged 6–8 years had one or more dental cavities in their primary and/or permanent teeth (1988–94)

Target: 42 percent

Baseline: 61 percent of adolescents aged 15 years had cavities in their permanent teeth 1988–94

Target: 51 percent

Issue: Lack of Treatment for Dental Decay
Objectives

Reduce the proportion of all Americans with untreated dental decay in primary and/or permanent teeth

Baseline: 16 percent of children aged 2–4 years had untreated dental decay in their primary teeth (1988–94)

Target: 9 percent

Baseline: 29 percent of children aged 6–8 years had untreated dental decay in their primary or permanent teeth (1988–94).

Target: 21 percent

Baseline: 20 percent of adolescents had untreated dental decay in their permanent teeth (1988–94)

Target: 15 percent

Baseline: 27 percent of adults aged 35–44 years had untreated dental decay (1988–94)

Target: 15 percent

Issue: Loss of Permanent Teeth
Objectives

Increase the proportion of American adults who have never had a permanent tooth extracted because of dental decay/cavities or periodontal disease

Baseline: 31 percent of adult Americans aged 35 to 44 years had never had a permanent tooth extracted because of dental caries or periodontal disease (1988–94)

Target: 42 percent

Reduce the proportion of older adults who had all their natural teeth extracted

Baseline: 26 percent of American adults aged 65–74 years had lost all their natural teeth (1997)

Target: 20 percent

Issue: Incidence of Periodontal Disease
Objective

Reduce the incidence of periodontal disease

Baseline: 48 percent of American adults aged 35–44 years had gingivitis (inflammation of the gum tissue)

Target: 41 percent (gingivitis)

Baseline: 22 percent of American adults aged 35–44 years had destructive periodontal disease (loose teeth, loss of gum and bone tissue)

Target: 14 percent

Issue: Early Detection of Oral Cancers
Objective

Increase the proportion of oral and pharyngeal cancers detected at the earliest stage

Baseline: 35 percent of oral and pharyngeal cancers (stage I, localized) were detected in 1990–95

Target: 50 percent

Increase the proportion of adults who, in the past 12 months, report having had an examination to detect oral and pharyngeal cancers

Baseline: 13 percent of adults aged 40 years and older reported having had an oral and pharyngeal cancer examination (1998)

Target: 20 percent

Issue: Strengthening Teeth
Objectives

Increase the proportion of children and adolescents who have dental sealant applied to their molar teeth

Baseline: 23 percent of children aged 8 years are treated with dental sealant

Target: 50 percent

Baseline: 15 percent of adolescents aged 14 years are treated with dental sealant

Target: 50 percent.

Increase the proportion of the U.S. population served by community water systems with optimally fluoridated water.

Baseline: 62 percent of the U.S. population was served by community water systems with optimally fluoridated water in 1992

Target: 75 percent

Issue: Use of the Oral Health Care System
Objectives
Increase the proportion of children and adults who use the oral health care system each year

Baseline: 44 percent of persons aged 2 years and older in 1996 visited a dentist during the previous year

Target: 56 percent

Increase the proportion of low-income children and adolescents who received any preventive dental service during the past year

Baseline: 20 percent of children and adolescents under age 19 years living at or below 200 percent of the federal poverty level received preventive dental service (1996)

Target: 57 percent

Increase the proportion of long-term care residents who use the oral health care system each year.

Baseline: 19 percent of all nursing home residents received dental services (1997)

Target: 25 percent

Increase the proportion of school-based health centers with an oral health component

Baseline and target statistics unavailable

Increase the proportion of local health departments and community-based health centers, including community, migrant, and homeless health centers, that have an oral health component

Baseline: 34 percent of local jurisdictions and health centers had oral health components (1997)

Target: 75 percent

Issue: Referral and Treatment for Cranial Facial Defects
Objectives
Increase the number of states and the District of Columbia that have a system for recording and referring infants and children with cleft lips, cleft palates, and other craniofacial anomalies to craniofacial anomaly rehabilitative teams

Baseline: 23 states and the District of Columbia have systems for recording and referring children with craniofacial anomalies (1997)

Target: All states and the District of Columbia

Increase the number of states and the District of Columbia that have an oral and craniofacial health surveillance system

Baseline: No states or the District of Columbia had oral and craniofacial health surveillance systems (1999)

Target: All states and the District of Columbia

Tribal, State, and Local Dental Programs
Objective
Increase the number of tribal, state (including the District of Columbia), and local health agencies that serve jurisdictions of 250,000 or more persons that have in place an effective public dental health program directed by a dental professional with public health training

Baseline: 29 states/full directors; 14 states/part-time directors; 9 states/no directors (1999); 153 local health agencies serving 80 million Americans had a dental program; 62 percent were directed by dentists; 22 percent by dental hygienists; 16 percent by non-dental personnel (1995)

Target: All

heartburn/reflux Gastroesophageal reflux disease (GERD), a situation in which the acidic contents of the stomach splash back (reflux) past the lower esophageal sphincter (LES), a muscle around the bottom of the esophagus, into the esophagus itself, and then into the mouth. GERD is a common condition. According to the National Institute of Diabetes and Digestive and Kidney Diseases:

- more than 60 million American adults have heartburn at least once a month
- more than one-third of American women aged 35–44 and slightly less than one-third of American men in the same age group have "frequent" heartburn (more than two incidents a week)
- As many as 25 million Americans, including one in four pregnant women, have heartburn at least once a day

Symptoms and Diagnostic Path

The characteristic symptom of reflux is pain in the esophagus (throat) after eating, when lying down, or when bending over. Oral/dental symptoms of persistent reflux include bad breath, sour taste, "water brash" (a sudden flush of saliva), inflammation of the gums, and in longstanding severe cases, erosion of the enamel surface of the teeth.

To confirm the diagnosis, the doctor or dentist may prescribe a course of medication. If the discomfort is relieved by the medication, it is reasonable to assume the cause to be reflux. However, because the pain of reflux may mimic that of a heart attack (and vice versa), it is essential to have any incident of sudden or continuing chest pain evaluated by a physician.

Treatment Options and Outlook

Left untreated, reflux may lead to erosion of the dental enamel, esophagitis (chronic irritation and inflammation of the lining of the throat), dysphagia (difficulty in swallowing), Barrett's esophagus (precancerous changes in the lining of the esophagus), and esophageal cancer.

The treatment to prevent these developments is determined by the frequency and severity of the condition. To treat intermittent reflux the

physician or dentist may prescribe a simple antacid such as calcium carbonate (e.g., Tums) to neutralize the acid in the liquid splashing back into the esophagus.

To treat persistent reflux, the physician/dentist may prescribe a histamine 2 receptor antagonist (H_2 blocker) such as cimetidine (Tagamet), famotidine (Pepcid), or ranitidine (Zantac) that reduces the amount of acid secreted by glands in the stomach making the reflux less acidic.

To treat severe persistent reflux, the physician or dentist may prescribe a proton pump inhibitor (PPI), such as omeprazole (Prilosec), lansoprazole (Prevacid), or esomeprazole (Nexium), that inhibits the activity of an enzyme that enables cells in the stomach wall to pump out stomach acids. PPIs are also used to heal tissue damage caused by the reflux, thus reducing the risk of esophageal cancer.

Risk Factors and Preventive Measures

The basic risk factor for reflux is a defect in the lower esophageal sphincter that prevents the muscle from closing tight enough to keep stomach contents from splashing back into the throat and mouth.

While the state of the muscle is an individual characteristic of a person's body structure, some lifestyle factors may worsen the condition. These factors include (but are not limited to) smoking, eating fatty or spicy foods, drinking alcohol, lying down soon after eating, or being overweight or pregnant so that the abdomen presses on the throat. Controlling one or more of these factors may reduce the incidence or severity of reflux.

heart disease   See SPECIAL-NEEDS PATIENTS.

hemifacial atrophy   A chronic condition that leads to progressive shrinkage of the tissues (skin, underlying fat, muscle, connective tissue, bone) on one side of the face, most commonly on the left side. Hemifacial atrophy may also be linked to darkened skin, loss of facial hair, facial nerve pain, and/or seizures. On rare occasions, the tissue shrinkage may spread down to the tissues of the torso, including the internal organs and the limbs (arm and leg) on the affected side.

Symptoms and Diagnostic Path

The most common early sign of hemifacial atrophy is a painless cleft (opening) at or near the imaginary center line dividing the two sides of the face or, more commonly, the forehead, along with a bluish tint to the skin on the affected side.

The damage done by hemifacial atrophy is evaluated via simple physical examination as well as radiological studies (CT scans), which are also useful in establishing a treatment regimen.

Treatment Options and Outlook

Hemifacial atrophy usually appears before age 10 and progresses over a period ranging from two to 10 years before stabilizing. Its course is uncertain; some patients have minimal damage; others suffer significant loss.

There is no known cure. The standard treatment is reconstructive dentistry and/or plastic surgeries such tissue transplants or injections of natural or synthetic fillers (substances that fill out the face) or the insertion of prosthetic devices such as a cheek implant to improve the facial structure and make it possible for the patient to speak clearly and eat easily.

Risk Factors and Preventive Measures

Hemifacial atrophy is a rare condition that occurs more frequently in females. There is no known cause and no known risk factors, and no preventive measures have been identified.

herpes, oral; herpes labialis From the Latin word *herpes* and the Greek word *herpein* meaning "to creep," and the Latin word *labi* meaning "lip." An infection also known as a *cold sore* or *fever blister* caused by the herpes simplex type 1 (virus), which accounts for as many of 80 percent of oral herpes infections, or the herpes simplex type 2 (virus), which accounts for the remaining 20 percent and is the virus that causes genital herpes. Herpes zoster (shingles) is an unrelated virus infection caused by a virus called varicella zoster.

The herpes virus is common; most people are infected by at least one version early in life, most commonly by coming in contact with a person who has an active infection. Touching an active sore allows the virus to enter the body through a break in the skin or mucous membrane, and it begins to reproduce itself, triggering sores or, more commonly, burrowing into a resting place in the body at the base of a spinal nerve. The virus lies dormant at the base of the nerve until some form of physical or emotional stress lowers the patient's resistance, enabling the virus to reactivate itself and trigger new symptoms, such as mouth sores. Once the infection recedes, the virus again becomes dormant until the next episode.

Symptoms and Diagnostic Path

The first signs of a herpes infection are itching, burning, tingling, or pain that precedes a sore (or sores) or a cluster of tiny blisters, clearly visible on the lips, tongue, and mucous membrane lining of the mouth, and possibly accompanied by fever and muscle aches.

If necessary, the diagnosis of herpes infection can be confirmed by a biopsy to identify the virus in a small sample of tissue taken from the mouth or via a blood test that reveals the presence of antibodies to the herpes virus.

Treatment Options and Outlook

For healthy people with a normal immune system, over-the-counter (OTC) pain relievers such as acetaminophen, aspirin, ibuprofen, or a topical anesthetic product containing lidocaine can ease the discomfort of oral herpes.

There are a number of antiretroviral prescription products that, when applied as soon as a patient experience signs of a herpes simplex infection such as itching or redness, can prevent eruption of the herpes or shorten the period of infection. In addition, in 2000, the Food and Drug Administration approved the use of the antiviral drug docosanol as an OTC antiviral medication. Docosanol, which is sold as a cream under the brand name Abreva to treat herpes simplex infections on the lips and face, stops the herpes virus from fusing with human cells, thus preventing the virus from replicating itself and spreading the infection.

Risk Factors and Preventive Measures

Any medical condition such as HIV/AIDS or cancer chemotherapy treatment that weakens the body's immune system may trigger and/or worsen a herpes infection.

HIV/AIDS See SPECIAL-NEEDS PATIENTS.

Hobbs, Lucy Beaman (1833–1910) The first woman to graduate from a recognized dental college in the United States. Orphaned as a child, Hobbs worked as a seamstress and school teacher before attempting to enter the Ohio College of Dental Surgery. After being rejected several times and practicing without a diploma in Iowa where she built a sterling reputation, she was finally admitted to the school in 1865 on the recommendation of members of the Iowa Dental Society who threatened to boycott any school that refused to let her in. Given her previous experience, she was able to graduate the following year. A few months later, in July 1866, she became the first woman to address a state dental society (the Iowa society, to which she read her paper "The Use of the Mallet"). In 1893, Hobbs served on the Woman's Advisory Committee for the World's Columbian Congress held in Chicago. One hundred years later, in 1993, the American Association of Women Dentists created the Lucy Hobbs Taylor Award in her name to recognize "significant service to dentistry and contribution to society."

home care See DENTIFRICE; FLOSS, DENTAL; MOUTHWASH; ORAL HYGIENE; TOOTHBRUSH.

hormones See GENDER AND ORAL HEALTH.

hyperhydrosis, hyperhidrosis From the Latin words *hyper* meaning "over" or "beyond" and *hidrosis* meaning "perspiration"; excessive perspiration.

Primary hyperhydrosis is excess perspiration due either to oversensitive sweat glands or to a malfunction of the nerves, which causes excessive amounts of a chemical that triggers perspiration. *Secondary hyperhydrosis* is excess perspiration linked to a medical condition such as cancer, an infection, a neurological disorder, or a spinal cord injury. *Masticatory hyperhydrosis,* excessive facial sweating while chewing, is a condition linked to an injury that damages the facial nerve.

Symptoms and Diagnostic Path

The most common signs of hyperhydrosis are excess sweating under the arms or on the palms of the hands.

Treatment Options and Outlook

The treatment for mild to moderate primary hyperhydrosis is over-the-counter or prescription antiperspirants. In more severe cases, the treatment may include surgery to reduce the activity of the nerves linked to the excessive sweating. The treatment for hyperhydrosis linked to a medical condition is to treat the underlying disease. The treatment for masticatory hyperhydrosis is to repair the damaged nerve, if possible.

Risk Factors and Preventive Measures

There is no known risk factor for primary hyperhydrosis. However, the excess perspiration may be triggered by emotional stress, warm weather, alcohol beverages, spicy foods, and certain medications including aspirin and other drugs that reduce fever. Avoiding the trigger may reduce or prevent the hyperhydrosis.

The risk factor for secondary hyperhydrosis is a specific medical condition. Successful treatment of the underlying condition should relieve the excessive perspiration.

hyperplasia An abnormal growth in the number of cells in a tissue or organ that may be a precursor to a malignancy.

Denture hyperplasia is the enlargement of soft tissue in the mouth due to irritation from an ill-fitting DENTURE. Focal fibrous hyperplasia is a small, hard growth on the tongue or the mucous membrane lining the lip and cheek caused by injury or irritation such as chewing on the tissue. Gingival hyperplasia is an enlargement of a part of the gum due to infection, inflammation, or irritation. Papillary hyperplasia is a collection of red bumps ("papillae") on the hard palate (roof of the mouth) usually due to irritation from a denture.

Symptoms and Diagnostic Path
Hyperplasia may be visible on examination of the mouth. If necessary, the dentist may take a small piece of tissue for a biopsy so as to rule out any malignancy.

Treatment Options and Outlook
The cause of the hyperplasia determines the treatment and predicts the outlook. Benign hyperplasia is most frequently treated by excising the lesion and then eliminating the source of the irritation to prevent a recurrence. Hyperplasia indicating a malignant tumor is treated as an ORAL CANCER.

For example, hyperplasia due to ill-fitting dentures is remedied by refitting the dentures. Hyperplasia due to an injury may heal on its own or can be simply removed; after that, avoiding injury or a bad dental habit such as chewing on the mouth should prevent a recurrence. The same applies to hyperplasia of the gum due to an infection or irritation. On the other hand, hyperplasia diagnosed as a malignancy may require surgery, chemotherapy, or radiation.

Risk Factors and Preventive Measures
The most common risk factor for a benign hyperplasia of the oral tissue is irritation. Avoiding the irritating factors or behavior avoids the hyperplasia. The risk factors for hyperplasia due to a malignancy are the common risk factors for oral cancer, primarily the use of TOBACCO and excess use of alcohol.

I

immune system The immune system governs the body's ability to fight off and recover from infection; for example, the infections that may occur due to periodontal disease or after a dental surgical procedure.

The immune system itself is composed of a group of organs, including a circulatory system (the LYMPHATIC SYSTEM) and specialized blood cells such as B cells and T cells whose primary function is to identify, isolate, and destroy foreign organisms and substances in order to protect the body from infection and/or disease, including the infections that may occur in PERIODONTAL DISEASE. A healthy immune system reduces the risk of these infections and facilitates quick and complete healing after dental/oral surgery.

Immunodeficiency is the complete or partial failure of the immune system, due either to a defect in the system such as an inability to produce specific disease-fighting cells or to an illness that injures a previously healthy immune system. For example, alcoholism, drug abuse, some forms of cancer, diabetes, HIV/AIDS, lupus, and tuberculosis, among others, may impair the immune system, leaving the patient more susceptible to infection. Medical treatments such as cancer chemotherapy and radiation therapy and medical drugs such as corticosteroids also impair the immune system.

An immunosuppressant is any natural or artificial substance that reduces the effectiveness of the immune response. Immunosuppressants are commonly used in medicine to prevent the body from rejecting new tissue after an organ transplant, a procedure rarely required in dentistry.

These drugs may also be used to treat an autoimmune disease such as rheumatoid arthritis or psoriasis in which the immune system mistakenly attacks some of the body's own tissues as foreign. Some common immunosuppressants are azathioprine (Imuran), cyclosporine (Neoral, Sandimmune), and tacrolimus (Prograf). The primary complication associated with taking one of these drugs is an increased susceptibility to infection.

Immunotherapy is medical treatment designed to change the function of the immune system, either to suppress its function so as to allow the body to accept foreign material such as a transplanted organ or to increase its activity so as to ameliorate the effects of allergens, disable disease-causing microorganisms, or destroy malignant tumors, including ORAL CANCERS. In each case, the aim is to sensitize the body to a disease-causing agent (antigen) in an attempt to trigger the production of protective substances (*antibodies*). Immunotherapy for bacterial or viral infections exposes the patient to vaccines containing small amounts of live or dead microorganisms, such as the polio virus, enabling the body to produce antibodies to attack the microbe.

The term immunotherapy is also used to describe a variety of proposed treatments for cancer, including cytokines (interferon and interleukin), monoclonal antibodies, and cancer vaccines.

Cytokines are proteins made naturally by white blood cells in response to infection or inflammation. One cytokine, interferon-alpha (IFN-alpha), the first to demonstrate an ability to activate the immune system and slow the growth of malignant tumors, is approved by the Food and Drug Administration for treating several cancers, including the skin cancer melanoma and the blood cell cancers chronic myelogenous leukemia (CML), hairy cell leukemia, malignant, and multiple myeloma. Another cytokine, interleukin-2 (IL-2) is used to treat kidney cancer and melanoma. Other cytokines, such as interferon-beta, are currently under investigation for their value as cancer treatments. The side effects of treatment with interferons and interleukins include a feeling of weakness and illness, with flulike symptoms. The severity of the reaction depends on the size of the dose.

Monoclonal antibodies (mABs) are artificial antibodies manufactured to target a specific biological substance such as a cancer cell or a cell associated with the production and/or growth of cancer cells, used in cancer diagnosis as well as treatment. Cells containing monoclonal antibodies can be injected to help treat certain cancers. For example, rituximab (Rituxan) is used in treating non-Hodgkin's lymphoma; trastuzumab (Herceptin) is used for some breast cancers. Enhanced monoclonal antibodies linked to cytotoxic (cell-killing) drugs can be used to deliver the drug to specific cells. Until the monoclonal antibody reaches the cancer cell, its parts remain bound together. Once inside the cancer cell, the cytotoxic drug separates from the antibody and attacks the cancer cell. As a result, the cancer drug does not harm healthy tissue, thus reducing the incidence of the side effects of traditional chemotherapy.

Cancer vaccines are similar to other vaccines; they contain an antigen (in this case, cancer-related material) designed to stimulate the immune system to produce antibodies to attack body cells containing the antigen. Most cancer vaccines are still being tested in animals; one, targeting melanoma, appears to be the first one proven effective in stimulating a human immune system response to a specific cancer.

See also IMPLANTOLOGY.

implantology The branch of dentistry dealing with implants, one component of an *osseous integrated* (integrated into the bone) dental device designed to hold removable or permanent teeth/dentures securely in place in the jawbone.

The implant is a small metal (commonly titanium) cylinder. During implant surgery, the implant is inserted under the gum tissue into the jawbone. Once the surgical wound has healed and the implant is secure, a second component, known as an abutment or an extension, is attached to the cylinder, and an artificial tooth (also known as a CROWN) is put onto the abutment, creating the illusion of a natural tooth.

Implants are safe and effective replacements for teeth lost to injury or PERIODONTAL DISEASE. In addition, by eliminating the bacteria-friendly surface where the natural tooth meets the gum/jawbone, an implant may also reduce the risk of infection linked to the loss of BONE associated with periodontal disease.

Procedure

Implant surgery usually proceeds in four distinct phases: planning the surgery, inserting the implant, adding the abutment, and attaching the crown (false tooth).

Planning the Surgery The first step in planning implant surgery is a thorough examination of the mouth that often includes the dental surgeon taking dental X-rays and creating an impression of the area where the implant will go. Before surgery, the surgeon reviews the patient's medical history, including all relevant medical conditions, as well as a list of any drugs the patient is currently using.

If the patient does not have sufficient bone in the JAW to accommodate the implant, the dental surgeon may perform a bone graft prior to implant surgery, inserting either synthetic material or bone tissue from the patient's own body to strengthen the jaw.

Inserting the Implant This surgery is usually performed in the dentist's office or as an outpatient procedure in the hospital, under local anesthesia to numb the area where the implant will be inserted, sometimes along with a light sedative to relax the patient.

When the area is numb, the dental surgeon cuts into the gum, exposing the jawbone. He drills into the bone to make space for the implant (cylinder), inserts the implant, and (most commonly) places the abutment on top of the implant cylinder, which is visible during the healing period. The dental surgeon then closes the gum tissue with either absorbable or nonabsorbable sutures. When the gum is closed, the surgeon puts a temporary replacement over the gap, a denture that can be easily removed for cleaning and when the patient goes to sleep.

The implant is then left undisturbed for up to six months to allow the jawbone to grow around and bond to it, a process called *osseointegration* that establishes a solid base for the implant. During this time, the patient continues to use the temporary denture.

Occasionally, the abutment is put on during a second surgery. If so, once again, the surgeon administers anesthetic and opens the gum, this time to expose the cylinder. The abutment is secured to the cylinder, and the gum tissue is pulled tight and sutured, leaving the top of the abutment visible above the gum. The patient waits several weeks for the gum to heal around the abutment and then returns for the final step in implant surgery.

Attaching the Crown (False Tooth)   When the gum has healed sufficiently to allow the implant to support an artificial tooth, the surgeon makes a new impression of the abutment area and the surrounding teeth and sends the impression to a dental laboratory, which manufactures the prosthesis.

The prosthesis may be either a removable crown/denture with several teeth on a metal frame that snaps on and off the abutment, or a permanent crown/denture, which is a single tooth that is cemented onto a single abutment.

The removable prosthesis is less expensive than the permanent prosthesis.

Risks and Complications

Common aftereffects of surgery include swelling and bruising of gums and face, pain, minor bleeding, and stiff facial muscles.

Other, less common complications may include infection around the implant, damage to nearby teeth or blood vessels, and nerve injury resulting in temporary or permanent pain or loss of sensation in the gums, LIPS, cheeks, or chin. Rarely, an implant in the upper jaw may protrude into the sinus cavity above the jaw, creating a risk of sinus infection.

In some cases, the bone in the jaw may fail to close tightly around the implant cylinder or the implant may loosen. If that happens, the implant must be removed and the entire process repeated several months later after the bone has healed.

Outlook and Lifestyle Modifications

For several days after each surgery, patients may need to switch to a soft-food diet. Nonabsorbable stitches are usually removed within 10 days after surgery.

To protect the long-term viability of dental implants, patients are advised to care for implants just as they would care for natural teeth and the surrounding gum:

- keep the implant crown (tooth) and the gum around it clean
- avoid hard foods that might crack the crown and seek treatment for persistent BRUXISM (tooth grinding)
- Do not use TOBACCO—both chewing tobacco and smoking tobacco can stain teeth, as can excess use of caffeinated beverages, particularly tea; in addition, smoking heats and injures gums

As a rule, dental implants are most successful for patients who do not wish to wear dentures and:

- have good oral health
- do not have a health condition that impedes healing
- have enough bone tissue to anchor the implant, or
- can tolerate bone GRAFTS to provide a base for the implant
- have the patience required to deal with a process that may take as long as 10 months to complete

See also BRUXISM; EMERGENCIES, DENTAL; IMPRESSION, DENTAL.

impression, dental The mold ("negative") from which the dentist makes a cast, a model of one or more parts of the inside of the mouth. The dental impression is used to diagnose dental irregularities or as a base on which to build a dental appliance such as a CROWN, DENTURE, VENEER, or other dental RESTORATION.

There are two basic types of dental casts: a master cast and a diagnostic cast.

A master cast is an accurate replica of the teeth and/or JAW on which a dental technician builds a dental restoration. A corrected master cast is a master cast modified to show areas where teeth are missing. A working cast is an accurate copy of a master cast, used in preliminary production of a restoration so as to avoid damaging the master cast.

A diagnostic cast is an impression used to diagnose dental problems. A diagnostic implant cast is one used to build a trial WAX model of a proposed restoration. A preextraction cast is one made before a tooth is removed. A preoperative cast is one made before dental surgery. A record cast is one made as a reference against which to measure future changes. An implant cast is a cast showing the exposed BONE in the jaw for which an implant is proposed.

The subcategories of dental impressions are listed in the following chart.

TYPES OF DENTAL IMPRESSIONS

Impression	Purpose
Anatomic	Shows the actual shape of the tissue in the mouth
Bridge	Serves as a mold on which to build a fixed (permanently attached) bridge, denture, or other dental restoration
Denture	Serves as a base on which to build either a full denture (full denture impression) or a partial denture (partial denture impression)
Functional	Shows the position and structure of the supporting tissue (gums, ligaments, bone) in the jaw
Mandibular	Serves as a model of all the teeth in the lower jaw
Maxillary	Serves as a model of all the teeth in the upper jaw
Preliminary ("snap impression")	Serves as a quick diagnostic tool
Surgical Bone	Serves as a mold for a model of exposed bone surface; used in planning and creating dental implants

Procedure

A dental impression is created in several stages.

First, the dentist fills a horseshoe-shaped dental tray with a liquid material, most commonly an alginate (a thickener also used in food products) or silicone, which is a semisynthetic compound often used in prosthetic restorations because it holds its shape when exposed to heat or cold, is water-resistant, and is unlikely to provoke any bodily reaction.

Second, the patient rinses his mouth to remove any stray food or other particles, and the dentist places the tray in the patient's mouth. He presses it firmly into place over the upper or lower teeth, eliminating any air bubble spaces and creating a vacuum that holds the tray tight against the teeth/jaw. He then waits a few minutes to allow the material to set.

Third, when the molding material has set sufficiently, the dentist moves the tray gently from side to side to break the vacuum holding it in place, lifts the tray out of the patient's mouth, and sets it aside to allow the material to harden into a negative impression, a hollow mold of the patient's teeth/jaw. When the tray is removed, the patient rinses once again, this time to remove any debris left by the molding material.

Finally, when the mold is firm, the dentist fills it with a cement mixture, one layer at a time, tapping the molding tray to eliminate any air bubbles. The cement hardens over a period of 12 hours or more into a positive impression, an accurate representation of the patient's teeth/mouth. The dentist peels away the dental tray, and the model is ready for use.

Risks and Complications

There are no health risks and/or complications associated with this procedure.

Outlook and Lifestyle Modifications

The impression is a useful tool that makes it possible to produce well-designed, well-fitting dental restorations.

incision and drainage Surgery to drain a dental abscess, a bacterial infection, under the surface of the gum that has not resolved on its own. The infection may be due to decay that has spread to the dental pulp and from there to the gum next to the root of the tooth (a periapical abscess) or it may be a periodontal problem arising from food's having been caught in the space between gum and tooth. The signs of a localized dental abscess are redness, swelling, and pain; an infection that has spread beyond the original site may cause systemic symptoms such as nausea, diarrhea, or vomiting, as well as chills and/or fever.

Dental abscesses are usually named for their location and/or the affected tissue. For example,

an apical abscess (a.k.a. an alveolar or periapical abscess) is an infection of the tip of the tooth root and surrounding bone; a gingival abscess is an abscess in the space between the tooth and the gum; a periodontal abscess is an infection of the tissues attaching the tooth to the jawbone resulting from PERIODONTAL DISEASE.

Procedure

The dentist cuts into the gum at the site of abscess, releasing the pus collected under the surface. The infection is drained; the site is packed with sterile absorbent material; and the incision is left to heal. In some cases, the dentist may put a hollow tube (drain) in the area to enable any infected material to continue to escape.

A dental abscess stretches the gum and may be extremely painful, but as a rule no anesthetic is injected directly into the area when a localized abscess is opened and drained because doing so might spread the infection. Instead, the dentist applies local anesthetic to numb the gum. Although the patient will feel a sudden prick when the abscess is cut, the pain disappears immediately as the infected material drains.

An infection associated with a CAVITY may require immediate endodontic (root canal) treatment to remove the infected PULP inside the tooth. In this case, the dentist administers a regional block (anesthesia to numb the part of the mouth served by the nerves in the tooth and the immediate surrounding area).

Risks and Complications

Bruising of the gum, slight bleeding, and mild discomfort are common, usually alleviated with mild analgesics, nonsteroidal anti-inflammatory products such as aspirin or ibuprofen. Infection is a less common complication. To reduce the risk, the dentist prescribes a short course of antibiotics.

Outlook and Lifestyle Modifications

If the abscess is due to periodontal disease, the periodontist may eventually perform surgery to tighten the gum tissue and reduce the space between tooth and gum (pocket) so as to reduce the risk of future infection arising from food's being caught in the pocket.

infection control   A term describing techniques designed to reduce the transmission of infection from person to person in a medical or dental setting.

The current infection control techniques are contained in *Guidelines for Infection Control in Dental Health-Care Settings*, published by the Centers for Disease Control and Prevention (CDC) in December 2003, and *Guideline for Isolation Precautions: Preventing Transmission of Infectious Agents in Healthcare Settings 2007*. Both reports address three areas of concern: office cleanliness, contact between dental personnel and patients, and patient health. To reduce the risk of infection transmission in these areas, both recommend the use of the Standard Precautions, a set of procedures based on the principle that "all blood, body fluids, secretions, excretions except sweat, non-intact skin, and mucous membranes may contain transmissible infectious agents." For maximum safety, the Standard Precautions are to be used for all patients, regardless of their known or suspected health status.

The *Guidelines for Infection Control in Dental Health-Care Settings* are available online at www.cdc.gov/mmwr/preview/mmwrhtml/rr5217a1.htm.

The *Standard Precautions* excerpted from *Guideline for Isolation Precautions: Preventing Transmission of Infectious Agents in Healthcare Settings 2007* are available online at www.cdc.gov/ncidod/dhqp/gl_isolation_standard.html.

Maintaining Office Cleanliness

To protect both the dental patient and the dental personnel, disposable instruments and materials should be used whenever possible; nondisposable dental instruments should be sterilized (cleansed of all microorganisms) and the dental furniture disinfected (cleansed of most, but not all, microorganisms).

Safe Injection Techniques   Ideally, all injection equipment—needles, tubes (cannulae), syringes—should be sterile and disposable, used for one patient only. They should not be reused, either for another patient or to draw fluid out of a second vial that might be used for another person.

Dental Instruments   All instruments other than disposable instruments, which are used once and discarded, must be cleaned and sterilized before each use.

Dental instruments made of materials that remain stable at very high temperatures are sterilized in:

- an autoclave—a self-locking, pressurized cabinet that sterilizes instruments with steam

STERILIZING DENTAL INSTRUMENTS	
Technique	**Instruments**
Wet heat (autoclave)	All instruments that are heat-stable, as probes, drills, and handpieces
Dry heat (convection)	Carbon steel instruments, dental burs, smoothing instruments, all heat-stable hand instruments except handpieces
Heated chemical vapors	All instruments that are heat-stable such as probes, drills, drill holders, burs, and bur holders
Cold sterilization (gluteraldehyde)	Items that are not heat stable, such as rubber bowls
Cold sterilization (bleach)	Nondisposable protective equipment such as goggles

Source: University of Washington School of Dentistry (www.dental.washington.edu/hazards/chapter-2/instrument-sterilization-protocols.htm).

heated to 217°F to 250°F (121°C to 138°C), or

- a dry-heat convection (forced air) oven that sterilizes with air at temperatures ranging as high as 306°F (170°C), or

- a pressurized cabinet that heats a chemical solution to release a sterilizing vapor.

Instruments or implements made of a material that is not heat-stable (i.e., rubber, some plastics) may be sterilized by immersion in a chemical solution such as 2 percent glutaraldehyde or 10 percent household bleach. This technique, known as cold sterilization, may take as long as 10 hours, depending on the chemical and/or the instrument.

Some examples of sterilization techniques and the dental instruments for which they are used are listed below.

Dental Furniture   In the dental office, all work surfaces must be cleaned and disinfected after each use with a hospital disinfectant approved by the U.S. Environmental Protection Agency. Medical waste, such as bloody tissues or disposable sharp instruments including hypodermic needles, must be discarded in a puncture-resistant, color-coded, and leak-proof container; liquid waste, into a drain connected to a sanitary sewer system. Unless returned to the patient, extracted teeth are treated as medical waste, kept in a leak-proof container if sent to a dental research laboratory, and/or heat sterilized before being used for teaching purposes.

Dentists who treat children should take care to choose toys and furniture that are easy to clean, avoiding fuzzy stuffed toys that are difficult to disinfect. Because children are likely to put toys in their mouths, all toys that have been cleaned should be rinsed in plain water after disinfection. Dirty toys should be stored in a bin separate from those that are clean and ready to use.

Contact between Dental Personnel and Patients

To reduce the risk of transmitting blood-borne diseases such as AIDS and hepatitis B between patients and dental workers, the guidelines and Standard Precautions emphasize hand hygiene and personal protective equipment (PPE).

Hand Hygiene   Simply put, the CDC recommends that dental personnel keep their hands clean. The situations and recommended procedures are listed below:

HAND HYGIENE

Procedure	Situation
Wash with soap and water*	Before and after treating each patient
	Hands visibly dirty
	After touching potentially infectious material, including blood and other bodily fluids
	After touching mucous membranes (inside mouth), broken skin, or wound dressings
	After touching potentially contaminated instruments or surfaces, such as a tray holding used instruments or dressings
	Before putting on sterile surgeon's gloves and after removing them
Clean with alcohol-based hand cleansers (or soap and water)	Hand not visibly dirty
	No contact with infectious material

*Plain or antimicrobial

Personal Protective Equipment   Ideally, all protective gear—surgical masks, eye and face shields, gloves, lab coats—should be changed between patients. Disposable protective gear such as gloves should be used for one patient only and discarded after use in a protected container similar to that used for disposable sharp instruments. Reusable gear such as plastic face shields should be cleaned with soap and water or disinfectant after every use; lab coats should be laundered.

Evaluating Patient Health

A number of health conditions such as diabetes, heart disease, HIV/AIDS, and chronic PERIODON-

TAL DISEASE may increase the risk of infection for a dental patient. In each case, the dentist may adopt special procedures such as prescribing antibiotics before treatment or suggesting a soft toothbrush to avoid irritating and/or inflaming the gums.

See SPECIAL-NEEDS PATIENTS.

infertility   See GENDER AND ORAL HEALTH.

inlay   An inlay is a RESTORATION that fills a cavity on the top of the TOOTH in the space between the cusps (top edges of the tooth). It is unlike a simple AMALGAM filling, for which the dentist drills into the tooth, cleans out the decay, and then inserts the soft amalgam to fill and harden in the cavity. The inlay is made of a hard material such as GOLD or tooth-colored porcelain shaped to fit a cast of the tooth that has a space left by DECAY or the loss of a previous restoration.

An onlay is a restoration similar in preparation and purpose to an inlay. The only difference is that where an inlay fills a cavity caused by decay in the space between the cusps, an onlay replaces one or more of the cusps themselves.

Procedure

To make and place an inlay, the dentist:

- cleans out the decay or removes the old restoration

- shapes and smooths the space left in the tooth

- makes a cast of the tooth and (commonly) the abutting teeth, perhaps with CAD/CAM (computer-aided design/computer-aided manufacturing) technology

- places a temporary filling into the cavity to protect the tooth until the inlay is ready

- sends the cast to a dental LABORATORY where a dental technician creates a restoration to fit tightly into the tooth

- places the inlay into the tooth and, if it fits tight and smooth, cements it in place (occasionally, the inlay will be returned to the laboratory for further trimming to ensure a secure fit)

Risks and Complications

There are no risks or complications associated with this procedure.

Outlook and Lifestyle Modifications

A well-made and well-fitted inlay requires no special care by the patient and may last as long as 30 years, all the while preventing further decay.

See also CROWN; IMPRESSION, DENTAL; ONLAY.

instruments   Dental instruments are tools used to prepare or adjust teeth during dental procedures. Dental instruments may be hand-powered tools such as a scaler (a metal rod with a sharpened tip used to remove CALCULUS) or they may be electrically powered tools such as the drill used to open a CAVITY. The following is a representative list of common dental tools.

- *Aspirator* A powered instrument that removes fluids and other material via vacuum suction; more commonly known as an ejector. For example, a saliva ejector is a tool with a replaceable tube tip used to remove liquid from the mouth so that the surface remains relatively dry during a dental procedure.

- *Broach* A broach is a smoothing tool, essentially a rasp (file). A barbed broach is a metal rod with barbs. It is used to clean out the pulp when preparing a tooth for ROOT CANAL TREATMENT. A smooth broach, also known as a pathfinder broach, has no barbs; it is used to find the opening of the root canal and the end of the root.

- *Bur* A bur is a powered cutting tool that accommodates different rotating heads (tips). Burs may be classified by their construction, the material from which they are made, or the jobs they do. A carbide bur is made of tungsten metal and carbon; it turns at very high speed to cut through metals. A crosscut bur has blades extending directly out from the shaft. An end cutting bur has blades only at the tip of the tool. An excavating bur is a tool used to clean out debris when preparing a cavity for filling. A finishing bur or a plug finishing bur has many blades placed very close together; it is used to shape and smooth metal or composite fillings and other restorations. An inverted cone bur has a head shaped like an upside-down cone, with the wider end at the top rather than the bottom. A round bur has a ball-shape tip. A straight fissure bur is topped with a smooth cylinder. A tapered fissure bur is topped with a head that comes to a blunt end.

- *Chisel* A dental chisel is a tool used to cut into hard tissue, such as bone. The tool is a metal post (shank) with a beveled (slanted) cutting edge on one side of the tip; the post fits into a powered handpiece. A contra-angle chisel is an instrument whose cutting edge meets the handpiece at an angle rather than straight up.

- *Curet, curette* A curet is a metal rod with a sharp blade at the tip used to scrape material off the tooth during periodontal treatment. Curets are made with tips designed to be used in specific areas; for example, the blade may be short

or long depending on whether the curet is to be used to remove calculus and debris from the visible tooth surface or the tooth surface under the gum.

- *Disk, disc* Also known as an abrasive disk; a flat circular ABRASIVE metal head attached to a powered handpiece. When the handpiece is turned on, the disk rotates. A separating disk is used to remove material, such as part of a tooth; a finishing disk is used to smooth and shape the surface of a tooth or a restoration. A diamond disk is an abrasive disk coated with diamond particles. A garnet disk is coated with garnet particles. A polishing disk is coated with very fine abrasive particles. A sandpaper disk is coated with sandpaper. A safe-side disk has abrasive on only one side.

- *Drill* A powered cutting instrument used to make a hole into the tooth.

- *Elevator* A dental instrument used to lift or reposition a tooth (dental elevator), a part of the cheek bone (malar elevator), or section of gum (periostal elevator).

- *Excavator spoon* A tongslike instrument with spoon-shape tips used to remove decayed material when preparing a cavity for a filling.

- *Explorer* A metal rod with a very thin tip used to examine and assess irregularities such as pits and cavities on the various surfaces of a tooth during a dental examination. In PERIODONTICS, the explorer is used to evaluate pockets (areas where the bone has receded and the gum is separated from the tooth). The shape of the explorer tip depends on the task for which it is intended. For example, a straight explorer has a short, sharp point used to examine cavities just under the edge of the gum, while an Orban No. 20 explorer has a longer angled tip suitable for finding irregularities on the surface of the tooth under the gum.

- *File* A metal tool used to smooth various dental surfaces. For example, a gold file is used to smooth gold restorations, while a root canal file is used to clean and shape the tooth canal after the nerve has been removed so as to provide a smooth surface to which the filling may adhere.

- *Hatchet* A small axe-shaped cutting instrument used to remove decay and create the shape of a cavity inside a tooth for filling.

- *Irrigator* A soft tube used to send liquid forcibly through an area in the mouth so as to wash away debris during a dental procedure.

- *Knife* Any one of several types of hand tools or powered surgical cutting tools. For example, an amalgam knife is a hand tool used to trim away excess AMALGAM and create smooth margins for a filling; a gold knife is used to trim gold metal restorations. An electronic knife is an electrically powered tool used to cut or shave away pieces of tissue, commonly gum tissue. Some knives are named for the person(s) who invented them. Examples of these dental tools include the Goldman-Fox knife, the Kirkland knife, and the Merryfield knife, three tools used to cut or shape gum tissue during periodontal surgery.

- *Mallet* A small hammer whose hard leather, rubber, or fiber head may be metal-covered; used to compact an amalgam filling or to push a restoration firmly into place.

- *Reamer* A metal rod with a slim, tapered, spiraled tip used to clean out and enlarge a root canal for filling after the nerve is removed.

- *Saw* A cutting tool with a serrated edge. In dentistry, a gold saw is a hand tool used to clean away excess metal around a gold restoration. Koeber's saw is a hand tool used to trim, contour, and finish a metal foil restoration. An oscillating saw and a *rotating saw* are electrically powered tools used to cut bone.

- *Scaler* An instrument used during periodontal treatment to removed calculus and debris from the teeth (SCALING).

- *Syringe* A glass, metal, or plastic cylinder with a plunger used to push a liquid such as an anesthetic through the skin or mucous membrane into the tissue underneath or to force air into an area of the mouth so as to clear away debris or dry the area.

See also ORTHODONTIC BRACES; ORTHODONTICS AND DENTOFACIAL ORTHOPEDICS.

Invisalign Created in 1997 by Stanford University graduate students Zia Chishti and Kelsey Wirth, Invisalign is a series of clear plastic aligners, trays similar to orthodontic retainers, that propose to move teeth into alignment without the use of metal ORTHODONTIC BRACES.

Like metal braces, the Invisalign treatment begins with the orthodontist's making impressions of the patient's teeth on which to build the Invisalign aligners for upper and bottom teeth, if required. A complete Invisalign treatment may require as many as 30 such aligners for each jaw; the aligners are worn at all times except when the patient is eating or drinking.

Cosmetically, the Invisalign system has an advantage over braces because it is nearly invisible on the teeth. However, a 2005 report in the *Journal of the American Dental Association* by two researchers from the University of Alberta, in Canada, concluded that the limited number of clinical studies at the time (two) made it impossible to evaluate the value of the aligners. With other manufacturers entering the market for orthodontic aligners, the authors suggested that more time and studies currently under way in the United States and Europe would eventually determine exactly which orthodontic patients and what degree of MALOCCLUSION would benefit from an aligner system.

irrigation In dentistry, the use of water or a water-based solution to cleanse debris from the oral cavity, specifically from a wound, a pocket between gum and teeth, or a root canal. Supragingival irrigation is an oral hygiene technique during which a person uses a powered device to send a pressured, pulsating stream of water into the mouth to wash away dental PLAQUE and debris on and between the teeth above the gum line. This technique is especially effective for patients with orthodontic appliances and restorations such as DENTURES, implants, and CROWNS that might otherwise impede normal brushing and flossing.

In 2008, University of Nebraska dental researchers conducted an 18-day trial with 105 volunteers in which one group used a manual TOOTHBRUSH and dental FLOSS, a second group used a manual toothbrush and the Waterpik Dental Water Jet—a dental irrigation device whose 1,200 pulsations per minute deliver a water stream measured at 55 to 90 pounds per square inch (abbreviation: *psi*)—and a third group used a sonic toothbrush and the Waterpik. The subjects were told to brush for two minutes, twice a day. Comparing data collected before the study began, two weeks into the study and two weeks after that, the researchers found that brushing plus irrigation removed debris more efficiently and eventually reduced bleeding from the gums more effectively than did a toothbrush and dental floss.

See PERIODONTAL DISEASE; ROOT CANAL TREATMENT.

jaw A set of two bones, the maxilla (upper jaw) and the mandible (lower jaw) that frame the oral cavity and hold the teeth.

Both the maxilla and the mandible are made of two types of bone: basal bone (the bone that forms the dental "skeleton") and alveolar bone (the bone that forms the socket around each tooth). Both the maxilla and the mandible are supplied with nerves and blood vessels that enter through openings in the bone called *foramina* (singular: *foramen*), from the Latin word *foro*, meaning "to pierce." The word *body* describes either the entire maxilla or the entire mandible, as in "the body of the maxilla" or "the body of the mandible."

The Maxilla

The maxilla begins as two separate bones, one on each side of the face, that fuse during fetal development to form the bony center of the face. Anatomically, the body of the maxilla is divided into four distinct processes (areas):

- *The zygomatic process:* From the Latin and Greek word *zygoma* meaning "to join." This is the part of the maxilla that abuts the cheekbone (zygomatic bone).

- *The frontal process:* This part of the maxilla arches up and back to form part of the side and bridge of the nose and the side of the orbit (the socket holding the eyeball), fusing to the frontal bone, the flat bone across the forehead.

- *The alveolar process:* This is the thickest part of the maxilla, a ridge created when the two maxilla fuse during fetal development to form the alveolar arch, the part of the maxilla that holds the upper teeth. Nerves and blood vessels enter the maxilla through an infraorbital foramen, an opening in the bone above the canine teeth. There are two infraorbital foramina (from the Latin word *infra*, meaning "beneath," and *orbita*, meaning "wheel," and the Greek word *foro*, meaning "to pierce"), one on each side of the maxilla under the orbit, the circular bone holding the eyeball.

- *The palatine process:* This area of the maxilla forms the bottom of the nose and the arched roof of the mouth, and joins the palatine bone to form the hard palate (the back of the mouth).

The Mandible

Like the maxilla, the mandible is made of two bones, in this case, hemimandibles, that form early in fetal development. Soon after birth, the hemimandibles fuse and lengthen to form the single curved bone of the lower jaw.

The structure of the mandible includes:

- *The alveolar process:* The ridge on the upper part of the mandible that holds the sockets for the lower teeth. Nerves and blood vessels exit through the mental foramina, one on each side of the mandible below the second molars.

- *The ramus:* From the Latin word meaning "branch." A triangular piece of bone rising up from either side at the back of the alveolar process. Nerves and blood vessels enter through the two lingular foramina, one on each ramus.

• *The condyle:* From the Greek *kondylos,* meaning "knuckle." A projection on top of each ramus that joins the mandible to the temporal bone (the flat bone on either side of the face) to create the temporomandibular joint (TMJ).

The mandible is the only bone in the face that moves via the temporomandibular joint, which enables the lower jaw to move up and down and side to side as a person chews his food. Chewing is an important part of the digestive process, during which the teeth grind food, breaking it into small, manageable pieces that can be easily swallowed. In addition, grinding the food breaks down indigestible fibers surrounding foods from plants (fruit, vegetables, whole grains) so that digestive enzymes can get to the nutrients inside.

The muscles that power the lower jaw and make chewing possible are:

• *The temporalis muscle:* This muscle, which runs from the lower part of the temporal bone (the flat bone at the side of the face) to the ramus, raises and lowers the mandible.

• *The masseter:* This muscle, which runs from the cheekbone to the ramus, raises the mandible.

• *The lateral pterygoid:* This muscle, which runs from an area of the upper jaw under the eye to the temporomandibular joint, moves the lower jaw forward.

• *The medial pterygoid:* This muscle, which runs from under the eye to the ramus at the angle of the lower jaw, lifts the lower jaw and moves it forward.

See also CHIN RECONSTRUCTION; CLEFT LIP AND/OR PALATE; GUIDED BONE REGENERATION; MALOCCLUSION; PERIODONTAL DISEASE.

jaw, fracture Broken JAW; a break in the mandible (lower jaw) due to a direct injury such as a blow or a fall.

Symptoms and Diagnostic Path

The most common symptoms of a fractured jaw are pain, swelling, bleeding inside the mouth and bruising outside, teeth knocked out or moved out of alignment, and difficulty in speaking due to the failure of the TONGUE and jaw to move normally. If the NERVE running through the lower jaw to the lower lip has been injured, the lip may be numb. If the jaw is fractured and cannot support the tongue, the patient may have trouble breathing, a situation requiring emergency treatment to maintain an open airway.

To assess the damage to the patient's jaw, the doctor will physically examine the jaw and look inside the patient's mouth for injury. Then he evaluates the patient's ability to move the lower jaw and may test the stability of the jaw by asking the patient to hold a plain wooden tongue depressor in place between his teeth; failure to do so indicates a fracture that makes it difficult for the patient to keep his teeth together. If warranted, he will order an X-ray or CT scan to confirm or rule out a fracture.

Treatment Options and Outlook

First aid for an injury such as a fractured jaw is an ice pack to reduce swelling and bruising on the way to the doctor or emergency room. If an X-ray or CT scan shows a fracture, an oral/maxillofacial surgeon may thread a WIRE into the lower jaw and attach it to the upper jaw to act as a kind of cast that keeps the jaw immobile as it heals. More serious fractures may require the use of a surgical plate (a flat piece of stainless steel or titanium) that is put in place across the fracture line with screws. Once in place, the plate may allow more movement than do wires, enable the patient to move the lower jaw normally so as to speak and eat. Once the jaw heals, the wire is removed; the plate may remain in place permanently.

Risk Factors and Preventive Measures

Most fractures of the jawbone result from accidents such as motor vehicle (automobile, motorcycle) crashes or sports injuries. Wearing protective helmets while participating in contact sports and driving more carefully or defensively may reduce the risk of this type of injury.

jawbone, loss of The most common cause of loss of bone in the JAW is PERIODONTAL DISEASE, which leads to repeated incidents of bacterial infection in pockets (loose spaces between tooth and gum) that eat away at the bone. However, as with other bones in the body, bone tissue in the jaw may also be weakened and lost due to osteoporosis, an age-related interruption in the natural process by which "old" bone is broken down and "new" bone built to replace it.

Symptoms and Diagnostic Path

The most common symptom of loss of jawbone is abnormal movement of the teeth. The diagnosis is confirmed with X-rays showing the precise area and amount of bone loss.

Treatment Options and Outlook

The common treatment options include GUIDED BONE REGENERATION accompanied by GUM RESHAPING.

Risk Factors and Preventive Measures

The primary illness-related cause of loss of jawbone is repeated infections associated with severe periodontal disease. A second illness-related cause of jawbone loss is severe MALOCCLUSION (failure of the teeth to meet properly), which reduces the natural impact of tooth-against-tooth that triggers normal bone growth. The use of removable dentures that are not anchored to the underlying bone may also lead to increased bone loss. On the other hand, replacing missing teeth with dental implants that act as artificial roots and stimulate the *alveolar bone* (the bone sockets in which teeth once sat) may prevent or reduce the risk of future bone loss.

Finally, osteoporosis may be considered a risk factor for bone loss in the jaw.

See also DENTURES; GUIDED BONE REGENERATION; IMPLANTOLOGY.

jaw restoration Oral plastic surgery to replace bone missing due to a birth defect or lost after an injury or surgery to remove a tumor.

Procedure

The procedures commonly used to replace missing jawbone are a bone graft, a bone-skin-artery graft, or an implant of a synthetic network to support new bone cells.

If the bone replacement procedure is done to strengthen the jaw for an implant, depending on the state of the patient's jawbone, the implant may be inserted right after the bone is put in place or the bone graft may be left in place for as long as nine months before enough new bone has grown to support a dental implant.

Bone graft The preferred replacement is an autograft, also known as an autogenous bone graft (a graft from the patient's own body). This graft, which is easily accepted by the patient's body, provides natural substances essential to the growth of new bone. An allograft (tissue harvested from another person, usually a cadaver) is not quite as good because it carries the risk of an immune reaction. In either case, bone most commonly used to rebuild the jaw is usually taken from the iliac crest (flat top) of the hip, from a rib, or from the clavicle (the flat shoulder bone).

Two other forms of bone used in bone grafts are bone paste, filler material prepared from powdered bone taken from either the patient or a donor, and a freeze-dried graft, bone preserved by dehydration and chilling.

Bone-skin-artery graft In some cases, the replacement of choice may be an osteocutaneous graft, a piece of tissue including skin and blood vessels along with bone, lifted from the patient's own body. The tissues most frequently taken for this type of graft are:

- *radius:* the bone in the forearm that runs from the elbow to the thumb
- *fibula:* the smaller of the two calf bones
- *scapula:* the flat bone that connects the humerus (upper arm bone) with the clavicle (collar bone)
- *iliac crest:* the flat top of the hip bone

The bone for grafting is removed from the original site in one surgery and inserted into the appropriate place in the jaw.

Synthetic scaffold   In this procedure, the dental surgeon implants a network or frame made of synthetic material to provide a scaffold on which the patient's own bone can grow. Once the new bone grows in, the synthetic material is absorbed by the body. The benefit of this technique is that the synthetic material is easily available; it does not provoke an immune reaction; and it has a low risk of infection.

Note: In 2006, researchers at the Regea Institute of Regenerative Medicine of the University of Tampere, in Finland, reported that they had replaced a 65-year-old patient's upper jaw, lost to cancer, with a bone transplant cultivated from stem cells taken from his own fatty tissue and grown inside his abdomen. The Finns isolated mesenchymal stem cells (stem cells than can mature into bone, muscle, or blood vessels) from the fat, grew the cells in a special nutrient broth that included the patient's own blood, and then attached the cells to a scaffold that was implanted in the patient's abdomen for nine months, during which time the cells produced a piece of bone and blood vessels. This material was then placed in the patient's skull and connected to the skull bone with tiny screws. The blood vessels were connected via microsurgery to arteries and veins in the patient's neck. As with all autogenous transplants, this one offers the virtue of tissue compatible with the patient's body.

Risks and Complications

Postsurgical pain and/or discomfort are common. As with any surgery, the most common serious complication is infection that may destroy tissue, causing the replacement to fail. A transplant of bone taken from a donor other than the patient himself carries the risk of tissue rejection.

See also BONE; GRAFT; GUIDED BONE REGENERATION; TEMPOROMANDIBULAR DISORDER.

Jones, Emeline Roberts (1835–1916)   Believed to be the first woman to maintain a dental practice in the United States, Jones was the wife of Connecticut dentist Daniel Albion Jones. She began her dental work by filling teeth her husband had extracted from his patients. Eventually, impressed by her skill, he allowed her to work as his assistant and then took her on as a partner in his practice. When Daniel Jones died in 1864, Emeline Jones moved to New Haven, Connecticut, to establish a practice of her own. In recognition of her success, she was appointed a member of the Women's Advisory Council of the World's Columbian Dental Congress in 1893, elected an honorary member of the Connecticut Dental Society in 1912, and awarded a complimentary membership in the nascent National Dental Association two years later.

Jordan, M. (Minnie) Evangeline (1865–1952)   The first American dentist to create a practice limited to the treatment of children. A graduate of the University of California School of Dentistry in 1898, Jordan began her practice as a general dentist but quickly turned to pediatric dentistry. She was selected to develop a lecture course, "The Care of Children's Teeth," at the University of Southern California in 1900, and in 1924 began publishing articles on pediatric dentistry, which, in 1927, formed the basis of the first American book on the subject. A colleague of Samuel Harris, the founder of the American Society of Dentistry for Children in 1927, Jordan was a founder and the first president of the Federation of American Woman Dentists in 1928 (later the Association of Women Dentists).

junction From the Latin word *jungere* meaning "to join." The specific junctions in the oral cavity include:

- The *cementoenamel junction.* The place where the crown of the tooth (the part of the tooth covered by enamel) meets the connective tissue (CEMENTUM) that covers the root of the tooth.
- The *dentiocemental junction.* This is the line showing where the cementum and DENTIN meet.
- The *dentinoenamel* (or *dentoenamel*) *junction.* This is the surface that serves as a common boundary between the ENAMEL and the dentin.
- The *dentogingival junction.* This is the place where the gum meets the tooth.
- The *mucogingival junction.* This is the line that separates the GINGIVA (the fibrous tissue surrounding the teeth) from the mucous membrane of the alveolar process.

Kells, C. Edmond (1856–1928) American dentist, graduate of the New York College of Dentistry, who is credited with a long list of dental innovations, including the use of compressed air to dry teeth during dental procedures, the suction pump used to remove saliva and other liquids from the mouth during dental surgery, and the introduction of an electric dental drill. Several sources credit him with being the first to take a dental X-ray on a live patient. In addition, Kells is believed to have been the first dentist to hire a female assistant, also the subject of his first dental X-rays. A prolific inventor, he registered more than 30 patents for things as varied as the fire extinguisher, the automobile jack, and components for brakes and starters on building elevators. Unfortunately, Kells's work with X-rays occurred before people knew about the danger of radiation exposure. As a result, he eventually developed cancer in his right hand, arm, and shoulder, leading to multiple amputations and then to his death by suicide at age 72.

Kennedy classification A system of four categories created by American dentist Edward Kennedy (1883–?) to describe the pattern of one or more missing teeth based on the position of the missing teeth in relation to the teeth that remain. The system is used as a basis for designing appropriate removable dentures to replace the missing teeth. The four Kennedy classes are:

Kennedy Class I A situation in which the patient is missing the back teeth on both sides of the upper or lower jaw. The replacement for the missing back teeth is called a bilateral distal extension. (*Distal* means "in back of".)

Kennedy Class II A situation in which the patient is missing back teeth on one side of the upper or lower jaw. The replacement for the missing back teeth is called a unilateral distal extension.

Kennedy Class III A situation in which the patient is missing teeth on one side of the upper or lower jaw but has natural teeth remaining in front and in back of the missing teeth. The replacement for the missing teeth is called tooth-borne because it rests on the remaining teeth.

Kennedy Class IV A situation in which the patient is missing teeth in the center front of the upper or lower jaw with natural teeth remaining in back of the gap on both sides of the mouth. The replacement for the missing teeth is called an anterior extension. (*Anterior* means "in front of.")

Kloehn headgear See APPLIANCE, DENTAL.

"knocked-out tooth" The common term for a tooth that is *avulsed* (or *evulsed*)—that is, accidentally torn from its socket. According to the American Association of Endontists (AAE), 80 percent of all knocked-out teeth are front teeth. Among adults, the most common cause of a knocked-out tooth is engaging in a contact sport such as boxing or football. For children, the most common cause for lost primary teeth is a fall, often while a toddler is learning to walk.

Symptoms and Diagnostic Path

The complete avulsion of a tooth following a facial injury is unmistakable. A tooth knocked to the side but not completely out of its socket is identified by its extreme mobility.

Treatment Options and Outlook

A knocked-out tooth is a dental emergency that requires first aid at the scene of the accident to preserve the tooth and immediate follow-up by a dental professional, commonly a dentist specializing in ENDODONTICS, to replant the tooth in the patient's JAW.

First Aid for a Knocked-Out Tooth The first steps after a tooth is knocked out of its socket are designed to preserve the viability of the tooth, which is living tissue, so as to maximize the chances of its being replanted successfully in the patient's jaw. To accomplish this, the AAE recommends the following:

- Find the tooth, which may have fallen to the ground.

- Do not attempt to clean the tooth; rubbing may damage living tissue on the root.

- Keep the tooth moist. If the patient is an adult whose tooth has been knocked loose from the jaw but not out of the mouth, she may be able to hold the tooth between the cheek and the gum while traveling to the emergency room or dentist's office. If the patient is unconscious or is a child, put the tooth in a container filled with milk. DO NOT PUT THE TOOTH IN A CONTAINER OF PLAIN WATER, WHICH CAN DAMAGE THE ROOT.

- Seek professional treatment as quickly as possible. The faster the dentist is consulted, the greater the chance that the tooth can be successfully replanted in the jaw.

Replanting the Tooth Like first aid at the scene, replanting a knocked-out tooth is a multistage process.

- If the patient is a child whose lost tooth is not completely developed, the wound will be treated but the tooth probably will not be replaced in its socket lest doing so interfere with the growth of the permanent teeth developing inside the JAWBONE.

- If the patient is an adult, the dentist or emergency room personnel will clean the tooth and replant it if possible.

- When necessary, the dentist may stabilize the replanted tooth by *splinting*, or securing the tooth to the adjoining teeth.

Once the emergency procedures are complete, the dentist will discuss further treatment. For example, adult permanent teeth, which are fully developed, usually require ROOT CANAL TREATMENT to clean out and refill the cavity inside the tooth once the injury has healed and the tooth is again firmly rooted in its socket. Older children, which AAE defines as those aged seven to 12, may have permanent teeth that are still developing. The PULP (soft material inside the tooth) may contain stem cells that encourage the growth of nerve tissue and blood vessels in the root as the injury heals.

In follow-up appointments, the dentist will evaluate the tooth and determine what treatment is required. In addition, the dentist will check to be certain that the roots of the knocked out tooth are not *resorbed*—that is, broken down by the natural processes of the body, thus once again destabilizing the tooth.

Risk Factors and Preventive Measures

Any situation that poses the risk of facial injury is a risk factor for a knocked-out tooth. Accidents are not always preventable, but the use of protective gear such as a MOUTH GUARD or helmet during contact sports or activities such as bicycle riding that often lead to falls can reduce the incidence of injury to the face and mouth.

Because a misaligned tooth is most vulnerable to this kind of injury, orthodontia to align the teeth properly may also reduce the risk of knocking out a tooth.

laboratory A dental laboratory is a facility staffed by dental technicians, professionals who fill prescriptions for dental devices (restorations and prostheses) such as DENTURES, bridges, CROWNS, caps, and VENEERS.

The first successful commercial dental laboratory in the United States opened in 1887 in Boston under the ownership of dentist William H. Stowe and his cousin, Frank F. Eddy, a toolmaker and machinist. As the use of effective restorations became more common, additional dental laboratories were established, staffed by personnel eventually called dental technicians. By the mid-20th century, the National Association of Dental Laboratories (NADL) was organized to promote the profession and standardize the education of dental technicians.

Certified Dental Laboratories

As of 2008, only a few of the states have enacted legislation specifically governing the operation of a dental laboratory. However, every state regulates dental health services, including those of commercial dental laboratories and their licensed staff. For example, the laboratories are required to have a dentist's prescription in order to make a dental appliance for a patient. Both state agencies and the federal Occupational Safety and Health Administration (OSHA) regulate the safety of the workplace.

Lacking specific legal standards, the National Association of Dental Laboratories has created its own rules and regulations for the designation Certified Dental Laboratory (CDL). The certification must be revalidated every five years.

All certified dental laboratories must:

- maintain good infection-control procedures, including regular personnel training in infection control
- maintain regular supervision of technical staff
- follow strict standards of quality and safety
- maintain a complete record of products used in the laboratory
- meet or exceed any applicable government regulations
- support a written policy to remake or reconstruct any defective restoration
- use a labeling system that shows the composition of every restoration/appliance made in that laboratory
- offer expertise in one or more specific areas of dental restorations

Further information regarding the certification of dental laboratories is available from NADL's Web site (www.nadl.org).

Certified Dental Technician

In 1954, NADL created the first certification program for dental technicians. The first Certified Dental Technician (CDT) tests were given in October 1958; the first CDT certificates were awarded in March 1959. To achieve certification after study at one of the more than 30 programs in the United States accredited by the Commission on Dental Accreditation, a candidate must pass three examinations within a four-year period: a written comprehensive examination of dental technology, a specialty practical examination, and a specialty written examination in one or more of the five specialties:

- complete dentures
- partial dentures
- crown and bridge
- ceramics
- orthodontics

By 2004, more than 6,000 technicians held active CDT certificates, which, to remain active, must be renewed annually.

Further information regarding the requirements for certification as a dental technician is available from the National Board for Certification in Dental Technology (www.nbccert.org).

A list of accredited programs in dental laboratory technology is available from the Commission on Dental Accreditation at the ADA (www.ada.org).

laser The word *laser* is an acronym for *l*ight *a*mplification by *s*timulated *e*mission of *r*adiation. Lasers work by emitting a powerful beam of light that produces intense heat. This heat can be used as a surgical instrument, cutting with heat as a scalpel cuts with steel. In 1997, the Food and Drug Administration approved the used of the erbium YAG laser (see below) to treat tooth decay. Today, dentists use lasers not only to clean out decay but also to prepare cavities for filling, to cut hard tissue such as teeth and bone to correct defects, and to disinfect periodontal pockets by killing bacteria that are the prime culprits in PERIODONTAL DISEASE.

Inventing the Laser

The first person to use the term *laser* was Gordon Gould, who built the first optical laser while a student at Columbia University in 1958. The first commercial laser was made in 1960 by Theodore A. T. Maiman, an engineer at Hughes Research. The first gas laser (helium and neon) was created at the Massachusetts Institute of Technology by physicist Ali Javan in 1960. Q-switching lasers were invented by physicists R. W. Hellwarth and F. J. McClung in 1962; the first carbon dioxide laser was built at the Massachusetts Institute of Technology in 1964 by physicist C. Kumar N. Patel.

How Lasers Work

There are two basic types of lasers: solid state lasers and gas lasers. Solid state lasers draw their energy from solid materials, commonly gemstones or silver-colored metallic minerals known as "rare earth elements." The latter commonly occur in nature together with nonmetallic elements in compounds such as phosphates (rare earth elements plus phosphorus), carbonates (carbon), fluorides (fluorine), and silicates (silica). Gas lasers are powered by gases.

Regardless of the source, lasers generate energy by using light or electrical current to "excite" the molecules in the mineral or gas inside a chamber. When the chamber opens, the energy escapes as a beam of high-intensity light.

- A continuous wave laser releases energy as a steady beam of light.
- A pulsed laser releases energy as a very short single burst on the order of a nanosecond (1 billionth of a second).
- A Q-switched laser releases energy in short (1 billionth of a second) bursts of intense light that can heat tissue to a temperature over 300°F. Although the energy released by Q-switched lasers is potentially hazardous to the eyes and skin, Q-switched lasers designed to operate with light that is eye-safe are used in dentistry to cut surfaces and to remove an amalgam tattoo, a stain on the gum caused by the silver in an AMALGAM filling.

Lasers Used in Dentistry

The lasers commonly used in dentistry are, in alphabetical order, the solid state argon gas laser, the CO_2 (carbon dioxide) laser, the diode laser, the Er:YAG laser and the Nd:YAG laser.

- Argon lasers are power by argon (Ar), one of the so-called noble gases, a group of elements that includes helium (He), neon (Ne), krypton (Kr), xenon (Xe), radon (Rn), and ununoctium (Uuo). Their group name reflects the fact that these elements are considered chemically unreactive.
- The CO_2 (carbon dioxide) laser is a high-power continuous wave laser.
- The diode laser is a small (less than 1 mm across), lightweight (less than a gram) device that emits low-intensity energy in the visible light or infrared spectrum when powered by a small amount of electricity (three to 12 volts). The diode laser does not damage soft tissue such as that inside the mouth.
- The Er:YAG laser draws energy from a crystal containing the elements yttrium and aluminum plus the semiprecious stone garnet, and erbium (Er), a gray-silver metal identified by the Swedish scientist Carl Mosander in 1843.
- The Nd:YAG laser (also known as the Q-switched laser) draws its energy from the same combination of yttrium, aluminum, and garnet plus the element neodymium (Nd).

See also CURING LIGHT.

leukoplakia A thick white benign patch that forms on the inside of the cheeks, on the gum, or on the TONGUE in response to irritations including (but not limited to) a badly fitting denture, or an unconscious habit of chewing on the inside of the cheek, or TOBACCO smoke.

Symptoms and Diagnostic Path
The white patch is clearly visible when the dentist examines the patient's mouth. Approximately three to four people in every 100 develop leukoplakia at some time. The overwhelming majority of these lesions are benign, but up to

20 percent become malignant. To confirm the diagnosis and rule out malignancy, the dentist may order a biopsy of a suspicious area such as one that is noticeably red and irritated.

Treatment Options and Outlook
Treatment for simple leukoplakia is to remove the source of the original irritation; for example, to repair or replace ill-fitting dentures.

Risk Factors and Preventive Measures
The primary risk factor for simple leukoplakia is irritation. Prevention dictates removing the source of the irritation. In cases of stress-related unconscious chewing on the inside of the cheek, the recommendation is a variety of methods to reduce stress.

lichen planus From the words *lichen*, a plant found on rocks and trees, and the Latin *planus*, meaning "flat." Lichen planus is a chronic inflammatory condition of the skin and mouth ("oral lichen planus"), with periods of active disease followed by periods of remission.

Symptoms and Diagnostic Path
Oral lichen planus causes one or more areas of fine white lines or dots, most commonly on the inside of the cheeks and tongue, less commonly on the gums and inside of the lips. The patches are usually painless, but in severe cases, the condition may cause painful sores or reddened or yellowish ulcers (deep sores).

Symptom-free, mild oral lichen planus is commonly identified during a routine dental checkup, after which the dentist may order blood tests and/or a biopsy of the tissue to rule out other conditions such as a bacterial infection, yeast infection (THRUSH), viral infection (canker sore, HERPES), or ORAL CANCER.

Treatment Options and Outlook
There is no cure for oral lichen planus. Mild cases may require no treatment. Cases in which the patient experiences pain or sores are treated with a variety of topical anesthetics to relieve

discomfort and systemic medication to speed healing.

To reduce irritation and discomfort, the patient with active lichen planus may be advised to avoid spicy foods, acidic foods such as citrus fruits, tomatoes, coffee, and soft drinks, and hard-edged foods such as chips and toast. Patients with lichen planus are at slightly increased risk of oral cancer. As a result, dentists (or dermatologists) treating oral lichen planus may recommend the patient return once or twice a year for a cancer screening.

Risk Factors and Preventive Measures

The cause of lichen planus is unknown and there are no known risk factors. The condition occurs most frequently in middle-aged adults, twice as commonly in women as in men. Some researchers believe that it may be an autoimmune disease, a condition in which the body attacks its own tissues (see IMMUNE SYSTEM), but that remains to be proven.

lip, cancer of   Malignant tumor of the lip, most commonly starting in the thin, flat squamous cells that line the lips and mouth.

Symptoms and Diagnostic Path

The common signs of cancer of the lip are:

- a sore that does not heal
- a lump that does not disappear
- an area that bleeds spontaneously or feels numb

The cancer may be identified during a routine dental visit. To confirm the diagnosis, the dentist (or dermatologist) will take a small piece of the affected area for a biopsy.

Treatment Options and Outlook

The treatment for cancer of the lip is surgical removal of the tumor along with some healthy tissue just beyond the margins (edges) of the tumor. If the cancer has spread from the lip to the underlying BONE or to lymph nodes in the neck, the surgeon will remove them as well. After surgery, some patients may be given RADIATION THERAPY to kill malignant cells that may remain hidden near the site of the original cancer.

Following the initial surgery, the patient may require plastic surgery to restore the appearance and function of the lip. The surgeon may choose to do this either with a skin FLAP or a skin GRAFT.

A skin flap is a piece of skin or mucous membrane, such as the lining of the mouth, with or without the underlying tissue (fat, blood vessels, muscle, bone), partially or completely lifted from one place on a patient's body (the donor site) and turned toward or transferred to another (the recipient site) to replace skin that has been damaged or entirely destroyed. Some common flaps used to repair the lip are:

- *lip-lip flap*: This flap is tissue from one lip (or from one side of the lip) used to repair the other lip (or other side of the same lip)

- *mustache flap*: This flap is hair-bearing skin lifted from the lower back part of the scalp and used to reconstruct the male upper lip

- *nasolabial flap*: This flap is lifted from the side of the nose, used to repair the area above the lip

- *over-and-out cheek flap*: This flap is lifted from the cheek and reversed, with the membrane side out and the skin side in, to repair the lip

A skin graft is a piece of healthy skin lifted from one site on the body and moved to another area of the body. Unlike a skin flap, a skin graft does not have its own blood supply; after the skin is transferred the blood vessels in the grafted skin are joined to those in the recipient site so that the graft is vascularized (attached to local blood vessels). A graft is said to *take* (fix in place) when new blood vessels and scar tissue form in the injured area. All grafting, including grafts taken from the patient's own body, cause scarring at both the donor and recipient sites.

Risk Factors and Preventive Measures

The known risk factors for lip cancer include tobacco use (smoking and chewing tobacco) as well as excess exposure to ultraviolet light (as in sunlight). The recent decline in the incidence of cancer of the lip is generally credited to the growing awareness of the danger of ultraviolet light and an increased used of protective clothing such as wide-brimmed hats that shade the face, and sunscreens, including colorless lip protectants and cosmetic lipsticks with a sun protective ingredient.

Patients who develop lip cancer may be at increased risk of a second tumor of the head or neck. Clinical trials in the United States and overseas are investigating the possibility that vitamin A derivatives called retinoids may be useful in reducing this risk. Information about ongoing clinical trials is available on the Web site of the National Cancer Institute (www.cancer.gov).

lips The lips are folds of tissue that protect the oral cavity.

The outer surface of the lips is covered with keratinized epithelial tissue (skin hardened with proteins). The outer contours of the lips are defined by the vermillion border, a ridge of collagen (connective tissue) at the point where the skin covering the lip meets the facial skin; the entire outer pink surface of the lip is known as the vermillion zone. The shiny tissue on the inside of the lips is the same mucous membrane that line the rest of the mouth.

The lip is attached to the center of the upper JAW by a small membrane tag called the upper labial frenum and to the center of the bottom jaw by a similar tag called the lower labial frenum. Both the outside and the inside of the lip are plentifully supplied with small blood vessels that give lips their naturally reddish color and cause them to bleed freely when injured. In addition, the blood vessels in the lips dilate and constrict in response to heat and cold, as well as emotional signals. For example, when a person is exposed to very hot weather or an emotional signal such as sexual arousal, the blood vessels in the lips dilate and the lips redden, while when exposed to very cold temperatures or an emotional signal such as fear, the blood vessels constrict and the lips become pale.

The upper lip's distinguishing feature is the *Cupid's bow,* two peaks at the center of the lip created by the philtrum, a vertical groove created by two ridges of collagen, one coming down from the inner edge of each nostril to the top of the lip. The lower border of the bottom lip is usually smoothly defined, with no natural indentations.

What the Lips Do

In a healthy mouth, the lips perform both physical and sensory tasks. They:

- keep the mouth closed to hold food and liquids in while a person eats and drinks
- help to hold the teeth and tongue in position
- transmit temperature signals from food
- facilitate speech by moving into shapes that form the specific sounds that build words

The lips are also a communicative tool that enables a person to display emotions. For example:

- a person may show anger by tightly pressing his lips together
- drawing the lips back so tight that one's teeth are visible suggests anger that has escalated to rage
- a fearful person may suck in his cheeks, showing the teeth on the side of the mouth but not in the front
- simply pursing one's lips indicates disgust
- conversely, the absence of expression—a "blank face" with the eyes open, the lips closed, and the facial muscles relaxed—suggests calmness or simply an intention not to interact with others

TABLE 1. MUSCLES CONTROLLING THE LIPS

Muscle	Site	Function
Buccinator	At the back corner of the jaws	Pulls lips inward
Caninus (levator anguli oris)	Upper jaw near canine teeth to lip	Pulls lip up and to side
Depressor labii inferioris	Chin to lower lip	Pulls lip down and to side
Mentalis	Front of lower jaw	Pushes chin up and curves lips in a "U"
Orbicularis oris	Circle around the mouth	Controls size and shape of the opening of the mouth
Risorius	Near the corner of the mouth	Pulls mouth to sides in smiles
Zygomatic major	From the cheekbone to the corner of the mouth	Lifts corner of the mouth
Zygomatic minor	From cheekbone to place between corner and center of top lip	Pulls up upper lip

The Muscles that Control the Lips

Table 1 lists the specific muscles that control the lips. If these muscles or other facial muscles or the nerves that power them are damaged, the patient may lose the ability to eat or speak properly as well as the ability to form facial expressions, a major bar to normal communication. Such damage may occur due to a developmental or neurological disorder, a disease (such as a tumor), an infection, an injury (including injury during surgery), or an adverse reaction to a medicine. Surgery to restore functioning of one or more of the facial muscles is known as facial reanimation.

See also CLEFT LIP AND/OR PALATE; JAW; MUSCLE; ORAL CANCER; TONGUE; TOOTH.

lymphatic system   The lymphatic system, a major component of the immune system, includes a group of organs and a circulatory system. The lymph organs—the tonsils, the adenoids, the spleen, and the thymus—"catch" and filter pathogens such as bacteria and viruses. The lymph circulatory system consists of lymph vessels (similar to blood vessels) and lymph nodes.

Lymph vessels carry clear-to-white fluid called lymph around the body. Lymph is composed of chyle (fluid released by the intestines after digesting food); red blood cells; and lymphocytes, specialized white blood cells that circulate through lymph vessels then leave the lymphatic system to travel through the bloodstream. As they travel, the lymphocytes identify and attack foreign bodies such as bacteria, fungi, viruses, and cancer cells and sweep up and eliminate debris such as worn-out red blood cells in the spleen. The most important lymphocytes are B cells, T cells, and helper T cells. B cells, which are made in the bone marrow, latch onto and "swallow" antigens (substances that trigger an immune response). T cells and helper T cells,* then hook onto the antigen/B cell fragment to release antibodies (substances that attack the antigens). T cells can also destroy diseased cells such as cancer cells.

Lymph nodes are bean-shaped nodules packed together in the neck, armpit, and groin. The nodes are filters that catch foreign matter such as microorganisms and cancer cells while producing extra white blood cells to fight infection.

See also IMMUNE SYSTEM.

---

*which are made in the thymus (a gland located behind the breastbone).

macrodontia/microdontia From the Greek words *macros,* meaning "long," and *donto,* meaning "tooth." Macrodontia is a rare dental disorder characterized by larger-than-normal teeth. The opposite of macrodontia is microdontia (from the Greek word *micro* meaning small), smaller-than-normal teeth. The medical term for a person with abnormally large teeth is macrodont; a person with abnormally small teeth is known as a microdont.

Macrodontia may occur as a result of *pituitary gigantism,* a condition in which the pituitary gland excretes abnormally large amounts of growth hormone producing an abnormally large body and larger teeth sized to fit into the larger JAWS. Macrodontia may also be one characteristic of a GENETIC disorder such as KBG syndrome, which causes malformations of the head and face, or Klinefelter's syndrome, a condition in which males have extra copies of the X or both the X and Y chromosomes.

Microdontia is most common among persons with dwarfism, whose smaller teeth are sized to fit into a smaller jaw. Alternatively, the smaller teeth may occur in normal-size jaws, or only one tooth may be involved, most commonly either the third molar or the lateral (side) incisor in the upper jaw.

Symptoms and Diagnostic Path
Macrodontia and microdontia are clearly visible upon physical examination of the mouth. The usual pattern is a full set of teeth larger or smaller than normal. Regional macrodontia (a group of larger-than-normal teeth) may be linked to a rare congenital condition called hemifacial hyperplasia, in which one side of the face is larger than the other. A macrodont may have one large tooth, most commonly a molar in the lower jaw, while a microdont may have one small tooth, either a molar or an incisor in the upper jaw. Diagnosis of an underlying inherited disorder is confirmed by genetic testing.

Treatment Options and Outlook
People whose teeth are larger or smaller than normal but proportionate to the size of their jaws do not require treatment. People with one or more larger- or smaller-than-normal teeth that do not meet correctly may find it difficult to chew food efficiently. The aim of treatment for these patients is to make it possible for the patient to eat without difficulty, often by extracting one or more teeth and replacing them either with an implant or a fixed denture. Patients with regional microdontia may be fitted with a removable denture that slides on over the teeth much like a MOUTH GUARD.

Risk Factors and Preventive Measures
Abnormalities in tooth size and shape arise from an error in fetal tooth development. A family history of such problems increases the risk of macro- or microdontia, but there is no known preventive measure.

See also DENTURE; IMPLANTOLOGY.

magnetic resonance imaging (MRI) This non-invasive diagnostic technique employs magnets and radio waves rather than RADIATION to create detailed images of soft tissue structures. For example, in dentistry, the MRI can give a clearer picture of structures such as the salivary glands than can other imaging techniques such as X-ray.

The MRI creates an image by stimulating the hydrogen atoms in the water molecules that make up nearly two-thirds of the human body, and then using strong magnets and pulses of radio waves to encourage the excited protons to release a burst of energy. A computer in the machine translates the bursts of energy into a picture that shows different kinds of tissue, enabling the radiologist to identify changes due to a disease. For example, the signals given off by protons in hydrogen cells in a tumor are more pronounced than those produced by protons in healthy tissue.

Procedure

The standard MRI is a tube-shaped machine with strong magnets in the walls and a table that slides in and out of the tube (an open MRI is an incomplete tube that is more comfortable for people who feel confined by the standard machine).

Once the patient takes his place on the table, the technician leaves the room, sends the table into the tube, and begins to collect images from the MRI scanner. During the scan, the patient must remain still for several seconds while the MRI creates its images, but he can relax between picture-taking sequences.

The entire scan may run for 15 to 45 minutes, depending on how many images are required and the size of the patient (it takes longer to capture images from a large body than from a small one). Occasionally, a patient may be asked to return to the scanner for additional pictures.

Risks and Complications

For some procedures, the radiologist may inject contrast material (dye) to highlight some tissues such as blood vessels. The contrast material used during an MRI scan is less likely to produce an allergic reaction than the dye used during X-rays and CT scans.

The strong magnetic field used for MRIs will attract substances such as iron, nickel, cobalt, and various mixtures of these materials. Dental fillings or braces are not magnetic; neither are dentures, glasses, hairpins, hearing aids, or most jewelry, but any of these may distort the MRI image and should be removed, if possible.

Some magnetic devices are safe in older, less powerful MRIs but not in the newest models. Therefore, to prevent injury during the scan, the patient must remove any clothing with metallic accessories, such as zippers and snaps, and inform the radiologist or technician about any implanted devices including (but not limited to):

- an artificial joint or heart valve
- pacemaker
- intrauterine device (IUD)
- implanted port or catheter (tubes to allow continuous administration of medicines)
- metal plates, pins, screws, or surgical staples
- shrapnel fragments or bullets
- tattoos (including permanent eyeliner) created with ink that may contain metallic dust

Outlook and Lifestyle Modifications

MRI is a useful diagnostic tool, used in dentistry to diagnose tumors such as cancer of the salivary glands. However, occasionally, it may not distinguish between tissue and edema (fluid collected in an area).

See also SALIVARY GLANDS, CANCER OF.

malocclusion Misalignment of the teeth so that the upper teeth do not sit slightly in front of the bottom teeth and the points of the upper molars (large back teeth) do not fit neatly into the grooves of the lower molars. There are three broad classes of malocclusion: Class 1 malocclusion, Class 2 malocclusion, and Class 3 malocclusion. EDWARD HARTLEY ANGLE first described these in 1899. The Angle categories of malocclusion are:

- *Class 1 malocclusion*: The teeth in the top jaw line up with teeth in the bottom jaw, but the teeth on top, on bottom, or in both places are turned or crooked, as though there are too many teeth for the space. Another name for this form of malocclusion is *crowded teeth*.

- *Class 2 malocclusion*: The teeth in the upper jaw protrude markedly past the bottom teeth. Other names for this form of malocclusion are overbite, over jet, and buck teeth. The terms *closed teeth* and *deep bite* describe an overbite in which the upper teeth cover the lower teeth when the patient bites down.

- *Class 3 malocclusion*: The teeth in the lower jaw sit in front of the teeth in the upper jaw. Other names for this form of malocclusion are *prognathism, intercession,* and *underbite.*

Other terms used to describe malocclusions are buccoversion (a tooth or teeth in one or both jaws closer than normal to the cheek), labioversion (one or more teeth closer than normal toward the lips), and *retroversion* (one or more teeth farther back than normal). The term crossbite describes a malocclusion in which some upper teeth are behind the lower teeth when the patient bites down.

One interesting but temporary form of malocclusion is the ugly duckling stage, the moment in an individual's dental development—usually between the ages of seven and 12—when the front teeth (incisors) on the upper jaw may temporarily slant away from each other to the side because the canine teeth have not fully erupted through the gum. The sideways slanting of the incisors may produce a gap between the two center teeth, a phenomenon first described in the mid-1940s by American orthodontic researcher B. HOLLY BROADBENT. As with many advances in physical development, the ugly duckling stage appears earlier in girls than in boys. In both girls and boys, the spacing of the upper teeth is often accompanied by crowding of the teeth in the lower jaw.

Symptoms and Diagnostic Path

The most obvious sign of malocclusion is an abnormal facial appearance due to protruding upper or lower teeth. Other signs of malocclusion include:

- difficulty in biting or chewing food
- a lisp or other speech problem caused by an inability to position the tongue correctly behind the teeth
- soreness due to the misaligned teeth hitting the inside of the cheek or the patient's accidentally biting the tissue
- Temporomandibular disorder, a muscle strain due to an attempt to force misaligned jaws into an effective position; occasionally, the continually tight muscles and clenched teeth may exert enough pressure to fracture a tooth

Malocclusion is commonly diagnosed during a dental examination and confirmed via dental X-rays.

Treatment Options and Outlook

Simple misalignment of the teeth is treated with orthodontics, most commonly with appliances inside the mouth that move the teeth into position. Occasionally, the orthodontic treatment may include removing a tooth to alleviate crowding and enable the other teeth to straighten. Orthodontic treatment is usually prescribed early in life primarily because bones are softer in childhood and adolescence so that the teeth can be adjusted more easily than in an adult jaw.

Other causes of malocclusion such as a birth defect (CLEFT LIP AND/OR PALATE), a badly healed fracture, an oral tumor, or an abnormally long or short jaw or unusually shaped jawbone may require corrective surgery.

Correcting any malocclusion has distinct benefits. Because the teeth are straight and therefore easier to clean, the risk of decay and periodontal disease goes down. Because the patient does not have to strain to make the teeth meet, the muscles relax and there is a lower risk of both TMD and a fractured tooth.

These treatment options apply only to natural teeth in natural bone. Mismade or badly fitting dentures or other restorations can also cause malocclusion that is treated simply by repairing the restorations.

Risk Factors and Preventive Measures

The common risk factors for malocclusion are hereditary traits (size and shape of the jaw and teeth), birth defects (extra teeth, fused teeth, missing teeth, cleft lip and/or palate), traumatic injury (a fracture of the jaw that does not heal properly), illness (tumor of the jaw), and behavior (THUMB SUCKING). Of these, only thumb sucking may be preventable.

See DENTURE; EXTRACTION; ORAL CANCER; ORTHODONTICS AND DENTOFACIAL ORTHOPEDICS; ORTHODONTIC BRACES; TEMPOROMANDIBULAR DISORDER.

mandible See JAW.

margin An edge. In dentistry, the free gingival margin is the edge of the gum beside the slight indentation in the tooth as it goes down to the root; the gingival margin is a term used to describe either the inner wall of a cavity nearest to the tooth root or the tip of the gum tissue.

The enamel margin, the place where the border of a restoration such as a filling meets the enamel surface of the tooth, is a potentially problematic area. Any imperfection in sealing the margin when the filling is inserted raises the risk of bacteria entering to cause a secondary decay requiring removal and replacement of the original filling. Even a perfectly sealed filling can be risky. To catch any problem early, the dentist will pay special attention to this part of the tooth during routine examinations; any change in

sensation at the site may signal new decay and should be reported quickly.

mastication See CHEWING.

maxilla See JAW.

McKay, Frederick S. (1874–1959) American dentist; attended Boston Dental College, the predecessor to the Dental School of Tufts University, and graduated from the University of Pennsylvania in 1900. In 1901, while spending time at his sister's home in Colorado Springs, McKay noticed a widespread incidence of dental staining and pitting accompanied by a paradoxical low incidence of CAVITIES, which came to be known as the "Colorado Brown Stain." Four years later, while practicing orthodontics in Saint Louis, McKay found the same phenomenon among his patients.

In 1908, having returned to Colorado Springs, McKay and a number of associates brought a patient to a Colorado Dental Association meeting to demonstrate the staining and pitting, but their presentation drew little interest among their peers. The following year, having set up a program to provide dental care for children, McKay identified the same staining and pitting in nearly 90 percent of the children, particularly among those living in the area around Pike's Peak. Other dentists offered many theories to explain the phenomenon—poverty, too much pork in the diet, spoiled milk, a calcium deficiency—but by 1917, working with several grants from various dental organizations, McKay tentatively linked the brown staining to large quantities of natural fluorides leeching out of the ground into the water supply in various western states.

In 1931, after more than 25 years of studying "brown stain," McKay was finally able to prove his theory, a discovery that led not only to the prevention of "brown stain" but also to the introduction of artificial fluoridation of the drinking water in the United States so as to reduce the incidence of dental DECAY among Americans.

See FLUORIDE.

membrane Thin tissue covering a body surface or the surface of an organ such as the inside of the lips and mouth.

There are three basic types of membranes covering body/organ surfaces: mucous membranes, fibrous membranes, and serous membranes.

Mucous membranes, the most prominent from a dental point of view, are a thin layer of pinkish-red mucosa tissue that covers the inside of the mouth, including the gums, TONGUE, and palate, and lines the inside of other body cavities opening to the air (nose, throat, vagina, penis, urethra, and rectum). Some, but not all, mucous membrane contains specialized glands that secrete mucus, a clear sticky fluid that keeps the membrane moist even when exposed to air.

In the mouth, some mucous membranes, or mucosa, are named for the places where they are located. For example, the buccal mucosa covers the inside of the cheeks; the labial mucosa covers the inside of the lips; the oropharyngeal mucosa covers the area where the back of the mouth enters the throat; the palatine mucosa covers the palate; and the periodontal mucosa is the membrane that covers the gums. Mucositis is an inflammation of the mucosa. A mucostatic agent is one that interferes with the mucosa's natural secretion of mucus.

Fibrous membranes are strong, protective membranes made of connective tissue. Examples of fibrous membranes include the periosteum (the membrane covering a bone such as the jawbone) and the dura mater (the membrane lining the inside of the skull).

Serous membranes such as the peritoneum (the membrane lining the abdominal cavity) release a watery fluid to moisten the membrane and keep it from sticking to other tissues, including organs.

In addition to the large membranes lining body cavities and/or enveloping organs and structures, each cell in the body is covered with a semipermeable membrane, a specialized tissue that allows some molecules, such as medical drugs, to be specifically designed to fit into and slip through the openings in membranes surrounding the cell in the body part for which the medicine is meant.

See also ENDODONTICS; PERIODONTICS.

menstrual gingivitis An inflammation of the GINGIVA (gums) and bleeding at the gum line (the place where the top of the gum meets a TOOTH) associated with normal hormonal fluctuations during the menstrual cycle, specifically increased levels of the female hormone progesterone. A similar condition occurs during pregnancy.

In the middle of the menstrual cycle, approximately 14 days after the start of menstrual bleeding, when ovulation (the release of an egg from the ovaries) occurs, progesterone secretion increases to prepare the uterus for the implantation of a fertilized egg. Higher progesterone levels increase the flow of blood to body tissue, including the gums, which may redden, swell, and bleed slightly.

If implantation does not occur, the levels of progesterone fall naturally, and menstrual bleeding occurs several days later as the uterus sheds the layer of tissue it had produced to support the fetus. This natural change in hormone levels resolves the inflammation of the gingiva until the cycle begins again.

Symptoms and Diagnostic Path
Redness and swelling of the gums, along with bleeding at the gum line, in the second half of the menstrual cycle; these symptoms usually resolve once menstrual bleeding starts and the hormonal balance shifts.

Treatment Options and Outlook

NSAIDs (nonsteroidal anti-inflammatory drugs) such as aspirin and ibuprofen (Advil) may reduce redness and swelling. Switching to a softer toothbrush and exercising care not to injure the gum while flossing helps avoid further irritations. If inflammation, pain, and/or bleeding at the gum line persist after menstrual bleeding, dental treatment may be required to avoid a progression to infection characteristic of PERIODONTAL DISEASE.

Risk Factors and Preventive Measures

The primary risk factor for menstrual gingivitis is being a woman of childbearing age. The best prevention is to practice good oral hygiene; that is, brushing and flossing after eating to keep the mouth as clean as possible.

See PREGNANCY AND DENTAL HEALTH; PREGNANCY GINGIVITIS.

mercury and mercury poisoning   See AMALGAM.

meth mouth   Term used to describe the dental problems caused by using the illegal drug methamphetamine.

Symptoms and Diagnostic Path

The dental consequences of regular methamphetamine use include stained teeth and extensive tooth DECAY due to both the acidic environment created by the drug and a drug-related craving for sugary foods. Methamphetamine use dries the tissues in the mouth ("dry mouth") and may promote jaw clenching and tooth-grinding, leading to TEMPOROMANDIBULAR DISORDER (TMD) and cracked or fractured teeth.

Methamphetamine use is also associated with gastric upset, cardiovascular problems (irregular heartbeat, hypertension), neurological disorders (brain damage, hallucinations, convulsions), and psychological symptoms (irritability, aggression, paranoia). In addition, according to the 2003 National Survey on Drug Use and Health from the Substance Abuse and Mental Health Services Administration, a division of the U.S. Department of Health and Human Services, more than 12 million Americans older than 12 may fail to follow an adequate diet and become malnourished due to methamphetamine use.

Treatment Options and Outlook

The dental treatment for meth mouth includes standard procedures such as filling CAVITIES, repairing teeth where possible, removing teeth too damaged to save, and alleviating dry mouth. If the drug use continues, the damage to the teeth will as well.

Risk Factors and Preventive Measures

The only risk factor for meth mouth is methamphetamine use.

To strengthen the teeth and reduce the incidence of decay, the dentist may apply fluorides or prescribe the use of fluoridated dental products (toothpaste, MOUTHWASH). She may also advise the patient to practice ORAL HYGIENE and avoid sugary foods and beverages. If the patient is willing, the dentist may refer him/her to a substance abuse professional or facility.

See also FLUORIDE; TOOTHBRUSH.

metric system   System of measurement used worldwide for all scientific measurements, including dental measurements such as the size of a tooth or the depth of a pocket caused by PERIODONTAL DISEASE. The defining characteristic of the metric system is the fact that all its units are related by factors of 10, so that converting from one measure to another within the metric system is simply a matter of multiplying or dividing by 10 (or a multiple of 10 such as 100 or 1,000).

In the metric system, the meter (m) is the basic metric unit of length; the kilogram (kg)

COMMONLY USED METRIC PREFIXES

Decreasing Amounts	Increasing Amounts
Deci (tenth) 1 decimeter is 1/10th of a meter	Deka (ten) 1 dekameter is 10 meters
Centi (hundredth) 1 centimeter is 1/100th of a meter	Hecto (hundred) 1 hectometer is 100 meters
Milli (thousandth) 1 millimeter is 1/1,000th of a meter	Kilo (thousand) 1 kilometer is 1,000 meters
Micro (millionth) 1 micrometer is 1/1,000,000th of a meter	Mega (million) 1 megameter is 1,000,000 meters
Nano (billionth) 1 nanometer is 1/1,000,000,000th of a meter	Giga (billion) 1 gigameter is 1,000,000,000 meters

CONVERTING FROM METRIC TO ENGLISH UNITS*

Length	Multiply by
Centimeters to inches	0.39
Meters to feet	0.32
Kilometers to miles	0.62
Weight	
Grams to ounces (dry)	28.6
Kilograms to pounds	2.2
Volume	
Milliliters to fluid ounces	28
Liters to quarts (liquid)	1.1
Liters to quarts (dry)	0.9

CONVERTING FROM ENGLISH TO METRIC UNITS*

Length	Divide by
Inches to centimeters	0.39
Feet to meters	0.32
Miles to kilometers	0.62
Weight	
Ounces to grams (dry)	28.6
Pounds to kilograms	2.2
Volume	
Fluid ounces to milliliters	28
Quarts to liters (liquid)	1.1
Quarts to liters (dry)	0.9

*Conversion figures are approximate. For example, the conversion figure for grams to ounces is given here as 28, but 100 grams is commonly considered equal to 3.5 ounces, which makes the exact conversion figure 28.571428.

is the basic unit of weight; and the liter (l) the basic unit of volume. Smaller and/or larger units are described by adding a specific prefix. The prefixes used in the metric system are shown in the following table.

The metric system is also the common system of measurement in all countries except the United States, which still uses the English system, whose standard measurements are the foot, the pound, and the quart.

minerals, dietary Like VITAMINS, dietary minerals are nutrients essential for the proper growth and development of the body and mind. Unlike vitamins, which are organic compounds (substances containing carbon, hydrogen, and oxygen), minerals are made of a single element such as calcium or iron or zinc. Minerals occur naturally in rocks and metal ores. The minerals found in plant foods (such as the calcium in dark green leafy foods) and the minerals in food from animals (such as the calcium in milk) are absorbed from the soil in which plants grow or from the plants the animals eat.

Minerals and Dental Health

From a dental point of view, the most important minerals for human beings are calcium and phosphorous, which promote healthy teeth and bones, including the jawbones, plus FLUORIDE, which hardens teeth and may also protect bones. Individuals who do not get sufficient amounts of calcium early in life may have a higher risk of osteoporosis as adults, including the loss of bone in the jaw due to PERIODONTAL DISEASE.

It is estimated that 95 percent of the ENAMEL outer covering of the teeth and 66 percent of the DENTIN that makes up the bulk of the tooth and its root are composed of minerals, primarily a compound called hydroxyapatite (crystals of calcium and phosphorus). Unlike bones, which are constantly losing and replacing the mineral

MAJOR MINERALS: RECOMMENDED DIETARY ALLOWANCES							
Age (Years)	Calcium (mg)	Phosphorus (mg)	Magnesium (mg)	Iron (mg)	Zinc (mg)	Iodine (mg)	Selenium (mg)
Males							
19–30	1,000	700	400	8	11	150	55
31–50	1,000	700	420	8	11	150	55
51–70	1,200	700	420	8	11	150	55
70+	1,200	700	420	8	11	150	55
Females							
19–30	1,000	700	310	18	8	150	55
31–50	1,000	700	320	18	8	150	55
51–70	1,200	700	320	8	8	150	55
70+	1,200	700	320	8	8	150	55

*The higher figure is for women taking postmenopausal estrogen supplements. Source: National Academy of Medicine reports, 2009.

calcium, the mineral content of teeth remains relatively stable.

Classifying Minerals

Dietary minerals are divided into three groups: major minerals (more than 5 grams stored in the body; more than 100 mg required each day for a healthful diet), trace elements (less than 5 grams stored in the body; less than 100 mg required each day), and electrolytes (positively charged mineral particles that facilitate the transmission of impulses from cell to cell in the body). The major minerals considered vital for human beings are calcium, phosphorous, magnesium, and sulfur. The trace elements considered vital are iron, zinc, iodine, selenium, copper, manganese, fluoride, chromium, and molybdenum. The electrolytes are sodium, potassium, and chloride. The following table shows the recommended dietary allowances for the major minerals.

mouth   See JAW; LIPS; TEETH; TONGUE.

mouth breathing   Breathing air in and out through the mouth rather than through the nose.

Symptoms and Diagnostic Path

Continued mouth breathing dries the mucous MEMBRANES inside the mouth and may lead to excessive growth of gum tissue or increase the risk of fungal infections.

Treatment Options and Outlook

The treatment for mouth breathing varies with the cause. For example, a temporary infection such as a cold, which makes tissues swell and blocks the nasal passages, will simply heal itself, while a deviated septum (the bone that separates the chambers of the nose), which blocks the nasal passages, may require surgery to straighten the bone, and misaligned teeth that keep the jaws ajar may require orthodontia.

Risk Factors and Preventive Measures

Risk factors for mouth breathing include an allergy, a upper respiratory infection, a sinus infection, or structural problems such as a deviated septum or misaligned teeth.

mouth guard   Mouth protector; a protective device worn over the teeth to prevent injury to the teeth, jawbones, and soft tissue inside the mouth.

Mouth guards are commonly prescribed for people with BRUXISM (tooth grinding), an important cause of tooth chips and breakage among older people. The use of a mouth guard is also strongly encouraged for people, especially children, who participate in physical activity that carries a risk of facial injury. These activities include but are not limited to contact sports (boxing, football, hockey) as well as sports such as gymnastics or bicycling that carry the risk of falling onto a hard surface.

How Mouth Guards Work

A well-designed mouth guard cushions the impact of any blow that might otherwise chip the enamel surface of the tooth or break the tooth or knock it loose from the gum, while it softens the impact of the teeth against the soft tissue of the tongue or the inside of the lips and cheek.

Ordinarily, the mouth guard fits over the top teeth. However, the dentist may advise a protector for the lower teeth as well for people who wear sharp dental appliances such as ORTHODONTIC BRACES or have breakable fixed RESTORATIONS (bridges, permanent DENTURES, or dental implants) on both upper and lower teeth/jaws. Some studies suggest that wearing a mouth guard may reduce the risk of concussion during contact sports by dissipating the impact of a blow to the face; this theory remains unproven.

A patient whose teeth are loose due to PERIODONTAL DISEASE should check with her dentist before using any mouth guard to be certain that the guard will not exacerbate the mobility of the teeth.

The Three Types of Mouth Guards

There are three basic types of mouth guards: stock mouth guards, mouth-formed or "boil and bite" mouth guards, and custom-made mouth guards.

Stock Mouth Guards   Commonly known as standard sports mouth protectors, these are standard-size (small, medium, large) plastic devices sold in sports equipment stores. The virtues of stock mouth guards are their low cost (typically less than $20) and wide availability. The drawbacks are their size, bulkiness, and poor fit. The stock guards cannot be adjusted; the large may not be large enough to cover the back teeth in a large mouth. These mouth guards do not fit snugly; to hold them in place, the athlete must keep his teeth clenched, which makes breathing difficult and natural speech virtually impossible. (To counter this, the guards have either a woven string or plastic tab that attaches to a helmet so that they can be taken out of the mouth without fear of their falling and being lost.)

Mouth-Formed Mouth Guards   Sometimes called "boil and bite" mouth guards, these are made of thermoplastic (from the Greek word *thermos,* meaning "hot," and *plastos,* meaning "formed") material that softens when heated and hardens when cooled. To use this protector, the patient immerses the guard in boiling water for a short period of time (usually 20 seconds), lifts it out, places it over his upper teeth, and bites down into the guard while using his fingers to push the edges of the softened guard up around the teeth. This creates a guard shaped to the user's teeth. If formed correctly it will remain securely in place without the user having to clench his teeth.

Like stock sports mouth guards, the "boil and bite" guards are relatively inexpensive ($14 to $25) and come in three standard sizes. The largest may not be large enough for a big jaw, but the guard can easily be cut down to fit a smaller jaw. The "boil and bite" guard is less bulky than the stock guard, which means it does not interfere with breathing, but it is also less protective for someone playing contact sports.

Custom-Made Mouth Guards   These are medical devices made either in a dental office or in a dental LABORATORY to specifications of the examining dentist. There are two basic types of custom-made guards: the vacuum mouth guard and the pressure laminated mouth guard.

The vacuum mouth guard is made of one layer of plastic molded onto a cast of the patient's mouth, allowed to harden, and then trimmed and polished so that it has no irritating edges. The pressure-laminated mouth guard is molded of several layers of plastic sheets that fuse chemically to create a smooth surface, thicker in some places and thinner in others.

The vacuum mouth guard has long been the standard for custom-made guards. But the pressure laminated mouth guard is gaining in popularity because it is more flexible than the vacuum mouth guard and more protective as its variable depths are built specifically to shield particularly vulnerable spots in the mouth such as a fixed denture.

However, both types of custom-made guards are less bulky and more comfortable than the standard sports mouth guard. They fit better and accommodate irregularities in an individual patient's mouth such as orthodontic appliances, fixed restorations, and missing teeth. They hold their shape through repeated use. Both are highly protective but do not interfere with breathing and are the least likely of the mouth guards to interfere with normal speech. Their major drawback is their price, which may range upward of $500.

Caring for a Mouth Guard

Mouth guards should be kept clean and checked regularly to keep them in proper working order. To protect the mouth guard:

- rinse the appliance with cool water daily or before and after each use
- if there is food debris in the guard, brush the guard clean with a soft TOOTHBRUSH and MOUTHWASH or a nonabrasive DENTIFRICE to avoid scratching the plastic surface to create niches in which debris or bacteria might collect
- at least once a week, wash the guard with warm, soapy water and rinse thoroughly

- after cleaning, dry the guard and store it in a clean container
- store the guard at room temperature, away from any heat source such as direct sunlight or a radiator so as to prevent distortion of the plastic
- check the guard regularly for damage such as holes in the plastic or any change in shape that might interfere with a close fit
- if the guard is custom-made, bring it to your regular dental appointment so that your dentist can check the fit and general condition of the appliance

mouth sores   See STOMATITIS.

mouthwash   Mouthwash is a water-based solution used to clean the mouth and/or treat several dental/oral conditions.

The first mouthwashes, created by the ancient Egyptians, Greeks, and Romans, were based on common liquids such as water or milk with added sweeteners and aromatic plants to freshen the breath. The first antiseptic mouthwash, formulated by the Romans, relied on naturally occurring ammonia in urine, a bodily liquid often credited with medicinal effects. (Modern mouthwashes also contain ammonia, but in the form of manufactured quaternary ammonium compounds, a class of antiseptic solvents and emulsifiers—chemicals that enable opposites such as oil and water to mix—such as benzalkonium chloride.)

The first effective commercial mouthwash, Odol, was introduced in Switzerland in 1892 by Karl August Lingner. Odol, which is still sold today, uses alcohol as an antiseptic. Listerine contains both alcohol and antiseptic essential oils. This mouthwash is named for British surgeon Joseph Lister, who did not invent the mouthwash but did pioneer the use of antiseptics during surgery. In fact, Listerine was introduced in

1879 as a surgical antiseptic. It was first sold to dentists during the mid-1890s, then, after World War I, the Warner-Lambert Company began selling it over-the-counter as the first commercial mouthwash in the United States. More sophisticated mouthwashes, containing ingredients to strengthen the teeth or reduce the incidence of PERIODONTAL DISEASE, became popular during the 1990s.

As a rule, modern mouthwashes fall into one of two general categories: nonmedicated mouthwash and medicated mouthwash.

Nonmedicated mouthwash, also known as cosmetic mouthwash, contains water, diluents (ingredient such as alcohol that dissolve other ingredients), astringents, flavors, colors, and sometimes foaming agents. Nonmedicated mouthwashes temporarily freshen breath by rinsing debris off the teeth and tongue and lowering the level of bacteria in the mouth for a short time. Because nonmedicated mouthwashes are classified by the Food and Drug Administration as cosmetics they cannot carry health claims on the label or in advertising. Table 1 lists some of the ingredients commonly found in nonmedicated mouthwashes.

Medicated mouthwash, also known as therapeutic mouthwash, contains the same diluents, coloring agents, flavoring agents, astringents, and preservatives found in nonmedicated mouthwash. In addition, medicated mouthwashes contain medically active ingredients considered safe and effective when used as directed. These ingredients are designed to reduce the formation of plaque on teeth and/or reduce inflammation of the gums and/or strengthen the teeth.

Because medicated mouthwashes have medical effects, the Food and Drug Administration classifies them as either over-the-counter (OTC) drugs (such as Listerine) or prescription drugs (such as Peridex), depending on the medically active ingredient and/or its concentration. Both OTC and prescription medicated mouthwashes may carry medical claims on the label or in advertising. One example is the statement "Kills germs that cause bad breath, plaque, and the gum disease gingivitis" printed on the Listerine label. Table 2 lists some of the medically active ingredients commonly found in medicated mouthwashes.

Procedure

Mouthwash is one component of a complete oral hygiene regimen that includes toothbrushing and flossing. Some people use mouthwash every day; others, only in certain medical situations.

Dentists are most likely to prescribe using mouthwash daily for patients who have:

- bad breath (see HALITOSIS)
- a history of repeated DECAY
- dry mouth (the failure to produce adequate SALIVA increases the risk of decay)
- a history of periodontal disease
- a physical or medical condition that makes it difficult to brush or floss
- a dental appliance such as ORTHODONTIC BRACES that is difficult to clean with brushes and floss

Dentists are most likely to prescribe mouthwash for short periods of time for patients who have:

- mouth sores, such as canker sores
- recent dental/oral surgery and cannot brush until the tissue heals

---

TABLE 1. INGREDIENTS IN NONMEDICATED MOUTHWASH

Ingredient Class	Examples
Antibacterial	Alcohol, thymol
Astringent	Citric acid, small amounts of alcohol
Coloring agent	FD&C* certified dyes, commonly blue and green
Deodorant	Sodium bicarbonate (baking soda)
Flavoring gel	Eugenol, menthol, methyl alicylate, peppermint
Preservative	Benzoic acid, sodium benzoate
Surfactant	Synthetic detergent, cleanser

*FD&C meaning food, drugs, cosmetics; colors labeled FD&C are safe for use in all three product types.

TABLE 2. ACTIVE INGREDIENTS IN MEDICATED MOUTHWASHES

Types	Medically Active Ingredient	Function
Anti-cavity agent	Fluoride	Strengthens tooth enamel to reduce risk of decay
Antiplaque agent (antibacterials)	Alcohol,* chlorhexidine gluconate, aromatic oils (thymol, eucalyptol, menthol, methyl salicylate)	Reduces bacterial activity and gum inflammation
Antiplaque agent (surfactant/ detergent)	Sodium lauryl sulfate, poloxamer 407	Loosens plaque so brushing removes it
Antiseptic	Cetylpyridinium chloride, chlorhexidine, domiphen, hydrogen peroxide, phenolic compounds	Reduces bacterial level in mouth; reduces mouth inflammation
Anti-tartar agent	Zinc citrate	Reduces buildup of tartar (hardened plaque)

*also in non-medicated mouthwashes.

- high risk of oral infection due to a medical condition such as an IMMUNE SYSTEM deficiency

In general, whether a patient uses mouthwash every day or only as a temporary measure, the proper procedure is to swish the undiluted solution around the mouth for about 30 seconds and then spit it out. To avoid adverse reactions (see below), young children must be taught to spit out mouthwash after swishing rather than swallow it.

Some patients may also be directed to gargle the solution so as to rinse away bacteria at the back of the tongue. After using certain medicated mouthwashes, such as a FLUORIDE solution, the patient may be asked to avoid eating or drinking for an hour or more to let the mouthwash settle on the teeth.

Risks and Complications

Some adverse effects occur even when mouthwash is used as directed. For example, chlorhexidine gluconate, an ingredient in antiplaque mouthwash, often leaves a bitter aftertaste, and the fluorides in mouthwashes meant to strengthen teeth may corrode the nickel WIRES used in orthodontic braces, reducing the braces' ability to move teeth and raising the risk of an allergic reaction when the damaged metal releases nickel, a potential allergen, into the mouth.

Mouthwash Problems for Adults Among adults, the most common adverse effects of mouthwash are due to overuse. Using mouthwash more frequently than directed on the label or by the dentist may cause the following reactions:

- *Teeth and dentures*: Stains due to the dyes in the mouthwash; increased sensitivity to heat and cold at the tooth root
- *Lips, tongue, and cheeks*: Burning sensation due to alcohol; mild irritation; erosion or ulceration of the tissue (rare)
- *Sense of taste*: Unpleasant aftertaste; changes in the ability to taste food and drink (uncommon)
- *Oral health*: Overgrowth of bacteria due to repeated use of antiseptics, a condition known descriptively as *black hairy tongue*

Mouthwash Problems for Children Among children, the most common serious problem with mouthwash is toxicity due to swallowing the mouthwash, particularly mouthwash containing alcohol.

The alcohol content of mouthwashes ranges from high (Listerine, 23 percent) to low (Viadent, 5–10 percent) to none at all (Alcohol-free Biotene or Rembrandt Dazzling Fresh). To put that in everyday terms, 5 ounces of a high-alcohol mouthwash contains approximately 35 grams of alcohol, the amount of alcohol in two drinks—that is, two 12-ounce regular beers, two five-ounce glasses of wine, or two 1.5-ounce servings of distilled spirits. This amount of alcohol is considered potentially lethal for a small child. In 1999, the results of a survey published the *British Medical Journal* showed that 12.5 percent of poisonings among children younger than six were due to "cosmetics, personal-care products or alcohol-containing products" including mouthwashes, and that 97 percent of the poisoning in this age group involving alcohol were due not to alcoholic beverages but to alcohol in cosmetics such as perfume and mouthwash. To prevent accidental ingestion of mouthwash, the U.S. Consumer Products Safety Commission ruled in 1995 that mouthwash must have childproof caps. Some signs of alcohol/mouthwash intoxication are listed below.

SIGNS OF ALCOHOL/MOUTHWASH INTOXICATION

Organ/Body System	Signs
Heart and lungs	Fast, shallow breathing, slow breathing, or no breathing; sudden low blood pressure (fainting)
Stomach	Pain, nausea, vomiting, diarrhea; excessive thirst
Central nervous system	Dizziness, drowsiness, loss of consciousness, convulsions, coma
Skin	Blue tint to skin, lips, and nails; excessive sweating
Kidneys	Inability to urinate
Muscles	Uneven gait, slurred speech

Outlook and Lifestyle Modifications

Used correctly, mouthwashes wash away debris, strengthen teeth, and/or reduce the incidence of decay. Those that do not contain alcohol may also help moisten the oral tissues.

See also CAVITY; GINGIVA; PLAQUE.

mucosa See MEMBRANE.

muscle Specialized body tissue that contracts and relaxes in response to electrical impulses from the nerves. The most important oral muscles are the muscles that control the LIPS, the JAW, and the TONGUE, an organ composed of muscle covered with mucous MEMBRANE. These muscles are all skeletal muscle, the type of muscle found attached to bones by strong fibrous cords called tendons. Skeletal muscles are also known as voluntary muscle, because a healthy person can move them at will; for example, to smile or frown or chew food. Skeletal muscle is composed of long thin cells called muscle fibers containing smaller units called myofibrils, some with light-colored protein strands (actin) and some with dark-colored protein strands (myosin). The fibers in skeletal muscle are arranged in distinct patterns that make the light and dark protein strands look like stripes, so skeletal muscle is sometimes called striated (striped) muscle. Skeletal muscles are extremely well supplied with nerves that transmit the messages that make the muscles move. For example, the muscles that shape the tongue for speech and chewing are connected to several cranial nerves that direct the tongue muscle's intricate movements during speaking and processing food.

The body contains two other types of muscle. Visceral muscle, also known as smooth or involuntary muscle, is found in the walls of hollow organ such as the bladder, the blood vessels, or the digestive tract. This second type of muscle is controlled by brain impulses, not deliberate movement. Cardiac muscle is found only in the heart, where it enables the contractions of the four chambers of the heart that pump blood out into the body. Like skeletal muscles, cardiac muscle looks striped; like smooth muscle, its actions are involuntary.

myofascial pain See TEMPOROMANDIBULAR JOINT DISORDER.

Nance, Hays N. (1893–1964) American orthodontist Hays N. Nance began his practice as
a general dentist in Arizona in 1919, then
moved to California. In 1930, Nance began the
research that eventually lead to his ground-
breaking paper, "The Limitations of Orthodontic Treatment: Mixed Dentition Diagnosis and
Treatment," published in the *American Journal of
Orthodontic Oral Surgery* in 1947. The article laid
out Nance's belief that an orthodontically treated
dental ARCH eventually returned to its original
width, an important observation as orthodontists
began to employ extraction rather than simple
movement of teeth to create a stable arch.

Nance is also the creator of the *Nance arch
length analysis,* a method for estimating the size
of the dental arch by measuring the difference
between the diameter toward the back of the
primary canine teeth and molars and the teeth
that grow in when they fall out. The analysis
is still used in planning orthodontic treatment,
as are several orthodontic treatment appliances
that bear his name.

See ORTHODONTICS AND DENTOFACIAL ORTHO-
PEDICS.

Nathoo Classification System See TOOTH
DISCOLORATION.

National Call to Action to Promote Oral Health
In 2003, three years after the publication of ORAL
HEALTH IN AMERICA, the U.S. Surgeon General
released a follow-up report, the "National Call
to Action to Promote Oral Health." Based on

the conclusions in the earlier report, this second report was designed to set parameters for a
national campaign to improve oral health in the
United States by:

- altering perceptions regarding oral health
  and disease so that oral health becomes an
  accepted component of general health
- accelerating the creation of the science and
  evidence base required to improve Americans'
  oral health
- building an effective health infrastructure that
  meets the oral health needs of all Americans
  and integrates oral health effectively into
  overall health
- removing known barriers between people and
  oral health services
- using public-private partnerships to improve
  the oral health of those with the least access
  to proper dental/oral health care

The report is organized by "Actions," five
specific steps to be taken at the local, state, and
national levels to accomplish these five goals.

Action 1. Change Perceptions of Oral Health

According to the Surgeon General, Americans
regard oral health as less important and separate from general health. The action to change
this perception is designed to increase public
awareness of the aspects of oral health so as
to facilitate informed decisions regarding the
prevention, early detection, and management
of diseases of the dental, oral, and craniofacial
structures. To implement the goals of Action 1,

the Surgeon General proposes the steps outlined in the following list.

Steps to Implement Action 1

- Enhance oral health literacy among all Americans.
- Develop messages that are culturally sensitive and linguistically competent.
- Enhance knowledge of the value of regular, professional oral health care.
- Increase the understanding of how the signs and symptoms of oral infections can indicate general health status and act as a marker for other diseases.
- Change policy makers' perceptions.
- Inform policy makers and administrators at local, state, and federal levels of the results of oral health research and programs and of the oral health status of their constituencies.
- Develop concise and relevant messages for policymakers.
- Document the health and quality-of-life outcomes that result from the inclusion (or exclusion) of oral health services in programs and reimbursement schedules.
- Change health providers' perceptions.
- Review and update health professional educational curricula and continuing education courses to include content on oral health and the association between oral health and general health.
- Train health care providers to conduct oral screenings as part of routine physical exams and make appropriate referrals.
- Promote interdisciplinary training of medical, oral health, and allied health professional personnel in counseling patients about how to reduce risk factors common to oral and general health.
- Encourage oral health providers to refer patients to other health specialists as war-

ranted by examinations and history; similarly, encourage medical and surgical providers to refer patients for oral health care when medical or surgical treatments that may impact oral health are planned.

Action 2. Overcome Barriers by Replicating Effective Programs and Proven Efforts

In improving the oral health of Americans, it is vital to have accurate data on disease and disabilities for various population groups available, to improve access to health care for those commonly limited by poverty, educational level, geographic isolation, age, gender, disability, or an existing medical condition, and to provide adequate reimbursement for oral health care procedures through both private and public insurance programs. To accomplish the goals outlined in Action 2, the Surgeon General proposes the steps in the following list.

Steps to Implement Action 2

- Implement science-based interventions appropriate for individuals and communities.
- Enhance oral health–related content in health professions school curricula, residencies, and continuing education programs by incorporating new findings on diagnosis, treatment, and prevention of oral diseases and disorders.
- Build and support epidemiological and surveillance databases at national, state, and local levels to identify patterns of disease and populations at risk; collect data on oral health status, disease, and health services utilization and expenditures, sorted by demographic variables for various populations—surveys should document baseline status, monitor progress, and measure health outcomes.
- Determine, at community or population levels, oral health care needs and system requirements, including appropriate reimbursement for services, facility and personnel needs, and mechanisms of referral.

- Encourage partnerships among research, provider, and educational communities in activities, such as organizing workshops and conferences, to develop ways to meet the education, research, and service needs of patients who need special care and their families.

- Refine protocols of care for special care populations based on the emerging science.

- Improve access to oral health care.

- Promote and apply programs that have demonstrated effective improvement in access to care.

- Create an active and up-to-date database of these programs.

- Explore policy changes that can improve provider participation in public health insurance programs and enhance patient access to care.

- Remove barriers to the use of services by simplifying forms, letting individuals know when and how to obtain services, and providing transportation and child care as needed; assist low-income patients in arranging and keeping oral health appointments.

- Facilitate health insurance benefits for diseases and disorders affecting craniofacial, oral, and dental tissues, including genetic diseases such as the ectodermal dysplasias, congenital anomalies such as clefting syndromes, autoimmune diseases such as Sjögren's syndrome, and chronic orofacial pain conditions such as temporomandibular disorders.

- Ensure an adequate number and distribution of culturally competent providers to meet the needs of individuals and groups, particularly in health-care shortage areas.

- Make optimal use of oral health and other health-care providers in improving access to oral health care.

- Energize and empower the public to implement solutions to meet their oral health–care needs.

- Develop integrated and comprehensive care programs that include oral health care and increase the number and types of settings in which oral health services are provided; explore ways to sustain successful programs.

- Apply evaluation criteria to determine the effectiveness of access programs and develop modifications as necessary.

- Enhance health promotion and health literacy.

- Apply strategies to enhance the adoption and maintenance of proven community-based and clinical interventions, such as community water fluoridation and dental sealants application.

- Identify the knowledge, opinions, and practices of the public, health-care providers, and policymakers with regard to oral diseases and oral health.

- Engage populations and community organizations in the development of health promotion and health literacy action plans.

- Publicize successful programs that promote oral health to facilitate their replication.

- Develop and support programs promoting general health that include activities supporting oral health (such as wearing oral facial protection, tobacco cessation, and good nutrition).

Action 3. Build the Science Base and Accelerate Science Transfer

In this action, the authors of the National Call to Action stress the requirement for biomedical and behavioral information drawn from basic research and clinical trials in creating stratagems to identify, diagnose, and treat primary oral and dental disorders and diseases, as well as the oral and dental complications of seemingly unrelated conditions ranging from malnutrition to heart disease. They note that a comprehensive research effort also requires statistical surveys to establish and monitor the oral health of specific risk groups and disease patterns and genetic studies to identify persons at risk. Finally, they recognize the necessity of open communication among researchers, clinicians, and the lay public. To implement the requirements described in Action 3, the Surgeon General proposes the steps in the following list.

Steps to Implement Action 3

- Enhance applied research (clinical and population-based studies, demonstration projects, health services research) to improve oral health and prevent disease.

- Expand intervention studies aimed at preventing and managing oral infections and complex diseases, including new approaches to prevent dental caries and periodontal diseases.

- Intensify population-based studies aimed at the prevention of oral cancer and oral-facial trauma.

- Conduct studies to elucidate potential underlying mechanisms and determine any causal associations between oral infections and systemic conditions. If associations are demonstrated, test interventions to prevent or lower risk of complications.

- Develop diagnostic markers for disease susceptibility and progression of oral diseases.

- Develop and test diagnostic codes for oral diseases that can be used in research and in practice.

- Investigate risk assessment approaches for individuals and communities, and translate them into optimal prevention, diagnosis, and treatment measures.

- Develop biologic measures of disease and health that can be used as outcome variables and applied in epidemiological studies and clinical trials.

- Develop reliable and valid measures of patients' oral health outcomes for use in programs and in practice.

- Support research on the effectiveness of community-based and clinical interventions.

- Facilitate collaborations among health professional schools, state health programs, patient groups, professional associations, private practitioners, industries, and communities to support the conduct of clinical and community-based research as well as accelerate science transfer.

- Accelerate the effective transfer of science into public health and private practice.

- Promote effective disease-prevention measures that are underutilized.

- Routinely transfer oral health research findings to health professional school curricula and continuing education programs and incorporate appropriate curricula from other health professions—medical, nursing, pharmacy, and social work—into dental education.

- Communicate research findings to the public, clearly describing behaviors and actions that promote health and well-being.

- Explore ways to accelerate the transfer of research findings into delivery systems, including appropriate changes in reimbursement for care.

- Routinely evaluate the scientific evidence and update care recommendations.

Action 4. Increase Oral Health Workforce Diversity, Capacity, and Flexibility

The aim of this action is simply to ensure that oral and dental health professionals provide services that meet the needs of their patients. In addition, because a provider's patient usually mirrors his/her own racial, ethnic, and/or economic background, the dentist/physician has a unique opportunity to serve as a liaison to specific communities, not only as a service provider but also as a mentor and recruiter bringing groups into the profession, thus enlarging and diversifying the population of dental and oral health care providers. To accomplish the goals listed in Action 4, the Surgeon General proposes the steps in the following list.

Steps to Implement Action 4

- Change the racial and ethnic composition of the workforce to meet patient and community needs.

- Document the outcomes of existing efforts to diversify the workforce in practice, education, and research.

- Develop ways to expand and build upon successful recruitment and retention programs, and develop and test new programs that focus on individuals from underrepresented groups.

- Document the outcomes of existing efforts to recruit individuals into careers in oral health education, research, and public and private health practice.

- Create and support programs that inform and encourage individuals to pursue health and science career options in high school and during graduate years.

- Ensure a sufficient workforce pool to meet health care needs.

- Expand scholarships and loan repayment efforts at all levels.

- Specify and identify resources for conducting outreach and recruitment.

- Develop mentoring programs to ensure retention of individuals who have been successfully recruited into oral health careers.

- Facilitate collaborations among professional, government, academic, industry, community organizations, and other institutions that are addressing the needs of the oral-health workforce.

- Provide training in communication skills and cultural competence to health-care providers and students.

- Secure an adequate and flexible workforce.

- Assess the existing capacity and distribution of the oral health workforce.

- Study how to extend or expand workforce capacity and productivity to address oral health in health-care shortage areas.

- Work to ensure oral health expertise is available to health departments and to federal, state, and local government programs.

- Determine the effects of flexible licensure policies and state practice acts on health-care access and oral health outcomes.

Action 5. Increase Collaborations

Finally, the Surgeon General's Call to Action on Oral Health proposes to provide the knowledge, expertise, and resources required to link the private and public sectors in the effort to improve dental and oral health. The aim is to enlist community members in promoting professional health-care recommendations, something as simple as convincing parents to insist that their children use protective mouth/face gear during athletic activities or as sophisticated as providing nutritional support for pregnant women and new mothers. To accomplish these goals, the Surgeon General proposes the steps in the following list.

Steps to Implement Action 5

- Invite patient advocacy groups to lead efforts in partnering for programs directed toward their constituencies.

- Strengthen the networking capacity of individuals and communities to address their oral health needs.

- Build and nurture broad-based coalitions that incorporate views and expertise of all stakeholders and that are tailored to specific populations, conditions, or programs.

- Strengthen collaborations among dental, medical, and public health communities for research, education, care delivery, and policy development.

- Develop partnerships that are community-based, cross-disciplinary, and culturally sensitive.

- Work with the Partnership Network and other coalitions to address the four actions previously described: change perceptions, overcome barriers, build a balanced science base, and increase oral health workforce diversity, capacity, and flexibility.

- Evaluate and report on the progress and outcomes of partnership efforts.

- Promote examples of state-based coalitions for others to use as models.

The complete text of the National Call to Action to Promote Oral Health is available online at www.surgeongeneral.gov/topics/oralhealth/nationalcalltoaction.htm.

National Institute of Dental and Craniofacial Research (NIDCR)   A division of the National Institutes of Health (NIH), established when the National Dental Research Act (Public Law 755) was signed into law by President Harry S. Truman. The agency's initial charge was to research the causes of dental DECAY, document the value of FLUORIDES in reducing the incidence of dental cavities, and investigate the role of bacterial infection in PERIODONTAL DISEASE.

Today, the NIDCR describes its mission as improving "oral, dental, and craniofacial health through research, research training, and the dissemination of health information," a goal it accomplishes by "performing and supporting basic and clinical research; conducting and funding research training and career development programs to ensure an adequate number of talented, well-prepared, and diverse investigators; co-ordinating and assisting relevant research and research-related activities among all sectors of the research community; and promoting the timely transfer of knowledge gained from research and its implications for health to the public, health professionals, researchers, and policy-makers."

The NIDCR serves as the lead agency for oral and dental health research projects. Operating with a budget approaching $400 million a year, the agency distributes research grants to universities, dental schools, and medical schools across the United States and occasionally in other countries as well. These grants fund basic research as well as clinical trials and epidemiological information documents such as the Surgeon General's 2000 *ORAL HEALTH IN AMERICA* and the NATIONAL CALL TO ACTION.

Through a Federal Coordinating Committee, the NIDCR exchanges information with other federal agencies such as the Department of Agriculture, Department of Education, Department of Justice, Department of Defense, Department of Veterans Affairs, and the Department of Energy while maintaining control of studies and programs covering a broad range of oral, dental, and craniofacial (head and face) diseases and disorders including, but not limited to, dental caries, orthodontics, birth defects such as CLEFT LIP AND/OR PALATE, and ORAL CANCERS.

The NIDCR and the U.S. Centers for Disease Control and Prevention cosponsor the National Institute of Dental and Craniofacial Research NIDCR/CDC Dental, Oral, and Craniofacial Data Resource Center (DRC). This joint agency provides much of the statistical and interpretive data required to create and support NIDCR clinical programs and policy programs and proposals such as the dental and oral health sections of Healthy People 2000 and *HEALTHY PEOPLE* 2010. Finally, NIDCR maintains a consumer-friendly Web site at www.nidcr.nih.gov.

necrosis   Destruction or death of body tissue, from the Greek words *nekros* meaning "dead body" and *nekrosis* meaning "dying" or "the process of dying."

Exanthematous necrosis is an acute incident of the death of tissue in the gums, jawbones, and soft tissue around both, a condition similar to NOMA. Gingival necrosis is the destruction of cells in the gum tissue as may occur during an episode of *necrotizing ulcerative gingivitis* (NUG) and *necrotizing ulcerative periodontitis* (NUP), acute PERIODONTAL DISEASE resulting in the loss of gum tissue and bone, leading to the loss of teeth. Interdental necrosis is the death of tissue between teeth. Necrotizing stomatitis is an inflammatory disease causing the destruction of connective tissue and bone, leading to the loss of teeth. Radiation necrosis is tissue death due to exposure to RADIATION, commonly during radiation therapy for a malignant tumor.

nerve block   See ANESTHETIC.

nerves   Nerves are cordlike structures made of multiple fibers built of nerve cells (neurons). The fibers transmit two kinds of impulses: (1) motor impulses, messages that move the body, such as the message to open and close the mouth or raise and lower the lower jaw, and (2) sensory stimuli, such as flavor messages to the taste buds on the tongue, back and forth between the brain and the body.

The Central Nervous System

The brain and spinal cord are the body's central nervous system. The nerves that come out from the lower surface of the brain are called cranial nerves; the nerves that come out from spaces between the vertebrae (bones in the spine) are called spinal nerves. Cranial nerves link the brain to the mouth and jaw, as well as the eyes, ears, nose, head, neck, and some sections of the upper body. Spinal nerves carry messages to and from various parts of the body.

There are two types of cranial and spinal nerves. Efferent nerves (from the Latin verb *efferre,* meaning "carry out") carry impulses from the central nervous system to the body. Afferent nerves (from the Latin ADFERENS, meaning "carry to") bring impulses from the body to the brain.

The Somatic (Voluntary) Nervous System

The somatic nervous system is a group of 12 pairs of nerves originating in the brain and 31 pairs of nerves originating in the spine that transmit messages to and from the muscles to control the voluntary movements of the body such as opening and closing the mouth and lower jaw and moving the tongue when speaking or eating. Somatic nerves also contain sensory fibers for taste as well as sight, hearing, smell, and touch.

The nerves that send motor and sensory impulses back and forth from the brain to the mouth and jaw are:

- *alveolar nerve, anterior superior alveolar nerve:* These nerves in the pulp and tissue around the teeth in the upper jaw send messages to the maxillary portion of the infraorbital nerve and the trigeminal nerve (see below)

- *buccal nerve:* This nerve, in the cheek, sends impulses from the gums on the side nearest the cheek

- *facial nerve:* This nerve sends motor impulses to muscles used to create facial expressions and sends sensory impulses (taste) to the tongue and palate

- *glossopharyngeal nerve:* This nerve sends motor impulses to the stylopharyngeus muscle, which controls the opening at the back of the throat, and sends sensory impulses (taste, feeling) to the tongue, palate, and pharynx (top of the throat)

- *hypoglossal nerve:* This nerve sends impulses from the brain to the muscles of the tongue

- *lingual nerve:* This sensory nerve impacts the lower jaw, tongue, and area under the tongue

- *mental nerve:* This nerve transmits messages from the tissue around the teeth nearest the lips and chin in the upper and lower jaw

- *trigeminal nerve:* This nerve sends motor impulses to the muscles that move the jaw and sensory impulses from the skin and mucous membranes of the head (face, mouth) and neck.

- *mandibular nerve:* This nerve is located in the mandibular (lower jaw) section of the trigeminal nerve

- *maxillary nerve:* This nerve is located in the maxillary (upper jaw) section of the trigeminal nerve.*
- *vagus nerve:* This nerve sends motor impulses to the palate and throat and sends sensory messages (taste, feeling) to the tongue and throat; the vagus nerve also carries hearing sensation to the ear

The Autonomic (Involuntary) Nervous System

The autonomic nervous system is made up of two complementary sets of nerves, the sympathetic nervous system (SNS) and the parasympathetic nervous system (PNS), that transmit messages back and forth between the brain and organs such as the heart, lungs, and blood vessels whose functions are usually considered beyond voluntary control, such as the secretion of material from glands. For example, the facial nerve and the glossopharyngeal (from the Greek words *glossa,* meaning "tongue" and *pharynx,* meaning "throat") nerve control the secretion of SALIVA from the salivary glands.

Messages from the autonomic nervous system travel via chemicals called neurotransmitters such as acetylcholine, epinephrine, adrenaline, and norepinephrine/noradrenaline secreted by the outer covering (cortex) of the adrenal gland, a small structure sitting atop the kidney.

The nerves of the sympathetic nervous system send signals that step up protective body responses such as a quickened heartbeat or blood vessel constriction to reduce blood loss should there be an injury. The parasympathetic nervous system, on the other hand, is a calming agent that does exactly the opposite, sending "slow down and relax" messages.

neuralgia   Neuralgia is pain that occurs along the path of one specific nerve. For example, TRIGEMI-NAL NEURALGIA is pain along the path of a major nerve on one side of the face. Other examples of dental and/or facial neuralgia are buccal neuralgia, a throbbing pain in the lips, jaws, gums, cheek, and nose; and glossopharyngeal neuralgia, a pain centered in the nerves to the tongue and pharynx (the opening from the back of the mouth and nose to the top of the throat).

Symptoms and Diagnostic Path

The symptoms of neuralgia include increased sensitivity and consistent or intermittent pain at the same site along the affected nerve; "trigger points" (places along the path of the nerve where any touch causes severe pain), and voluntarily impaired movement to avoid discomfort—for example, restricted movement of the jaws in a patient with facial neuralgia.

While the dentist can rule out some common causes of facial pain such as an infected tooth, there are no specific tests to diagnose neuralgia. However, imaging techniques such as X-ray or magnetic resonance imaging (MRI) may be employed to identify possible causes of pain such as a tumor pressing on a nerve.

Treatment Options and Outlook

All treatments for neuralgia, including dental neuralgias, aim to provide adequate pain relief and, if possible, identify the cause of the problem. If the latter appears to be pressure on a specific nerve, treatment may involve surgery to move or remove the source of the pressure; for example, a blood vessel or a tumor.

In addition, there is a broad list of medications that may relieve nerve pain, including, but not limited to, antidepressants, antiseizure drugs, nonprescription oral and topical analgesics, prescription painkillers, and injectable anesthetic drugs. As with many conditions or injuries, neuralgia may improve or disappear over time even without treatment; however, if the pain is intractable, the dentist may refer the patient to a pain control specialist.

---

*When the maxillary nerve enters the area around the eye socket (orbit), it is known as the infraorbital nerve.

Risk Factors and Preventive Measures

While neuralgia occurs in people of all ages, it is more common among the elderly. In most cases, the precipitating cause is never identified. However, the known triggers may include an infection, an infectious disease such as shingles, a chronic disease such as diabetes, a physical irritation, the pressure of a tumor or body structure on a nerve, or some medical drugs.

See PRESCRIPTION.

nevus A pigmented spot on the skin or mucous membrane. From the Latin word *naevus,* meaning "birthmark." Nevi in the mouth are called oral nevi.

Symptoms and Diagnostic Path

Oral nevi are usually symptom-free. A small percentage of patients report feeling a mass or pain at the site, but most oral nevi are discovered by accident during a routine dental exam. Nevi on the skin (including the skin of the lips) are sometimes associated with the development of melanoma, a malignant tumor of pigmented cells. There is no such link between nevi inside the mouth and melanoma, but to rule out malignancy the dentist may take a piece of tissue for biopsy.

Treatment Options and Outlook

No treatment is required for benign oral nevi. Malignant melanoma of the lip is surgically removed; follow-up chemotherapy, radiation, or plastic surgery to replace the excised tissue may be required (see LIP, CANCER OF).

Risk Factors and Preventive Measures

Oral nevi occur among persons of all ages. They are slightly more common among women than among men. Although some studies show them to be more common among white Americans (55 percent of cases) than in African Americans (23 percent), Asians (14 percent), or Hispanics (7 percent), researchers suggest that the differ-

ence in identifying nevi may be due to a difference in the frequency of dental examinations among the three groups.

noma Also known as *cancrum oris* or gangrenous STOMATITIS; a type of gangrene (tissue death due to the loss of blood supply) affecting the mucous membranes of the mouth. The exact cause of noma, which is most common in malnourished children, remains unknown, but the condition is often attributed to a bacteria also linked to trench mouth.

Symptoms and Diagnostic Path

The primary sign of noma is a sudden, virulent inflammation of the gums and lining of the cheeks progressing quickly to ulcers and death of soft tissue inside the mouth. Unchecked, the infection moves to bones and facial skin, eventually leaving gaping holes in the face. The infection is diagnosed by these signs and the identification of the bacteria.

Treatment Options and Outlook

Noma is treated with antibiotics and nutritional therapy to provide an adequate diet. In severe cases, the patient may require plastic surgery to cut away dead tissue, including bone, and then to rebuild the facial structure so as to restore jaw function.

In rare cases, noma heals spontaneously without treatment; the more likely course is that it will continue to progress, to disfigurement and sometimes to death.

Risk Factors and Preventive Measures

Noma occurs most frequently in malnourished young children, who do not get sufficient amounts of protein, are living in unsanitary conditions, and may have already contracted another infectious illness such as measles, scarlet fever, or tuberculosis.

Preventive measures include adequate sanitation, a protein-rich, nutritionally balanced diet, clean water, and inoculations to reduce the risk of common childhood infectious diseases.

See also NECROSIS; PERIODONTAL DISEASE.

notch An indentation in a surface.

In dental anatomy, the coronoid notch is an indentation on the ramus, the flat BONE that rises up from the back of the lower jaw. The mandibular notch is an indentation on lower jaw that accommodates nerve and muscle fibers. The pterygomaxillary notch is a narrow groove at the place where the upper jaw meets the sphenoid bone at the side of the face. The sigmoid notch is an indentation on the ramus.

In dental prosthetics, a buccal notch is an indentation in the side of a DENTURE to make room for the buccal frenum (a fold in the tissue attaching the inside of the cheek to the upper and lower jaw). The labial notch is the indentation in the front of an upper or lower denture that makes room for the labial frenums, the tissue folds that attach the inside of the lip to the upper or lower jaw.

nutrition   See MINERALS, DIETARY; VITAMINS.

occlusion From the Latin word *occludare,* meaning "to close"; the term used to describe how the upper and lower teeth fit against each other, specifically how the *occlusal surfaces*—the tops of the back teeth that come together to cut and grind food—meet when the teeth are closed. The *occlusal plane* is an imaginary line showing where the teeth meet. An *occlusal X-ray* is a picture showing all the teeth in the dental ARCH (the curve formed by the teeth in the jaw).

In an ideal situation, otherwise known as an *ideal occlusion*:

- the upper teeth are all slightly in front of the lower teeth
- the cusps (pointed tips) of each molar fit into the grooves of the opposing molar
- all teeth are straight and spaced evenly with no tooth crossing over into another's space

To get a picture of a patient's occlusion for an *occlusal analysis,* the dentist may ask the patient to bite into a wax wafer, leaving an impression of the upper and lower teeth in each part of the dental arch.

Occlusal irregularities are known collectively as MALOCCLUSION.

See also ORTHODONTICS AND DENTOFACIAL ORTHOPEDICS.

odontogenesis See TOOTH.

onlay A restoration that fills the space caused by a cavity that includes one or more of the cusps (the raised tips on the biting surface of a tooth). Unlike a simple amalgam filling, for which the dentist drills into the tooth, cleans out the decay, and then inserts the soft amalgam to fill and harden in the cavity, the onlay is made of a hard material such as gold or tooth-colored porcelain shaped to fit a cast of the tooth that has space left by decay or the loss of a previous restoration.

An inlay is similar in preparation and purpose to an onlay, the difference being that the inlay fills a cavity occupying only the space between the cusps.

Procedure

To make and place an onlay, the dentist:

- cleans out the decay or removes an old restoration
- shapes and smooths the space left in the tooth
- makes a cast of the tooth and (commonly) the abutting teeth
- places a temporary filling into the cavity to protect the tooth until the inlay is ready
- sends the cast to a dental LABORATORY where a dental technician creates a restoration to fit tightly into the tooth
- places the onlay into the tooth and, if it fits tight and smooth, cements it in place
- if necessary, the onlay will be returned to the laboratory for further trimming to ensure a secure fit

Risks and Complications

Mild pain and sensitivity to heat and cold are common for a short time after the onlay is put in place. If the discomfort lasts longer than a few weeks, the onlay should be rechecked by the dentist.

If the onlay is not fitted properly, moisture may seep in to disturb the connection to the tooth, raising the risk of further decay. Should this occur, the onlay may have to be removed and either remade or reapplied.

Outlook and Lifestyle Modifications

A well-made and well-fitted onlay can last as long as 30 years, all the while preventing further decay.

See also CROWN; IMPRESSION, DENTAL; INLAY.

oral and maxillofacial pathology   One of the nine dental specialties approved by the AMERI-CAN DENTAL ASSOCIATION Council on Dental Education and Licensure. Oral and maxillofacial pathologists are dentists who have completed a postgraduate, in-hospital course in pathology (the study of the nature and causes of disease). These specialists diagnose and treat health conditions of the mouth, upper jaw, and face, including birth defects such as CLEFT LIP AND/OR PALATE and work with other medical and dental specialists such as plastic surgeons and pediatric dentists to identify links between oral conditions and systemic disease. A board certified oral and maxillofacial pathologist has met the requirements of the American Board of Oral and Maxillofacial Pathologists, passing qualifying examinations in

- surgical oral and maxillofacial pathology (diagnosis via microscopic slides)
- clinical and radiographic oral and maxillofacial pathology (diagnosis via clinical and radiological images)
- oral and maxillofacial pathology
- general, systemic, and clinical pathology (written exam on pathology, tissue chemistry, cell biology, and basic science)

See also DENTISTRY; ENDODONTICS; ORAL AND MAXILLOFACIAL RADIOLOGY; ORAL AND MAXILLO-FACIAL SURGERY; ORTHODONTICS AND DENTOFACIAL ORTHOPEDICS; PEDIATRIC DENTISTRY; PERIODONTICS; PROSTHODONTICS; PUBLIC HEALTH DENTISTRY.

oral and maxillofacial radiology   One of the nine dental specialties approved by the AMERI-CAN DENTAL ASSOCIATION Council on Dental Education and Licensure. Oral and maxillofacial radiologists are dentists who have completed a postgraduate, in-hospital residency in radiology. They use the entire panoply of imaging techniques including conventional X-rays, digital imaging, CT scans, MRI (magnetic resonance imaging), and radiation therapy to diagnose and treat illnesses of the mouth, head, and neck. A board certified oral and maxillofacial radiologist, a specialist most likely to practice in a recognized medical center or hospital, has passed the examination administered by the American Board of Oral and Maxillofacial Radiology.

See also DENTISTRY; ENDODONTICS; ORAL AND MAXILLOFACIAL PATHOLOGY; ORAL AND MAXILLO-FACIAL SURGERY; ORTHODONTICS AND DENTOFACIAL ORTHOPEDICS; PEDIATRIC DENTISTRY; PERIODONTICS; PROSTHODONTICS; PUBLIC HEALTH DENTISTRY.

oral and maxillofacial surgery   One of the nine dental specialties approved by the AMERI-CAN DENTAL ASSOCIATION Council on Dental Education and Licensure. Oral and maxillofacial surgeons are graduates of a four-year dental school who have completed (at a minimum) a four-year, in-hospital, postgraduate surgical residency. They are trained to diagnose and perform reconstructive surgery to repair soft tissue and bone defects caused by injury, tumors, or birth defects. They are also trained in pain control, may treat facial pain, and may perform dental procedures such as the extraction of impacted wisdom teeth. A board-certified oral and maxillofacial surgeon has successfully completed written and oral examinations administered by the American Board of Oral and Maxillofacial Surgery.

See also DENTISTRY; ENDODONTICS; ORAL AND MAXILLOFACIAL PATHOLOGY; ORAL AND MAXILLOFACIAL RADIOLOGY; ORTHODONTICS AND DENTOFACIAL ORTHOPEDICS; PEDIATRIC DENTISTRY; PERIODONTICS; PROSTHODONTICS; PUBLIC HEALTH DENTISTRY.

oral cancer   Malignant tumors of the mouth and throat including the lip, tongue, gum, cheek, palate, salivary glands, and esophagus.

Symptoms and Diagnostic Path

The common symptoms of oral cancer include (but may not be limited to):

- white patches (*leukoplakia*) or red patches (*erythroplakia*) on the lips, mouth, gum, or inside of the cheek; the red patches are more likely than the white patches to become malignant
- a sore that does not heal
- unexplained bleeding from the oral tissues
- difficulty or pain while swallowing
- unexplained pain when wearing dentures
- swollen lymph glands in the neck
- unexplained earache
- unexplained change in OCCLUSION (the way the teeth meet when closed)

According to the American Association of Oral and Maxillofacial Surgeons, the most reliable tool for detecting early oral cancer is the basic dental checkup, during which the dentist visually and manually examines the lips, inside and out; the gums; the inside of the cheeks; the surface of the tongue; the tissues and glands under the tongue; the roof of the mouth; the area under the lower jaw. If the dentist discovers any irregularity in these areas, he is likely to perform a biopsy, taking a small sample of the tissue to be examined for signs of malignancy.

Treatment Options and Outlook

Most oral cancers are treated surgically, after which the patient may undergo RADIATION THERAPY to destroy any remaining cancer cells. In some cases, the patient may be treated with chemotherapy, which are drugs known to kill cancer cells. The side effects of treatment for oral cancer and the outlook vary with the type and stage of the cancer.

Oral cancers, like other forms of cancer, are *staged* according to three characteristics: *T*, the size of the tumor and the tissues in the mouth to which it has spread; *N*, the location and numbers of nodes to which the cancer has spread; and *M*, the number of *metastases* spread to other organs in the body.

The following list provides the American Cancer Society descriptions of the stages of an oral cancer.

Stages of Oral Cancer
Stage 0/Tis, N0, M0: The cancer is *in situ* (*is*). It is confined to the outer layer of tissue in the mouth or throat. It has not penetrated to deeper layers and has not spread to any other parts of the mouth, or the lymph nodes, or other parts of the body.
Stage I/T1, N0, M0: The same as Stage 0, except that the tumor may be as large as 2 centimeters (cm)/0.78 inch across.
Stage II/T2, N0, M0: The tumor is 2 cm/0.78 inches to 4 cm/1.5 inches wide but still has not spread to other areas of the mouth or to the lymph nodes or to distant sites in the body.
Stage III/T3, N0, M0: The tumor is larger than 4 cm/3 inches, but still has not spread.
Stage III/T1, N1, M0 or T2, N1, M0 or T3, N1, M0. The tumor may be small or large, has not spread to other tissues in the mouth or throat or to distant sites in the body, but it has spread to one lymph node on the same

side of the head or neck and the metastasis is smaller than 3 cm/1.18 inches.

Stage IV A/T4, N0, M0 or T4, N1, M0: The tumor, of any size, has invaded other tissues in the mouth. It has either not spread to the lymph nodes or it has spread to one lymph node on the same side of the head or neck (the metastasis is smaller than 3 cm/1.18 inches). The tumor has not spread to distant sites in the body.

Stage IV A/Any T, N2, M0: The tumor, of any size, may or may not have spread to other tissues in the mouth; it has not spread to other parts of the body but it has spread to either one lymph node on the same side of the head and neck or one lymph node on the opposite side of the head and neck or more than one lymph node on either side, all metastases smaller than 3 cm/1.18 inches.

Stage IV B/Any T, N3, M0: The tumor is any size and may or may not invade nearby structures. It has spread to one or more lymph nodes; the metastasis is larger than 6 cm/2.3 inches across. The tumor has not spread to distant sites.

Stage IV C/Any T, Any N, M1: The tumor is any size, and it may or may not have spread to lymph nodes, but it has spread to distant sites in the body, most commonly the lungs.

Source: Adapted from American Cancer Society, "Detailed Guide: Oral Cavity and Oropharyngeal Cancer. How Are Oral Cavity and Oropharyngeal Cancers Staged?" Revised September 28, 2007. Available online. URL: www.cancer.org/docroot/CRI/content/CRI_2_4_3X_How_is_oral_cavity_and_oropharyngeal_cancer_staged_60.asp.

Risk Factors and Preventive Measures

The risk factors for oral cancer include age and gender, tobacco use and excess use of alcohol, exposure to the virus known to cause cervical cancer (HPV-16), and exposure to sunlight.

Age and Gender Approximately 95 percent of the nearly 30,000 cases of oral cancer detected each year in the United States occur in people older than 40, more commonly in men than in women.

Tobacco Use The most common risk factors for oral cancer is tobacco, either smoked or chewed. Some types of oral cancer are tied to specific uses of tobacco. For example, pipe smoking is commonly linked to cancer of the lip, while chewing tobacco is most firmly linked to cancer inside the mouth.

Alcohol Beverages Excess use of alcohol, particularly in combination with tobacco use, is a risk factor for oral cancer.

Human Papilloma Virus (HPV-16) In May 2007, researchers at the Johns Hopkins Kimmel Cancer Center reported that a significant number of cases of oral cancer (esophagus) may be linked to oral sex that exposes the participant to HPV-16, the virus known to cause cervical cancer. The risk rises with the number of partners; the Johns Hopkins figures suggest that persons with multiple partners of oral sex have a risk of HPV-related cancer more than 8 percent higher than persons who are not exposed to the virus.

Frequent Exposure to Sunlight As with any cancer of the skin, exposure to sunlight is a risk factor for cancer of the lip.

See also LIP, CANCER OF; SALIVARY GLANDS, CANCER OF; TONGUE CANCER.

Oral Health in America: A Report of the Surgeon General

In May 2000, then–Surgeon General David Satcher released *Oral Health in America*, the first-ever Surgeon General report on the relationship between oral health and overall good health. The report identified a "silent epidemic" of dental and oral conditions such as tooth DECAY, PERIODONTAL DISEASE, mouth sores, oral birth defects, chronic facial pain, and ORAL CANCER that "may interfere with vital functions such as breathing, eating, swallowing, and speaking. The burden of disease restricts activities in school, work, and home, and often significantly diminishes the quality of life."

The Organization of the Report

The report is organized into five multichapter sections, each section addressing various aspects of one major question of oral health practice and policy.

Part One: What Is Oral Health? Chapter 1 discusses the link between oral health and general health. Chapter 2 provides a guide to the structure and development of the organs and tissues of the face and head, explaining the role each plays in maintaining essential body functions such as speech and nutrition.

Part Two: What Is the Status of Oral Health in America? Chapter 3 is a guide to the common disease and disorders affecting the craniofacial complex. Chapter 4 offers a report on the oral-health status and dental habits of people in the United States; where possible, the chapter adds information regarding specific groups such as children, adults, and certain ethnic groups.

Part Three: What Is the Relationship Between Oral Health and General Health and Well-being? Chapter 5 focuses on the way in which the health of the mouth reflects or predicts the health of the body. Chapter 6 lays out the relationship between oral health and quality of life, including the effects of poor oral health on such basic physical and psychological functions as appearance, speech, nutrition, education, self-esteem, and interaction with others.

Part Four: How Is Oral Health Promoted and Maintained and How Are Oral Diseases Prevented? Chapter 7 is a review of studies detailing the effectiveness of health promotion and disease prevention, particularly community-based efforts to prevent oral and dental disease such as tooth decay and tooth loss. Chapter 8 looks at the ways in which individual consumers and health-care providers can promote measures to improve oral health. Chapter 9 focuses specially on the pragmatic roles played by dental professionals, other health-care providers, and public

health agencies in providing and paying for oral health care.

Part Five: What Are the Needs and Opportunities to Enhance Oral Health? Chapter 10 evaluates the use of oral and dental health care in various social groups at different stages of life. Chapter 11 details the possibility of scientific discovery in promoting dental and oral health care, with special emphasis on recent advances in genetics and molecular biology. Chapter 12 reviews the themes of the report to set forth eight major categories of findings and proposals.

Major Findings

The importance of *Oral Health in America* is that the report brought the Surgeon General to draw specific conclusions regarding oral health among Americans. These conclusions are designed to enable laymen, professionals, and government policymakers to draw up proposals for implementing changes in their approach to improve oral health as the nation entered the 21st century.

Among the most important findings in the report are the following:

Dental Decay

- Tooth decay ranks high on the list of common childhood disease, five times as common as asthma and seven times as common as hay fever among American children aged five to 17 years.

- By age 17, nearly 80 percent of young Americans have developed at least one cavity.

Periodontal Disease

- Nearly half of all Americans age 35 to 44 have had gingivitis (inflammation of the gums); nearly a quarter have developed periodontal disease serious enough to destroy gum or bone tissue.

- Among adults aged 45–54, most have symptoms of gingivitis or periodontal disease. Nearly 15 percent have periodontal disease severe enough to have caused loss of the attachment of the gum tissue to the tooth producing a "pocket" 6 mm deep.

- Nearly a quarter of Americans aged 65 to 74 have similarly severe periodontal disease.
- At all ages, men are more likely than women to have severe periodontal disease.

Tooth Loss

- By age 17, 7 percent of young Americans have lost at least one permanent tooth.
- Nearly seven of every 10 Americans age 35 to 44 had lost at least one permanent tooth.
- Approximately three of every 10 Americans older than 65 had lost all natural teeth. Although high, this number is 16 percent lower than it was in 1980.

Other Oral Health Issues

- Nearly 20 percent of American adults aged 25 to 44 have had an oral viral infection (*Herpes labialis*/cold sores) or an oral ulcer (canker sore).
- 22 percent of American adults have experienced oral/facial pain in the past six months from a condition such as TRIGEMINAL NEURAL-GIA, facial shingles (post-herpetic neuralgia), or TEMPOROMANDIBULAR JOINT DISORDER (TMD).
- A significant number of cancer patients who do not have oral cancer experience oral symptoms from medication or radiation therapy for their disease.
- Patients whose immune system has been weakened by an HIV infection or medication for an organ transplant are at higher than normal risk for an oral fungal infection.

Economic Issues

- More than 108 million Americans did not have dental insurance.
- For every child without medical insurance, there are 2.6 children without dental insurance.

For every adult without medical insurance, three were also without dental insurance.

- Fewer than one of every five children covered by Medicaid had a single dental visit in a year.
- American children lose more than 51 million school hours a year and American adults lose more than 160 million work hours a year due to dental illness.

Recommendations of the Report

Having outlined the problems, the Surgeon General then called for a national effort to improve oral health among Americans by changing perceptions regarding oral health and disease among the public, their health care providers, and government policymakers on every level so as to make maintaining oral health an accepted component of any public health regimen.

In addition, the report:

- advocated programs to teach Americans about common preventive tactics, including personal daily oral hygiene habits such as brushing with a fluoride toothpaste and flossing daily
- urged health-care providers to practice interventions such as the use of dental SEALANTS to protect teeth and examinations to check for cancer of the mouth and throat
- suggested putting into effect expanded community-based programs such as water fluoridation and tobacco cessation
- recommended expanding and speeding up the scientific research required to identify the relationship between chronic dental disorders such as periodontal disease and general health problems such as diabetes; pinpoint the people most at risk for serious oral health conditions; translate current research findings into targeted and effective health problem prevention methods; and promote their adoption by the public and the health professions
- remove social and economic barriers to oral health services and, when applicable, use pub-

lic-private partnerships to facilitate treatment for those in need

This entry represents a précis of *Oral Health in America* (2000). The entire report is available online at www.surgeongeneral. gov/library/oralhealth.

See also NATIONAL CALL TO ACTION TO PROMOTE ORAL HEALTH.

oral hygiene The preventive and proactive regimen designed to strengthen the surface of the teeth and clean the mouth so as to reduce the build up of dental PLAQUE, thus lowering the risk of dental DECAY, PERIODONTAL DISEASE, and tooth loss.

The techniques and tools used to accomplish this include (but are not limited to):

- brushing teeth twice a day
- flossing daily (or when required) to remove debris between teeth
- regular use of fluoridated toothpaste and mouthwash as prescribed by the dentist, in amounts appropriate to the age of the patient
- use of an antiseptic mouthwash or rinse, as prescribed by the dentist
- use of fluoridated drinking water (or fluoride supplements *only* as prescribed by the dentist)
- regular professional dental and periodontal examinations including SCALING (removal of dental plaque); evaluation or the oral cavity; dental X-rays where required; and application of dental SEALANTS

According to the American Dental Association's "2003 Public Opinion Survey: Oral Health of the U.S. Population," women were more likely than men to brush their teeth after every meal and also more likely to visit a dentist on a regular basis (see GENDER AND ORAL HEALTH). In addition, a comparison between the previous ADA survey

in 1997 and the 2003 survey whose subjects included 1,014 adults older than 18 who identified themselves as the head of household shows a clear increase in the number of Americans practicing good oral hygiene measures.

For example:

- the percentage of those brushing twice a day rose from 75.4 in 1997 to 78 percent in 2003
- the percentage of those brushing after every meal rose from 11.5 in 1997 to 24.8 percent in 2003
- the number of those using dental floss or another method to clean between the teeth rose from 48.2 in 1997 to 50.5 percent in 2003

See FLUORIDE; MOUTHWASH; TOOTHBRUSH.

oral moisturizers See SALIVA SUBSTITUTES/STIMULANTS.

oral surgery See BIOPSY; JAW, FRACTURE; TEMPOROMANDIBULAR JOINT DISORDER.

oral tumors See LIPS, CANCER OF; ORAL CANCER; PREGNANCY GRANULOMA; SALIVARY GLANDS, CANCER OF; TONGUE CANCER.

orthodontic braces Orthodontic braces are metal appliances that may include ceramic or plastic components bonded to the surface of the tooth (orthodontic bracket) or cemented around the entire tooth (orthodontic band). The entire system works to apply increasing amounts of pressure to correct a MALOCCLUSION by moving crooked or crowded teeth into a more effective and attractive alignment.

Procedure

Once the orthodontist has determined the patient's need for braces, the process of attaching the braces begins.

- *Step One:* The orthodontist or her assistant checks the teeth for CAVITIES and then cleans the teeth so as to reduce the risk of future cavities under the orthodontic appliances and to insure that the components of the braces will fit perfectly onto each tooth.

- *Step Two:* The orthodontist or her assistant will measure the teeth and four farthest back teeth (used to anchor the archwire) to find the appropriate size band for the teeth. Each band has a buccal tube (a small tube on the cheek side of the teeth) through which the archwire will be threaded and anchored.

- *Step Three:* Once the teeth are cleaned and dried, and the appropriate bands have been chosen, the orthodontist will coat the inside of the bands with cement and then push the bands onto each of the back teeth and ask the patient to bite down on a tool called a bite stick to force the band into place. Once the bands are in place on the back teeth, the orthodontist will ask the patient to bite down on a cotton pad to hold the bands in place while the adhesive cement hardens firmly. Once the cement hardens, the orthodontist uses a *scaler*—a sharp instrument commonly used during periodontal treatment to remove CALCULUS from the teeth—to scrape away excess adhesive.

- *Step Four:* The orthodontist will bond small brackets to the front and side teeth. The brackets are used to hold the archwire next to the teeth. For bonding, the teeth are dried and then etched to rough the surface so the brackets will hold securely.

- *Step Five:* When the brackets are securely in place the archwire is placed in the brackets and anchored through the buccal tubes on the bands on the back teeth.

Risks and Complications

Getting braces put onto the teeth is uncomfortable but not painful. As with any dental procedure, there may be some pain afterward and for a few days or weeks as the teeth adjust to the new pressure. In addition, the appliances may rub against the inside of the lips and cheeks as well as the tongue.

The discomfort usually responds to simple over-the-counter pain relievers such as aspirin or acetaminophen (Tylenol). The orthodontist often provides a waxy coating that can temporarily cover any rough edges that need to be trimmed and smoothed when the patient returns for a visit a few weeks later.

Outlook and Lifestyle Modifications

The patient returns to the orthodontist every few weeks to have the archwire tightened or changed as the teeth begin to move into their new position. Eventually, the teeth settle into place, the braces are removed, and the patient is given a *retainer* to wear at night as the jawbone

COMPONENTS OF ORTHODONTIC BRACES

Component	Purpose
Archwire	Metal wire that moves the teeth
Band	Flat metal ring on the back teeth that anchors the archwire
Bracket	Metal or ceramic "hook" that holds the archwire against each tooth
Buccal tube	Metal tube on the outer, cheek side of a banded tooth that anchors the archwire
Ligature module	Doughnut-shaped plastic part used to hold archwires in brackets
Lip bumper	An archwire attached to a molded piece of plastic; used to push the molars in the lower jaw farther back so as to make more room for other teeth
Retainer	Wire and plastic or all-plastic device that holds teeth in place after braces are removed and the bone settles firmly into its permanent position
Separator	Plastic or metal device used to create space between adjoining teeth so that bands fit comfortably

TOOLS USED ON ORTHODONTIC BRACES

Tool	Purpose
Band remover	Small plierslike tool to remove bands
Bite stick	Tool on which the patient bites to force bands into place
Cheek retractors	Plastic brackets used to hold back the lips and cheeks so the orthodontist has a clear view of the mouth while putting the braces on
Curing light	Bright blue light used to cure (harden) the adhesive used to attach brackets to the teeth
Distal end cutter	Small pliers used to cut archwires threaded through the bands on the back (distal) teeth
Interproximal stripper	Instrument that shaves off very small amounts of enamel from the tooth surface to create more space between teeth.
Scaler	Tool commonly used to remove debris during periodontal treatment; used in orthodontics to scrape away excess adhesive and check for spaces

hardens to hold the teeth in place. When this process is complete, the patient can discard the retainer.

Successful treatment with orthodontic braces produces a normal occlusion that enables the patient to chew and speak effectively. In addition, the new alignment of the teeth has beneficial cosmetic effects, producing a more attractive appearance.

See also INVISALIGN.

orthodontics and dentofacial orthopedics The term *orthodontics,* coined by French dentist Joachim LeFoulon in 1841, comes from the Greek words *ortho-,* meaning "straight" and *dont-* or *donto-,* meaning "tooth." The term *dentofacial orthopedics* refers to the development of the bones of the face and JAW.

Orthodontics and dentofacial orthopedics, one of the nine dental specialties approved by the AMERICAN DENTAL ASSOCIATION Council on Dental Education and Licensure, is concerned with the defects in the alignment of the teeth and jaws as well as the development of the facial structure. A modern orthodontist is a dentist who has graduated from an accredited dental school and then a two-to-three year orthodontist-supervised graduate residency program in the specialty of orthodontics. A board-certified orthodontist has passed the American Board of Orthodontics qualifying written and clinical examinations.

The primary treatment offered by orthodontists is the use of braces and appliances such as a FACEBOW to exert force that moves crooked teeth into a more normal alignment. If the teeth are crowded together, orthodontists may also extract teeth to provide the space for a normal dental ARCH. If the arch itself is very narrow, they may use an EXPANDER to widen it. In addition to correcting MALOCCLUSION, orthodontists may also treat TEMPOROMANDIBULAR JOINT DISORDER.

According to the American Association of Orthodontists, mummified remains suggest that the Greeks and early Romans attempted to straighten teeth with a metal band pulled together with threads or material such as catgut (see SUTURE), and later, gold WIRE. It was not until the 19th century, however, that orthodontics began to evolve into a recognized branch of dentistry.

Among the dates important to the evolution of orthodontics as a dental specialty are:

- *1728:* French dentist PIERRE FAUCHARD publishes *The Surgeon Dentist* with the first known chapter on methods used to straighten teeth, specifically with his own invention, a device called a *bandeau* or *bandolet,* an early dental expander.

- *1757:* French dentist Etienne Bourdet publishes *The Dentist's Art* with a chapter on straightening teeth and the various appliances available to do so. (Bourdet was also the first to have recommended extracting back teeth to provide room for other teeth in the jaw and the first to offer scientific proof of the growth pattern of the human jaw.)

- *1771:* British surgeon John Hunter publishes the first English text on orthodontics, *The Natural History of the Human Teeth.*

- *1843:* Gum elastic bands (made of natural rubber) introduced for braces; rubber bands were introduced in 1850.

- *Late 1800s:* Eugene Solomon Talbot becomes the first person to use X-rays to diagnose malocclusion and plan orthodontic treatment.

- *1880:* Norman W. Kingsley, one of several "fathers of orthodontics," publishes *Treatise on Oral Deformities,* a classic work on orthodontics and facial development.

- *1888:* J. N. Farrar, a "father of modern orthodontia" and the first to suggest tightening braces periodically to increase the force used to move teeth into position, publishes his two-volume *A Treatise on the Irregularities of the Teeth and Their Corrections.*

- *1889:* J. H. Guilford publishes the first textbook on orthodontia for dental students.

- *1901:* EDWARD ANGLE, another "father of orthodontics," organizes the American Society of Orthodontics, later the American Association of Orthodontia.

- *1900s:* Gold, platinum, silver, steel, gum rubber, the mineral vulcanite, wood, ivory, zinc, copper, and brass are all used to create orthodontic appliances.

- *1920s:* Orthodontic appliances are formally christened "braces."

- *1927:* Stainless steel braces and orthodontic wires are introduced.

- *1929:* The American Board of Orthodontics, the first dental specialty board, is established.

- 1994: The American Dental Association approves the name Orthodontics and Dentofacial Orthopedics for the specialty of orthodontics.

- *1945:* Some orthodontics begin to use a series of plastic "aligner trays" instead of metal braces to create small adjustments in the alignment of teeth.

- *1955:* First bonding of orthodontic appliances directly to teeth.

- *1970s:* Introduction of clear ceramic or porcelain orthodontic appliances.

- *2000:* Introduction of INVISALIGN, a modern system of plastic trays designed to move teeth into alignment without metal braces.

In modern dentistry, instant orthodontics is a term used to describe various cosmetic dentistry techniques that appear to alter the shape or placement of a tooth without the use of braces. For example, the dentist may apply a VENEER to bring the surface forward into line with the teeth on either side or use a CROWN to make a tooth look straight. Instant orthodontics is practical only for patients whose teeth are slightly crowded or out of line; those with more serious abnormalities, such as buck teeth, will still require standard orthodontic treatment to alter the tooth placement.

See also DENTISTRY; ENDODONTICS; ORAL AND MAXILLOFACIAL PATHOLOGY; ORAL AND MAXILLOFACIAL RADIOLOGY; ORAL AND MAXILLOFACIAL SURGERY; PEDIATRIC DENTISTRY; PERIODONTICS; PROSTHODONTICS; PUBLIC HEALTH DENTISTRY.

osteoporosis   See BONE.

overbite   See MALOCCLUSION.

pain Pain is a sensation triggered when body tissue is injured, either accidentally or during medical or dental procedures such as drilling into a tooth to fill a CAVITY or trimming and repositioning gum tissue during periodontal surgery.

The Mechanism of Pain Reactions

When body tissue is damaged, it releases histamines and cytokines, IMMUNE SYSTEM chemicals that manage the inflammatory response (redness, swelling, and heat at the site of the injury). The histamines and cytokines hook onto nerve fibers, transmitting electrical impulses that travel along the nerve fibers to the spinal cord. In response, the spinal cord releases chemical signals that transmit a message to the brain, which identifies the message as pain of one sort or another. Analgesics and anesthetics alleviate pain by interrupting one or more of these reactions.

The Types of Pain Reactions

There are several types of pain reactions, each classified either by the cause of the pain or by the nerves or area of the body it affects or by how long it lasts.

- *Central pain* is pain originating in the central nervous system (brain and spinal cord). Examples are pain from a spinal cord injury or from an illness such as multiple sclerosis that attacks the central nervous system.
- *Neuropathic pain* (*neuropathy*) is pain originating in a nerve, triggered by a traumatic injury to a nerve or an illness that attacks the nerves

and nerve endings at the skin. One example is the pain due to the herpes virus infection shingles. Another is TRIGEMINAL NEURALGIA, a.k.a. *tic douloureux,* a disorder of the trigeminal nerve whose name derives from the fact that it divides into three branches: the optic nerve, the maxillary nerve, and the mandibular nerve. Trigeminal neuralgia produces severe pain in the lips, jaws, nose, eyes, forehead, and scalp.

- *Nociceptive pain* (from the Latin *nocere,* meaning "to injure") is a response to an injurious stimulus such as heat. An example of dental nociceptive pain is the temporary sensitivity to temperature changes such as very hot or very cold food that occurs after a tooth is filled, or the longer-lasting sensitivity to these stimuli that occurs when gum recession exposes the root of a tooth.
- *Peripheral pain* (from the Greek *peri-,* meaning "around," and *phero,* meaning "carry") is nociceptive pain arising from an injury to the periphery of the body, that is the parts farther away from the trunk such as the arms, legs, hands, and feet. *Visceral pain* (from the Latin word *viscera,* meaning "internal organs") is nociceptive pain originating in an internal organ such as the stomach or gallbladder. *Persistent pain* is a long-lasting sensation usually associated with damage to muscles and/or bones; for example, the pain that lingers after a broken jaw. Persistent pain may actually change the way the body perceives and responds to pain signals, increasing the amount of chemicals released when a pain signal reaches a nerve ending or encouraging

the growth of new nerves at the place on the spine where pain signals are received, so that persistent pain spreads out along nerve fibers causing discomfort in parts of the body not directly related to the injury.

- *Phantom pain* is pain at the site of a missing body part. One example of dental phantom pain is phantom ondontalgia, discomfort in the area from which a tooth has been extracted. Interestingly enough, phantom pain may be eased with the same analgesics and anesthetics that relieve other kinds of pain. Relaxation techniques such as biofeedback may also be useful.

- *Referred pain* is pain that originates in one part of the body but whose signals travel via nerve pathways to be perceived elsewhere. For example, pain due to a cavity in a molar in the upper jaw may be referred to the lower jaw so that the ache seems to come from there.

Measuring the Intensity of Pain

To evaluate a person's perception of the severity of his pain, doctors use a pain measurement scale. As a rule, adults are asked to rank their pain on a scale from 0 (no pain) to 10 (the worst possible pain). Children are asked to choose one of six pictures or drawings of faces whose expression ranges from smiling and happy to contorted as if in severe pain. To assess pain levels in patients who cannot speak, pain experts observe vital signs (heart rate, respiration, pulse, and temperature) along with the patient's general level of calm versus restlessness or agitation, the latter being more common when people are in pain.

pain measurement scale   See PAIN.

Parmly, Levi Spear (1790–1859)   American dentist, the first to identify a causative link between debris on the surface of the tooth and dental problems such as DECAY and PERIODONTAL DISEASE. Born in Vermont, Parmly practiced in New York and London before settling in New Orleans. His great contribution to dentistry was the idea that oral cleanliness would prevent dental disease. In 1819, well before the discovery of the activity of oral bacteria or the effects of dental plaque, Parmly published *A Practical Guide to the Management of the Teeth,* in which he listed three tools for oral cleanliness: toothbrush, dentifrice, and his own innovation, a silk thread to be drawn between the teeth thus removing debris the toothbrush could not reach. Parmly was innovative in other areas, as well. As an article in the August-November 1945 issue of the *Washington University Dental Journal* notes, in his book *Natural History of the Teeth* (1820), Parmly offered to teach dentistry to "ladies and gentlemen of liberal education," thus becoming one of the earliest Americans seeking to bring women into the dental profession.

pediatric dentistry   One of the nine dental specialties approved by the AMERICAN DENTAL ASSOCIATION Council on Dental Education and Licensure. A pediatric dentist is a professional specializing in the dental care and treatment of children from infancy through adolescence, as well as patients with special health-care needs.

A pediatric dentist has completed four years of dental school and a two-year residency in pediatric dentistry at an accredited dental school whose courses include oral pathology, advanced diagnostic and surgical procedures, including the management of oral and facial injuries and defects; radiology; sedation and anesthesia; along with child psychology and development, the use and effects of medicines in children, management of oral/facial trauma, and care for patients with special needs. A board-certified pediatric dentist has successfully completed this training and passed the American Board of Pediatric Dentistry's voluntary examination in the field.

See also DENTISTRY; ENDODONTICS; ORAL AND MAXILLOFACIAL PATHOLOGY; ORAL AND MAXILLOFACIAL RADIOLOGY; ORAL AND MAXILLOFACIAL SURGERY; ORTHODONTICS AND DENTOFACIAL ORTHOPEDICS; PERIODONTICS; PROSTHODONTICS; PUBLIC HEALTH DENTISTRY.

periodontal disease From the Latin prefix *perio-*, meaning "around," and *denta-*, meaning "tooth." Gum disease; inflammation and/or infection caused by bacteria in PLAQUE, a sticky colorless film that forms naturally on teeth. The bacteria excrete a toxin that inflames and eventually destroys the supporting gum and bone tissue.

Symptoms and Diagnostic Path

The common symptoms of periodontal disease are bleeding gums, pockets, recession, BONE loss, and tooth mobility.

Pockets All healthy teeth have a rim of gum tissue called a sulcus, a cufflike structure one to three millimeters deep. Bacteria present in the pocket causes the bone around the tooth to degenerate so that the gum pulls away from the tooth creating *pockets,* spaces between the tooth and the top of the gum that are more than three millimeters deep. The more severe the periodontal disease, the deeper the pockets will be.

Recession Gum recession is the disappearance of gum tissue. The recession may be due to a number of factors including periodontal disease, as well as BRUXISM, overaggressive toothbrushing, genetic predisposition, or movement of the teeth during orthodontic treatment. The extent of the recession is measured as the distance of the edge of the top of the gum from the cementoenamel junction (CEJ), the place where the ENAMEL covering the top of the tooth meets the CEMENTUM covering the tooth root.

Bone loss Bone loss is the destruction of bone due to periodontal disease. The amount of bone loss is measured by the ability to insert the periodontal probe into various sites on a tooth, as well as the appearance of the bone on radiographic images.

- Grade 1 bone loss allows the dentist to insert the probe into the groove between the tops of the roots on a multi-root tooth.
- Grade 2 loss allows the dentist to insert the probe into actual area of division between the roots.
- Grade 3 bone loss allows the dentist to insert the probe between the roots, from one side of the tooth to the other.

Tooth mobility As bone is lost, the teeth become less stable. To measure the amount of mobility, the dentist will use two blunt instruments to move the tooth back and forth or from side to side.

- Class I mobility is movement up to one millimeter.
- Class II mobility is movement between one millimeter and two millimeters.
- Class III mobility is movement greater than two millimeters and is depressible.

The American Academy of Periodontology (AAP) has developed a system for identifying and categorizing the stages of periodontal disease using broad descriptions based on easily observable criteria.

Table 1 shows the AAP classifications for stages of periodontal disease.

Treatment Options and Outlook

The first step in treating early periodontal disease is to establish a maintenance plan that includes (1) rigorous home care between dental visits and (2) periodic professional cleaning (SCALING) to remove plaque from the teeth and monitor the progress of the condition,

Progressive periodontal disease may require one or more of the following reconstructive surgeries:

TABLE 1. AMERICAN ACADEMY OF PERIODONTOLOGY TYPES OF GUM DISEASE

Disease Stage	Characteristics
Gingivitis	The mildest form of periodontal disease, characterized by reddened, mildly swollen gums that bleed easily during toothbrushing
Aggressive periodontitis	An active form of periodontal disease in people who are otherwise healthy, characterized by sudden, rapid loss of gum and bone tissue
Chronic periodontitis	The most common form of periodontal disease, characterized by continuing gum inflammation, formation of spaces (pockets) between tooth and gum, continuing gum recession (shrinkage), and loss of supporting bone
Periodontitis/ Chronic illness	Periodontal disease triggered by another chronic medical condition, commonly diabetes, heart disease, or respiratory problems
Necrotizing periodontal disease	The most severe form of periodontal disease, characterized by the necrosis (death) of gum tissue; commonly associated with medical conditions that weaken or destroy the immune system such as HIV/AIDS, malnutrition, or the use of immunosuppressant drugs after organ transplant

Source: American Academy of Periodontology, "Types of Gum Disease," *Perio.org*. Modified May 8, 2008. Available online. URL: www.perio.org/consumer/2a.html.

- *Pocket reduction:* Surgery to cut away loose gum tissue, reattach the gum to the tooth, and thus reduce the area in which bacteria flourish.

- *Bone replacement:* Addition of natural or synthetic material to act as a scaffold on which the natural bone can regenerate.

- *Soft tissue grafts:* Use of tissue lifted from the adjacent gum or the palate to cover areas where the original gum has been lost.

Patients who lose teeth to periodontal disease may be candidates for dental implants, small devices inserted into the remaining jaw as anchors for replacement teeth. Note: Once a tooth is removed, the periodontal disease at that site ceases; it does not resume if a false tooth is inserted but progressive periodontal disease on adjacent teeth may affect the stability of the implant.

Risk Factors and Preventive Measures

Periodontal disease often runs in families; the most common risk factor is a genetic susceptibility that may affect as many as one in every three adults in the United States.

Several medical factors influence the progress and intensity of periodontal disease. Fluctuating levels of estrogen at puberty, during menstruation, and during pregnancy can contribute to temporary local inflammation and deterioration, because unlike testosterone, which builds new bone, estrogen plays a role in breaking down old bone. Emotional or physical stress can reduce the effectiveness of the immune system, making gums more susceptible to bacteria. Other factors include specific illnesses such as diabetes, and certain drugs including (but not limited to) oral contraceptives, antidepressants, and some drugs used to treat heart disease.

Other risk factors for periodontal disease include tobacco use; in particular, smoking heats the gum tissue, making it more susceptible to bacterial injury; and clenching the jaws or grinding the teeth, especially while sleeping, puts extra pressure on the teeth and may hasten bone loss.

See also BONE; DENTURE; GRAFT; GUIDED BONE REPLACEMENT; GUM RESHAPING; JAW.

periodontics, periodontology From the Greek prefix *peri-*, meaning "around," and the word *odonto*, meaning "tooth." Periodontics is the branch of dentistry that specializes in the treatment of conditions affecting the tissues (gums, bone) that support and nourish the teeth, one of the nine dental specialties approved by the AMERICAN DENTAL ASSOCIATION Council on Dental Education and Licensure.

A periodontist is a graduate of an accredited dental school who has completed an accredited two to three years of postgraduate residency in periodontal dentistry. A board-certified periodontist has successfully completed the American Board of Periodontology qualifying examinations.

See also DENTISTRY; ENDODONTICS; ORAL AND MAXILLOFACIAL PATHOLOGY; ORAL AND MAXILLOFACIAL RADIOLOGY; ORAL AND MAXILLOFACIAL SURGERY; ORTHODONTICS AND DENTOFACIAL ORTHOPEDICS; PEDIATRIC DENTISTRY; PERIODONTAL DISEASE; PROSTHODONTICS; PUBLIC HEALTH DENTISTRY.

pH A system created by Danish biochemist Søren Peter Lauritz Sørensen in 1909 to quantify the acidity of water-based solutions such as coffee, various household chemicals, and the body fluids SALIVA, blood, and urine.

Sørensen's system equates acidity with the presence of particles called hydronium ions (hydrogen ions), hence the formal name *pondus hydrogenii* (the Latin for *potential hydrogen*), abbreviated as pH. The pH scale runs from 0 to 14, with the most acidic solutions at the lower end and their chemical opposites, the most basic (formerly alkaline) solutions at the higher end. For example, stomach acid (a solution of hydrochloride acid—HCl) is rated at 1 while a sodium hydroxide (NaOH), a.k.a. lye-based liquid drain cleaner is rated at 14, and pure (distilled) water is 7, the neutral center of the pH scale.

Human body fluids are also in the neutral range. For example, saliva is normally 6.5–7.5, a pH that facilitates the activity of enzymes required for digesting food while protecting the enamel surface of the teeth and the mucous membrane of the esophagus by neutralizing any stomach acids that may flow back into the esophagus (throat) during an episode of acid reflux.

The following table shows the pH of some well-known water-based solutions grouped into commonly accepted ranges of pH. For example, lemon juice (2.3) and vinegar (2.9) are both listed as 2.

PH OF SELECTED WATER-BASED SOLUTIONS

pH	Solution
0	Hydrochloric acid (HCl)
1	Stomach acid
2	Lemon juice, vinegar
3	Orange juice, grapefruit juice, beer, wine, cola drinks
4	Tomato juice, whiskey
5	Black coffee
6	Urine
7	Pure (distilled) water, human blood, saliva
8	Seawater
9	Baking soda solution
10	Milk of magnesia
11	Household ammonia
12	Household bleach
13	Oven cleaner
14	Liquid drain cleaner (sodium hydroxide/lye/NaOH)

piercing, oral Cosmetic procedure that involves puncturing the skin or mucous MEMBRANE in or around the mouth with a hollow needle to make a hole into which the patient may insert a piece of jewelry through the LIPS, TONGUE, or cheek.

Procedure

The site to be pierced is cleaned with an antiseptic, pierced, and cleaned again with an antiseptic. A temporary post (small metal rod) is inserted to keep the hole open as it heals.

In tongue piercing, the rod is typically placed at the front of the tongue through the groove in the middle. Placement on lip or cheek is a matter of the patient's aesthetic preference. Once the pierced area has healed, a process that may take several weeks, the temporary post is removed and the patient is able to insert a piece of jewelry into the opening.

Risks and Complications

Pain, swelling, or scarring around the pierced area are common, as in an increase in the flow of saliva. Allergic reactions may occur if the post or jewelry is made of nickel or brass rather than nonreactive titanium, 14-carat (or finer) gold, or surgical-grade steel. The pierced area may also become infected.

Complications specific to a dental (lip, tongue) piercing may include chipped teeth, receding gums, irritation under the tongue, excess scar tissue, and NEURALGIA triggered by the stud's irritating a nerve under the tongue connected to the trigeminal nerve. Finally, the lips and tongue are supplied with multiple blood vessels through which an infection may spread to major organs. In addition, the National Institutes of Health has identified body piercing as a possible source of transmission of blood-borne disease such as hepatitis and HIV/AIDS via nonsterile instruments or procedures.

Regardless of the piercing site, complications from body piercing are least likely to occur when a surgeon or another trained professional does the procedure. Currently, 43 states have legislated regulations for training nonmedical persons who perform piercing and the facilities in which they work and/or requirements for parental consent for body piercing for minors.

Outlook and Lifestyle Modifications

Pierced skin or mucous membrane commonly heals within two months or less; to speed healthy healing, patients are advised to avoid handling and moving the jewelry.

plaque Dental plaque is a biofilm, a thin sticky layer of microorganisms and other natural material that forms on the surface of a body part such as teeth and gums. Dental plaque is composed primarily (97 percent of the weight) of bacteria, primarily streptococcus organisms, plus components of SALIVA and other natural materials such as blood cells and minerals, all held together in a matrix (network) of proteins, fats, and complex carbohydrates. Plaque forms first as a soft film. If it is not cleaned from the teeth, it picks up minerals, primarily calcium, and hardens into a substance called CALCULUS, which is more difficult to remove.

Plaque is categorized in three ways: by its place on the tooth in relation to the top of the gum, by how it relates to the surface of the tooth, and by whether the majority of the bacteria in the plaque is likely to cause illness.

- *Gum position* Supragingival plaque is plaque on the tooth above the gum line. Subgingival plaque is plaque between the tooth and gum. The bacteria in plaque release acidic compounds that damage the tooth and other tissues. The accumulation of supragingival plaque (plaque above the gum line) increases the risk of dental DECAY. Subgingival plaque (plaque and calculus below the gum line) releases compounds that trigger inflammation and increases the risk of periodontal disease.

- *Tooth surface* Attached plaque is plaque tightly stuck on the surface of the tooth in a pocket between the tooth and gum. Unattached plaque, also known as epithelium associated plaque, is only loosely attached to the surface of the tooth.

- *Bacterial composition* Health-associated plaque and disease-associated plaque are differentiated by the primary bacteria component: that is, whether the bacteria in the plaque are likely to trigger illness.

Symptoms and Diagnostic Path

At home, a patient can perform a rudimentary diagnosis simply by running his tongue over his teeth. Clean surfaces are smooth; surfaces with plaque feel rough. A second home diagnostic aid is a test using a disclosing tablet or disclosing solution that contains red dye that stains bacteria. To perform this test, the patient chews the tablet and lets it mix with saliva or takes a small amount of a disclosing solution into his mouth. The he swishes the saliva-tablet mix or the solution over teeth and gums, spits out the solutions, rinses with cool water, and examines his teeth for pink stains. Then he brushes the stained areas until the dye (and the plaque) are gone. (Note: Because the dye stains bacteria, there may be some pink spots on lips, tongue, and gums.)

During a periodontal examination, plaque above the gum line is visible to the periodontist, dentist, or dental assistant. Plaque under the gum is detected by scaling the teeth, that is, inserting a dental probe between the tooth and the gum to scrape away plaque and calculus. The probe is a slim dental tool used to explore a dental cavity such as an area of decay or the space between the tooth and gum.

A manual probe is a simple hand tool that measures the depth of the space from the tip of the probe to the gingival margin (the place where the gum meets the tooth). An ultrasonic probe projects a narrow beam of high- frequency ultrasonic energy waves into the space between tooth and gum and measures the depth of the space by analyzing the energy waves bouncing back at the instrument. A furcation probe and a Nabers furcation probe are instruments that measure the amount of bone lost from the groove (furcation) between the roots on teeth with more than one root.

Treatment Options and Outlook

The treatment for plaque is to remove it from the teeth with conscientious home brushing and flossing plus regularly scheduled professional periodontal cleaning. In some cases, the periodontist or dentist may recommend a dental SEALANT to protect the surface of the tooth from the acidity of the bacteria in plaque.

Risk Factors and Preventive Measures

The most common risk factor for dental plaque is the failure to keep teeth clean.

See PERIODONTAL DISEASE.

porcelain See CROWN.

post See CROWN.

pregnancy and dental health When a woman is pregnant, she faces several challenges to her dental health, some driven by changes in her body, others by consideration for the fetus.

Diet

It is a myth that pregnant women lose a tooth for every pregnancy due to the fetus drawing calcium from the mother's teeth. A nutritious diet with adequate amounts of calcium meets the requirements of both mother and child. If the diet is lacking in calcium, the fetus may draw calcium from the mother's bones, but not the teeth.

Oral Hygiene

During pregnancy, a woman's body produces larger amounts of the female hormones estrogen and progesterone. The latter increases blood flow through the body, including to the gums, increasing the risk of inflammation and infection. It is important to counter this risk with home care and professional checkups.

Home Care To reduce the risk of PERIODONTAL DISEASE during pregnancy, dental professionals recommend brushing twice a day with a fluoride toothpaste to remove PLAQUE and cleaning between the teeth with dental FLOSS and a small brush called an interdental. The dentist may also recommend an antibacterial MOUTHWASH. If episodes of nausea ("morning sickness") influence the sense of taste, making it difficult to maintain oral hygiene, the dentist may recommend a bland toothpaste and/or mouthwash.

Dental Examinations Dental professionals recommend maintaining a regular schedule of dental and periodontal examinations and cleaning to remove plaque and other irritants. Any obvious changes in the gums—redness, swelling, bleeding—should be reported immediately to the dentist/periodontist.

Dental Treatment Unless there is an emergency—for example, a dental infection or a "KNOCKED-OUT TOOTH"—the Department of Dentistry at the Cleveland Clinic recommends avoiding dental procedures during the first trimester of pregnancy when the fetal organs are forming and during the second half of the third trimester to avoid the discomfort of sitting in the dental chair and/or any possibility of triggering premature delivery. As a rule, elective procedures, such as bleaching the teeth or applying cosmetic VENEERS, should be put off until after delivery.

Dental Medicines Some medications used to treat dental problems can cross the placenta and affect the developing fetus. Perhaps the best known example is tetracycline antibiotics, which may stain fetal teeth. The authoritative guide to the use of medications for pregnant women is the U.S. Food and Drug Administration classification of prescription drugs by the risk they pose to the fetus. The first FDA risk categories were created in the late 1970s and updated several times since then. In 2008, the FDA Center for Drug Evaluation and Research (CDER) proposed consideration of several changes in these listings:

- An explanation of the categories to make it clear that drugs in different categories may pose similar risks.

- Language to clarify the distinction between risks to animals and risks to human beings.

- A suggestion to replace the A, B, C, D, and X categories with three statements for each class of drugs: A one-sentence summary of the risk to the fetus; a list of clinical considerations such as dosing instructions and the risk of the condition the drug is used to treat; and a section with specific information about the tests on which a risk assessment is based, such as the species of animals used in the studies and the exact nature of any fetal abnormalities associated with the drug.

CURRENT CATEGORIES FOR DRUG USE IN PREGNANCY

Category	Description
A	Adequate, well-controlled studies in pregnant women have not shown an increased risk of fetal abnormalities.
B	Animal studies have revealed no evidence of harm to the fetus; however, there are no adequate and well-controlled studies in pregnant women.
	or
	Animal studies have shown an adverse effect, but adequate and well-controlled studies in pregnant women have failed to demonstrate a risk to the fetus.
C	Animal studies have shown an adverse effect and there are no adequate and well-controlled studies in pregnant women.
	or
	No animal studies have been conducted and there are no adequate and well-controlled studies in pregnant women.
D	Studies, adequate and well-controlled or observational, in pregnant women have demonstrated a risk to the fetus. However, the benefits of therapy may outweigh the potential risk.
X	Studies, adequate and well-controlled or observational, in animals or pregnant women have demonstrated positive evidence of fetal abnormalities. The use of the product is contraindicated in women who are or may become pregnant.

Source: Meadows, Michelle, "Pregnancy and the Drug Dilemma," *FDA Consumer Magazine,* May/June 2001. Available online. URL: www.fda.gov/fdac/features/2001/301_preg.html.

These changes have not yet been implemented. The table above shows the current categories for drugs used during pregnancy.

Dental X-Rays Although modern dental X-rays are extremely safe for both mother and fetus, most dental experts recommend avoiding the procedure except in an emergency such as a fractured jaw.

See also EATING DISORDER; EROSION, DENTAL; PREGNANCY GINGIVITIS; PREGNANCY GRANULOMA.

pregnancy gingivitis An inflammation of the GINGIVA (gums) associated with increased levels of the female hormone progesterone during pregnancy. The progesterone, which is essential to a successful pregnancy:

- develops the endometrium (the surface of the uterus in which the fertilized egg implants) and keeps it thickened throughout pregnancy
- enables the placenta to support the developing fetus
- bulks up the mucus plug covering the cervix (the opening from the uterus) to prevent the entrance of harmful microorganisms
- prevents the uterus from contracting until it is time for birth
- stimulates the growth of breast tissue while preventing lactation until the baby is born

However, the higher progesterone levels increase blood circulation throughout the body, including to the gums, which may be red and swollen, a condition known as pregnancy gingivitis and is similar to MENSTRUAL GINGIVITIS, a condition that occurs when progesterone levels peak midway through the menstrual cycle. Higher progesterone levels may also lower a woman's resistance to bacteria normally present in the mouth, thus raising the risk of inflammation and infection.

Symptoms and Diagnostic Path

Redness, swelling, and bleeding at the gum line (the place where the top of the gum meets a tooth). They can start as early as the second month. The condition tends to peak around the eighth month and then taper off after the baby is born. Pregnancy gingivitis most commonly occurs in the gums at the front of the mouth.

Treatment Options and Outlook

Switching to a softer TOOTHBRUSH and exercising care not to injure the gum while flossing helps avoid further irritations.

Risk Factors and Preventive Measures

The primary risk factor for pregnancy gingivitis is being a pregnant woman. The best prevention is to practice good oral hygiene. In addition, it is valuable to schedule regular dental/periodontal visits during pregnancy for professional cleaning to prevent gingivitis and treatment with the appropriate medication to prevent gingivitis from escalating to PERIODONTAL DISEASE.

See PREGNANCY AND DENTAL HEALTH; PREGNANCY GRANULOMA.

pregnancy granuloma   Pyrogenic granuloma, pregnancy tumor; a benign nodule (bump) on the gum, occurring in up to 10 percent of all pregnant women, most frequently in women whose gums are already inflamed due to PREGNANCY GINGIVITIS.

Symptoms and Diagnostic Path

These growths, which are attached to the gum by a slim piece of tissue, typically show up in the second trimester of pregnancy. They bleed easily and may either form a crust or develop into an ulcer on the gum.

Treatment Options and Outlook

Pregnancy granulomas disappear naturally once a woman has given birth. If the nodule makes it difficult to talk or eat, the dentist/periodontist may remove it before a woman gives birth, but there is no guarantee that it will not return.

Risk Factors and Preventive Measures

The list of risk factors for pregnancy granuloma includes injury to the tissue, hormonal swings during pregnancy, blood vessel malformations, and viral infections. However, there is no conclusive evidence for any of these. Many women with granulomas also have gingivitis, so keeping the mouth as clean as possible may be beneficial.

See GINGIVA; MENSTRUAL GINGIVITIS; PERIODONTAL DISEASE; PREGNANCY AND DENTAL HEALTH.

prescription From the Latin words *prae,* meaning "before," and *scribere,* meaning "to write," because a prescription is written before a medicine is made or given to the patient. The symbol for a prescription, *Rx,* comes from *recipe,* the past participle of the Latin verb *recipere,* meaning "to take."

With a few exceptions, such as D.A.W., the abbreviation for "dispense as written" (used when the dentist prefers the pharmacist to give the patient the brand name version of a drug), the directions on a prescription are usually written as abbreviation of Latin words in recognition of Latin's place as the first universal language. The following table shows some of the abbreviations used as common prescription directions.

ABBREVIATIONS USED IN PRESCRIPTIONS		
Abbreviation	**Latin Words**	**English Translation**
q4h, q.4.h.	*quaque quarta hora*	every four hours
qid, q.i.d.	*quater in die*	four times a day
q3h, q.3.h	*quaque 3 hora*	every three hours
tid, t.i.d	*ter in die*	three times a day
bid, b.i.d.	*bis in die*	two times a day
qh, q.h.	*quaque hora*	every hour
qd, q.d.	*quaque die*	every day
a.c.	*ante cibum*	before meals
p.c.	*post cibum*	after meals
p.o.	*per os*	by mouth
ut.dict.	*ut dictum*	as directed
ad lib	*ad libitum*	at will (i.e., as much as desired)
p.r.n.	*pro re nata*	"for the thing born," i.e., as required

pressure, bite See OCCLUSION.

process In dentistry, the word *process* has two definitions. The first defines an anatomical prominence (raised projection) on a bone. The second defines a specific stage in embryonic development.

One example of the first meaning of the word is the alveolar process, the ridge on the upper or lower jaw in which the teeth sit to create the dental ARCH. Other dental prominences include the condyloid process and the coronoid process, the two bumps at the top of the ramus, the flat bone that points upward from the back of the lower jaw toward the temporal bone (the flat bone at the side of the skull).

Two examples of the second dental meaning of the word process are the maxillary process and mandibular process. Each is a stage in the development of the mammalian embryonic structures, when the branchial arches come together to form, respectively, the upper and lower jaws. Failure of these arches to join correctly may lead to birth defects that require surgical repair.

prognathism An extremely prominent lower JAW (mandible) and overdeveloped lower lip resulting from a misalignment of the facial bones. The practical result is that the surfaces of the teeth do not meet properly, making it difficult for a person to chew or speak properly.

Symptoms and Diagnostic Path
Prognathism is obvious upon visual examination.

Treatment Options and Outlook
Modern dental techniques such as orthodontics and surgery such as CHIN RECONSTRUCTION can ameliorate some forms of prognathism by moving the teeth to improve the bite or reducing the size of the chin and lower jaw and/or moving the jawbone backward.

Risk Factors and Preventive Measures
Prognathism may be inherited as a family trait or arise later in life as the result of a medical condition such as acromegaly, a disorder in which the body produces excess amounts of growth hormone. The inherited form of prognathism, once commonly known as Hapsburg jaw, is reported to have originated with a Polish princess who married a member of the Hapsburg family, a European dynasty prominent in Spanish and Austrian/German royalty after the Renaissance.

See CHIN RECONSTRUCTION; MALOCCLUSION; OCCLUSION.

prosthodontics   From, the Greek word *prosthesis,* meaning "an addition." One of the nine dental specialties approved by the AMERICAN DENTAL ASSOCIATION Council on Dental Education and Licensure. Prosthodontics is the dental specialty dealing with the restoration and/or replacement of teeth using devices such as bridges, caps, CROWNS, dental implants, DENTURES, and VENEERS.

A prosthodontist is a dentist who has graduated from dental school and completed a two-to-three-year program in prosthodontics accredited by the American Dental Association. A board-certified prosthodontist is a dentist who has successfully completed a postgraduate course in prosthodontics and passed the written and oral examinations of the American Board of Prosthodontics. To maintain his certification, he must retake the examinations every eight years.

See also DENTISTRY; ENDODONTICS; ORAL AND MAXILLOFACIAL PATHOLOGY; ORAL AND MAXILLOFACIAL RADIOLOGY; ORAL AND MAXILLOFACIAL SURGERY; ORTHODONTICS AND DENTOFACIAL ORTHOPEDICS; PEDIATRIC DENTISTRY; PERIODONTICS; PUBLIC HEALTH DENTISTRY.

public health dentistry   One of the nine dental specialties approved by the American Dental Association Council on Dental Education and Licensure, public health dentistry focuses on practices listed by the American Association of Public Health Dentistry as the Ten Essential Public Health Services. These activities, listed on the AAPH Web site (www.aaphd.org/docs/ABDPH-brochure.doc), are:

- Monitor health status to identify community health problems
- Diagnose and investigate health problems and health hazards in the community
- Inform, educate, and empower people about health issues
- Mobilize community partnerships to identify and solve health problems
- Develop policies and plans that support individual and community health efforts
- Enforce laws and regulations that protect health and ensure safety
- Link people to needed personal health services and assure the provision of health care when otherwise unavailable
- Assure a competent public health and personal health-care workforce
- Evaluate effectiveness, accessibility, and quality of personal and population-based health services
- Research into new insight and innovative solutions to health problems

A public health dentist is a professional who has completed four years of study at an accredited dental school plus a two-year postgraduate course of study in public health. A board-certified public health dentist has successfully completed the qualifying examinations of the American Board of Dental Public Health.

See also DENTISTRY; ENDODONTICS; ORAL AND MAXILLOFACIAL PATHOLOGY; ORAL AND MAXILLOFACIAL RADIOLOGY; ORAL AND MAXILLOFACIAL SURGERY; ORTHODONTICS AND DENTOFACIAL ORTHOPEDICS; PEDIATRIC DENTISTRY; PERIODONTICS; PROSTHODONTICS.

pulp, dental   Dental pulp is a body organ composed of soft tissue that fills the hollow interior of the TOOTH from the pulp chamber (the inside of the top, or crown, of the tooth) down through the root canal(s). The pulp in the pulp chamber is called the *coronal pulp,* from the Latin word *corona,* meaning "crown." The pulp that extends from the middle of the tooth down to the root is called the radicular pulp, from the Latin word *radix,* meaning "root."

The dental pulp connects to the tissue around the tooth through the apical foramen (from the Latin words *apex,* meaning "tip," and *forare,* meaning "to pierce"), an opening at the tip of the root. Note: Some roots have more than one apical foramen and some teeth also have very small pathways that run sideways through the tooth to the surrounding tissue.

The Composition and Structure of Dental Pulp

Dental pulp is constructed in three layers. The innermost layer contains cells that develop into connective tissue (fibroblasts and mesenchymal stem cells). The second layer is an area (zone of Weil) packed with blood vessels and nerves. The top layer, next to the DENTIN, is filled predominantly with odontoblasts (cells that produce dentin).

A human being who has all her teeth will have 52 dental pulps, 20 in her primary teeth and, later, 32 in her permanent teeth. The longest dental pulp is in a cuspid, that is, the canine tooth. As a person ages, the pulp continues to deposit dentin on the inside of the tooth, and as the dentin layer grows thicker and the pulp is compressed, the tooth may take on a characteristic yellowish color.

The Functions of the Dental Pulp

The healthy dental pulp has four primary functions:

- It contains cells that form dentin, the hard, bonelike layer underneath the enamel covering the top of the tooth and the CEMENTUM covering the root.
- It provides nutrients and moisture to the tooth.
- It acts as a sensory organ that perceives changes in temperature and pressure, as well as injury to the tooth.
- It repairs the tooth, when possible, by forming new dentin.

A functioning dental pulp is essential until the tooth and its root(s) are fully formed and developed with enamel/dentin walls strong enough to withstand the force exerted during chewing and during dental procedures and treatments such as orthodontics. Once the tooth is mature, healthy pulp continues to lay down small amounts of dentin, but a mature tooth gets nourishment from the surrounding tissue and thus can remain firmly in the jaw even without its pulp. In other words, an injured or disease pulp can be removed during root canal treatment, the tooth filled, and the patient still keep the tooth in his mouth.

Note: To test the vitality (health) of the dental pulp before proceeding with treatment, the dentist may use an electrical current to stimulate the nerve between the suspect tooth and its neighbor or she may expose the suspect tooth to extremes of heat and cold.

Disorders of the Dental Pulp

Conditions affecting the dental pulp include, but are not limited to:

- *Pulpitis,* an inflammation and/or infection of the dental pulp; in serious cases, pulpitis requires root canal treatment to remove the pulp
- *Pulp stone,* also known as a denticle, this is a hard lump of dentin in the pulp chamber that may have no effect on the health of the tooth
- *Pulp mummification,* a condition in which an injured or diseased pulp dries and shrivels

Common treatments for problems with the dental pulp, other than ROOT CANAL TREATMENT, include:

- *Pulpotomy,* also known as pulp amputation; this is, the removal of the dental pulp in the upper part of the tooth
- *Pulp capping,* a procedure to cover exposed dental pulp

Note: When the dental pulp is injured, either through decay or a physical trauma, prompt treatment is essential to keep the pulp healthy and intact.

See DENTIN; ENAMEL.

Q-switch   See LASER.

quantitative light-induced fluorescence (QFL)
Fluorescence is the phenomenon that occurs when a substance, such as the enamel surface of the teeth, is exposed to radiation, such as a high-intensity light, and in response emits radiation. QFL makes use of this phenomenon by exposing the teeth to high-intensity blue light from a xenon lamp. In response, the surface of the teeth emits green light. Because the strength of the emission depends on the mineral content of the enamel surface, a lower emission of the green light at one or more points on the enamel indicates a loss of mineralization—that is, a possible cavity.

To obtain the QFL measurement, the dentist uses a handpiece that transmits light signals to a computer that assembles and displays a picture of the tooth surface on-screen. Although the accuracy of the measurement may be adversely affected by the presence of saliva or plaque, it can be increased by staining the teeth with a disclosing solution.

Because QFL can differentiate tooth-colored restorations (fillings) from natural enamel, it is also useful for forensic dentists who are attempting to obtain a complete picture of a person's teeth, RESTORATIONS and all, in order to identify a cadaver. In fact, QLF is primarily a research technique, not an instrument used in clinical practice.

See FORENSIC DENTISTRY.

radiation Radiation is energy in the form of high-speed submicroscopic particles and electromagnetic waves. In dentistry and medicine, radiation is used to power machines that produce X-ray images, which identify various defects such as CAVITIES in the teeth and loss of bone from the JAW due to PERIODONTAL DISEASE.

Ionizing radiation is radiation with enough energy to disrupt particles in an atom and cause damage to body tissues or, conversely, to heal by destroying malignant tissue such as a tumor of the jaw. The unit of energy absorbed from ionizing radiation either deliberately (in treatment) or by accident is called a radiation absorbed dose (RAD). Nonionizing radiation such as microwaves and visible light does not disrupt atoms, but it may produce sufficient heat to damage tissue. For example, some studies suggest that air traffic controllers sitting in front of radar screens for hours at a time have a higher than normal incidence of infertility or loss of sperm quality due to nonionizing radiation emitted by the screens.

radiation therapy Radiation therapy is RADIATION used to treat cancer, including some forms of head and neck cancer, a group of diseases that include ORAL CANCERS such as cancer of the jaw, lip, palate (top of the mouth), and tongue.

There are two basic types of radiation therapy: External radiation therapy, also known as external beam radiation therapy, and internal radiation therapy.

External radiation therapy is radiation delivered from outside the body via a device called a linear accelerator that sends a beam of radiation through the skin and underlying body tissues directly to the tumor. One important form of external radiation is stereotactic radiosurgery, the use of high-energy, precisely directed beams of radiation.

Internal radiation therapy is radiation delivered via a source placed into the body. Brachytherapy, from the Greek word *brakys,* meaning "short" or "close," is a technique that implants radioactive particles directly into the tumor. Other ways to deliver internal radiation therapy include having the patient swallow a pill or a liquid containing radioactive material or injecting the liquid via an intravenous needle.

Procedure: External Radiation Therapy
The first step in external radiation therapy is simulation, the use of imaging studies to pinpoint the exact location and dimensions of the tumor. One important imaging technique is conformal radiotherapy (3DCRT), which uses CT scans to enable the radiologist to visualize a tumor in three dimensions rather than the flat image provided by an X-ray. The resulting image is fed into a computer, which creates a plan that controls the delivery of precise doses of radiation to specific areas within the tumor while reducing the damage to the healthy tissue around the lesion, a process known as intensity modulated radiation (IMRT).

One form of IMRT is sterotactic radiation surgery (from the Greek word *stereos-* meaning "solid" and *taxis* meaning "arrangement"). Sterotactic, or radiosurgery, delivers a highly concentrated, precisely focused beam of radiation to an inoperable tumor; it is also used to eliminate tumor tissue remaining after conventional surgery and to obliterate congenital "tangles" of blood vessels known as arteriovenous malformations (AVM). Sterotactic radiosurgery typically involves one to three sessions; multiple smaller doses of radiation over a period that may stretch for several weeks are described as fractionated sterotactic therapy.

Locating and picturing the tumor allows the radiologist to define a treatment port or field, the site at which the radiation will be aimed. The port may be tattooed or marked with permanent ink to ensure the radiation's being delivered to the same spot each treatment. This precise targeting also helps reduce the risk of damage to healthy tissue. For example, in treating a tumor of the tongue, the radiologist will plan the delivery of radiation to spare the salivary glands if possible.

If treatment requires total stillness, immobilization devices such as molds may be used to keep the patient in the correct position during the radiation treatment. The treatment itself delivers a series of small doses of radiation separated by a rest period to protect healthy cells and tissues; the typical schedule for external radiation treatment is five days a week for several weeks.

The exact dose and timing of the radiation treatments depend on the size, site, and type of the tumor, as well as the patient's general health. During the treatment, the patient sits or lies on a special chair or treatment table positioned so as to enable the radiation to reach the treatment port. Depending on the site, the therapist may put shields on the patient's body to make sure that the radiation hits only the treatment port. The therapist then leaves the room to deliver the radiation from a nearby site that allows him to monitor the patient via television or through a window in the wall of the treatment room. The session may last as long as 30 minutes to allow for the patient to arrive, change clothes, and be positioned correctly, but the actually delivery of radiation takes only one to five minutes at most.

Procedure: Internal Radiation Therapy

To perform brachytherapy, the radiation oncologist (a radiologist specializing in treating cancer) uses a special applicator to insert a tube into the patient's body at the site of the tumor and then inserts narrow plastic tubes containing radioactive particles through the catheter directly into the tumor.

During low dose rate (LDR) brachytherapy, the applicator and the radioactive implants remain in place for up to a week and are then removed. The treatment may require the patient to remain in the hospital.

During high dose rate (HDR) brachytherapy, the radioactive material remains in place for up to 20 minutes at a time and is then removed. The treatment is repeated twice a day for up to five weeks. The patient may remain in the hospital or come in daily for the treatments.

During permanent brachytherapy, the radioactive material is inserted and the catheter is removed. The material remains in place permanently but the radiation strength diminishes naturally each passing day, eventually disappearing completely.

Risks and Complications

External radiation therapy The most common side effects of external radiation therapy are skin irritation, burns, or increased sensitivity to sunlight; lower-than-normal levels of red blood cells, white blood cells, or blood platelets (small particles that enable blood to clot); and fatigue.

The specific adverse effects for external radiation therapy for cancers of the head and neck are an increased risk of decay and bone loss; reduced secretion of saliva or very thick saliva; mouth sores; sore or dry mouth and throat; difficulty in swallowing; an altered sense of taste; and hair loss on the part of the face/head being treated. External radiation therapy does not make the body radioactive.

Internal radiation therapy During brachytherapy, the body gives off some radiation, but body fluids (urine, sweat, saliva) do not. With internal radiation therapy that requires a pill or liquid radioactive material, the body fluids are radioactive. The amount of radioactivity emanating from the body and body fluids depends on the dose of the radiation in the therapy. If the dose is very high, the patient may be sequestered in a private room and visitors (if permitted) will be required to follow strict safety rules such as checking with doctors or nurses before entering the patient's room even for short visits. Some safety precautions may be required after the patient leaves the hospital; in addition, the patient may need a medical clearance if traveling across borders with radiation detectors.

Outlook and Lifestyle Modifications

The outlook for successful radiation therapy is destruction of the tumor. Before, during, and after radiation therapy for head or neck cancer, the patient is advised to practice good oral hygiene to reduce the risk of decay and/or infection and PERIODONTAL DISEASE.

relaxation techniques See BIOFEEDBACK.

replantation, reimplantation See "KNOCKED-OUT TOOTH."

research study See EVIDENCE-BASED DENTISTRY.

resin A resin is a natural or synthetic plastic compound. Natural resins, clear or translucent saplike substances from plants, are used in a variety of products such as varnishes, plastics, and medicines. Some dental resins are made of synthetic thermoplastic materials (substances that soften when heated and harden when cooled).

The most common dental resin is composite resin, a mixture of acrylic resin (a lightweight plastic made from acrylic acid) plus fillers such as silica. Composite resin can be colored to match the teeth. This is an aesthetic improvement over dental AMALGAM, which may be one explanation for the fact that dental composite resin is now used in an estimated 90 percent or more of fillings in the front teeth as well as 50 percent of those in the less visible back teeth. Dental composite resin is also used to create a clean, smooth tooth surface (see BONDING), as material to fill small gaps between teeth, for minor reshaping of a tooth, and for a partial crown on one tooth.

The disadvantages of composite resin are its shorter life versus dental amalgam, its tendency to shrink after placement, and the likelihood that it will change color and stain over time, requiring periodic cleaning and/or replacement.

Composite resins are also used in medicine. For example, orthopedic surgeons use composite resins strengthened with fiber to make implants and anchor screws used to attach a replacement to a bone. Hydroxyapatite resin, a composite resin reinforced with calcium and other minerals, is used as a cement to stabilize fractured bones and to fix bone screws, particularly in older patients or those with osteoporosis.

resorption The first step in the process by which the body breaks down old BONE and, in normal circumstances, builds new bone. Like all body tissues, bone is constantly being replaced as old cells are resorbed by specialized body cells called osteoclasts and new cells are produced by a second kind of specialized cells called osteoblasts.

In dentistry, the term *resorption* is used to describe the loss of bone without replacement by new bone in the JAW or the loss of tissue at the root of a tooth. Loss of bone in the jaw occurs most commonly after an injury or an infection or when a tooth has been missing for a long period of time and the jawbone remodels, that is, adapts to fill the space. Loss of tissue from the tooth root is triggered by a third kind of specialized cell called cementoclasts that break down CEMENTUM, the bonelike tissue covering the outer surface of the tooth root. The destruction of the tooth from the outside is usually caused by a condition affecting the surface of the tooth such as an injury, including movement of the tooth during orthodontic treatment. Destruction from inside the tooth is usually due to a problem affecting the dental PULP.

See ENDODONTICS; ORTHODONTIC BRACES; PERIODONTAL DISEASE; ROOT CANAL TREATMENT.

restoration   In dentistry, an umbrella term that covers virtually every type of filling, CROWN, DENTURE, or other prosthetic used to restore or replace a part of a tooth or one or more whole teeth.

A direct restoration is a simple filling, a repair put into the tooth right after the cavity is cleaned and prepared rather than being made from a cast of the tooth. An indirect restoration is just the opposite, a restoration such as an INLAY, ONLAY, or crown made in a dental laboratory to fit a cast of the tooth. (Indirect restorations such as crowns or inlays require at least two visits, one for preparing the tooth and a second for placing the restoration, which has been created in a dental LABORATORY. An implant restoration is a crown for one or more teeth or a BRIDGE that replaces one or more teeth.

When preparing a restoration, dentists and dental laboratories strive to make one that fits precisely onto and into the area to be restored, a process that may require more than one "fitting." An overcontoured restoration is one that is too large for the tooth; an undercontoured one is too small.

retainer   An orthodontic device used to keep the teeth in position as the teeth and gums adjust to changes in bone structure after treatment to correct MALOCCLUSION (irregularities in the bite).

The Hawley retainer, first introduced in the mid-19th century and named after American orthodontist C. A. Hawley, is a metal WIRE anchored to a molded plastic base that fits up against the roof of the mouth. The wire, which fits close against the teeth, is designed to keep the teeth from moving apart after orthodontic treatment. The Hawley retainer is generally worn only at night.

The Essix retainer, sometimes called the invisible retainer, is a clear plastic shield that fits over the teeth and up against the roof of the mouth. The Essix retainer may be worn 24 hours a day. However, some orthodontists prefer not to use the Essix retainer because it prevents the tooth surfaces from meeting, something considered necessary if the teeth are to settle into a correct position after orthodontic treatment. Essix retainers are also less durable than Hawley retainers, especially for patients who clench and grind their teeth.

A fixed retainer is simply a wire bonded (glued) to the inside of the teeth, the side nearest the tongue. These retainers, which cannot be removed by the patient, are generally prescribed after orthodontic treatment that has produced dramatic changes in the bite. The benefit of the fixed retainer is that, like braces, it can be tightened or loosened as the teeth settle. The drawback is that, again like braces, the wire may support an increased buildup of tartar on the teeth leading to an increased risk of gingivitis or PERIODONTAL DISEASE.

Ricketts, Robert M.   (1920–2003) American orthodontist, celebrated for his advocacy of treating "faces, not teeth." To that end, he is credited with developing the first measurements of the head and face that made it possible for orthodontists to compare the development of their patients' facial and cranial features with persons of the same gender, age, and race, to project the results of specific therapies when planning orthodontic treatment, to project the eventual growth of the jaws, and to advance the use of computer simulations in these tasks. He developed methods for estimating the orthodontic force required to move the teeth safely, and created a plethora of innovative orthodontic appliances, including the quad helix and various forms of headgear. A graduate of the School of Dentistry at Indiana University and the University of Illinois Graduate School in Orthodontics, Ricketts held professorships at numerous universities, including Loma Linda University, the University of Illinois, the University of California in Los Angeles, and the University of Southern California, while authoring more than 300 articles, books, chapters, and texts on orthodontics.

ridge A long, narrow upper edge or crest; in dentistry, commonly the alveolar ridge, the bone top edge of the upper or lower jaw into which the teeth are set. The residual ridge is the part of the alveolar ridge remaining once a tooth has been extracted and its alveola (socket) disappears.

Some teeth have characteristic ridges. For example, the central labial ridge is a groove across the middle of a canine tooth on the side closest to the cheek. The transverse ridge runs from the buccal (cheek) side to the lingual (tongue) side of a molar. The triangular ridge is a higher line on the top of a back tooth running from the tip of the cusp (the elevated point[s] on the tooth corner) into the center of the top surface of the tooth. The marginal ridge is the elevated part of the enamel on a tooth's occlusal surface, the surface that meets the tooth above or below when a person is chewing or closes his jaws.

root canal treatment ENDODONTIC procedure to remove injured or diseased dental PULP, the soft tissue that extends from the pulp chamber (the large hollow inside the upper part of the tooth) down to the root canal (the narrow channel inside each tooth root). If the injured pulp is left untreated, it may become infected, and the infection may spread from the tip of the tooth to the bone that holds the tooth in place. Successful root canal treatment halts this process by removing the pulp, cleaning and sealing the pulp chamber and root canals, and (in most cases) saving the tooth.

Procedure

Once the endodontist has numbed the affected tooth, he may stretch a RUBBER DAM across the patient's mouth to keep saliva, which contains bacteria, from entering the mouth and tooth. Next, he will drill an opening into the top of the tooth to gain access to the pulp chamber and root canals.

Once he has drilled an opening into the tooth, the dentist uses a series of small instruments called root canal files to remove the pulp and then to shape and smooth the sides of the pulp chamber and root canals. The files may be manipulated by hand or the endodontist may attach them to a dental handpiece, which rotates the files mechanically. While cleaning out the pulp chamber and root canals, the dentist may take an X-ray picture with a file in place to make certain that he has reached the bottom of the root canal.

When the pulp chamber and root canals are clean and shaped, the endodontist usually inserts an antibacterial medication and then a filling. The material most frequently used to fill a tooth after root canal treatment is GUTTA-PERCHA, a rubber compound made from the sap of trees native to Southeast Asia. The gutta-percha may come in cones sized to match the diameter of the files used to clean out the tooth or it may be applied with an applicator that squeezes the paste into the tooth. The gutta-percha is held in place inside the tooth with a paste called a *sealer* that is either painted on the outside of the cones or spread over the inside surface of the pulp chamber and root canals. Once the gutta-percha is securely in place, the endodontist places a simple filling in the hole through which he entered the tooth.

This procedure is often completed in one visit. However, depending on the endodontist's evaluation of the tooth, the first visit may end with the endodontist inserting a temporary filling that is removed a week to 10 days later when the tooth is cleaned again and a permanent filling is put in place. If a significant portion of the top surface of the tooth has been destroyed, the patient's own dentist may restore the tooth after the treatment with a gold or porcelain CROWN or ONLAY.

Risks and Complications

Mild discomfort is common, along with temporarily increased sensitivity to heat and cold. Severe pain or sudden swelling are unusual and should be reported to the endodontist.

If the endodontist inserted a temporary filling, some of the filling material may flake off in the period between the first and second visits.

Outlook and Lifestyle Modifications

A successful root canal procedure gives the patient a healthy tooth that can last as long as his other natural teeth.

See ENDODONTICS.

rubber dam Also known as an oral dam. This is a small, thin, square sheet of latex or silicone with a hole punched in the appropriate place to enable the dentist to see the tooth on which he is working. The dam, which is held in place by clamping it to the teeth, is used during endodontic procedures such as ROOT CANAL TREATMENT or, occasionally, when filling a tooth. The dam helps hold back the lips and cheeks, thus giving the dentist a clear view of the tooth on which he is working. It keeps the affected tooth dry and free of bacteria found naturally in saliva, a vital consideration when the tooth is opened for root canal work. Finally, it protects the patient's airway from any flying debris such as particles of the tooth or of the material used to fill it.

saliva From the Latin word *saliva,* meaning "spittle." A water-based liquid containing minerals, proteins, digestive enzymes, antibacterial compounds, and mucus; secreted by the two types of salivary glands, the major salivary glands and the minor salivary glands. Both are controlled by the autonomic (involuntary) nervous system, which determines how much saliva each gland secretes and when the saliva is released.

Note: The Greek word *sialon,* which also means "saliva," is used in compound medical terms such as *sialagogue* (something that increases the flow of saliva), *sialitis* (inflammation of the salivary glands), *sialadenitis* (inflammation of the salivary glands due to an infection), *sialogram* (an X-ray of the salivary glands), and *sialorrhea* (excess salivation).

The Major Salivary Glands

There are three pairs of major salivary glands:

- the *parotid glands,* located at the hinge of the jaw, in front of the ear in the cheek on each side of the head; they secrete serous saliva, a mucus-free watery fluid similar in color and texture to blood serum
- the *sublingual salivary glands,* located under the tongue at the front of the mouth; they secrete *mucus saliva,* a thicker fluid than serous saliva
- the *submandibular (submaxillary) salivary glands,* located under the tongue toward the middle of the mouth; they secrete both serous and mucus saliva

Together, the parotid and the submandibular (submaxillary) saliva glands secrete as much as 90 percent of the approximately 1,500 milliliters of saliva normally produced each day in a healthy mouth. The rest of the saliva is secreted by the sublingual salivary glands plus the minor salivary glands.

The Minor Salivary Glands

The minor salivary glands, present not in pairs but by the hundreds, are:

- the palatine salivary glands, set under the surface of the palate
- the buccal salivary glands, set inside of the cheeks
- the labial salivary glands, set under the inside of the lips
- the minor lingual salivary glands and the sublingual glands, set under the tongue

The palatine salivary glands secrete only mucus saliva. The other minor salivary glands secrete mostly mucus saliva plus some serous saliva.

Saliva and Dental Health

Saliva lubricates the inside of the mouth, flushes away debris and bacteria, and strengthens teeth by depositing minerals on the surface of the dental enamel and laying down a protein coating that slows the enamel's natural loss of minerals and bathes the teeth in a mix of compounds such as lysosomes, lactoperoxidase, and lactoferrin (which contain enzymes that damage bacteria).

Saliva and the Digestive Process

Saliva dissolves food, compressing and binding it into a mass (bolus) that can pass down through the esophagus without injuring the tissues. In addition, the enzymes (amylases) in saliva begin the digestion of carbohydrates. The two basic salivary disorders are secreting too much saliva or secreting too little. The first leads to drooling; the second, to dry mouth and a higher risk of decay and PERIODONTAL DISEASE. The following table lists various medical conditions and lifestyle situations known to cause either excessive or insufficient secretion of saliva.

Saliva as a Diagnostic Tool

Like other bodily fluids, saliva can be analyzed to identify and quantify various substances in the body such as medicines and drugs (alcohol, nicotine, cocaine, opiates), hormones, environmental toxins, infectious agents (antibodies to HIV, hepatitis A and B, *Helicobacter pylori*), and is currently under study as a replacement for blood tests to diagnose and monitor chronic illnesses, including those affecting dental health.

- In 2005, scientists at the Forsyth Institute in Boston suggested that elevated levels of *Capnocytophaga gingivalis, Prevotella melaninogenicay, and Streptococcus mitis,* three types of bacteria normally found in the mouth, were associated with an increased incidence of oral squamous cell carcinoma (cancer).

- Three years later, in 2008, researchers from the University of California in Los Angeles published data in the journal *Clinical Cancer Research* reporting that a simple test for specific proteins in saliva could be used to detect the cancer.

- In November 2007, the AMERICAN DENTAL ASSOCIATION reported that researchers at the University of California in Los Angeles and the University Medical Center Groningen in The

CAUSES OF EXCESS OR INSUFFICIENT SALIVATION

Condition	Cause
Excess saliva (sialorrhea)	Medical conditions:
	• difficulty in swallowing
	• sore or swollen throat
	• mouth sores
	• infection such as tonsillitis
	• esophageal stricture (narrowing of the passageway)
	• oral cancer
	• emotional distress (anxiety, fear)
	Diet or lifestyle:
	• eating sour foods
	• anticipating various foods
Insufficient saliva	Medical conditions:
	• arthritis
	• bacterial or viral infections
	• chronic conditions such as Parkinson's disease, diabetes, and Sjögren's syndrome
	• swelling of the salivary gland due to blockage caused by a mucocele (mucus swelling in the gland)
	• salivary stone (*sialolith*; hardened mineral deposit in a duct in the gland) or a tumor
	• emotional distress
	Medical drugs/treatment:
	• some psychiatric drugs including some antidepressants
	• antihistamines
	• some antihypertensives
	• cancer chemotherapy
	• diuretics ("water pills")
	• sedatives
	• radiation treatment for head/neck cancer
	Diet or lifestyle:
	• natural aging
	• dehydration
	• mouth breathing
	• smoking

Netherlands had identified potential biomarkers for SJÖGREN'S SYNDROME in saliva.

See also DECAY; PERIODONTAL DISEASE; SALIVA SUBSTITUTES/STIMULANTS; XEROSTOMIA.

salivary glands, cancer of A malignant tumor of one or more of the salivary glands, the glands that secrete saliva.

Symptoms and Diagnostic Path

The most common sign of a tumor of the salivary gland is painless lump or swelling in the mouth or neck or near the jaw. Other possible signs of cancer of the salivary glands are facial numbness, muscle weakness, and/or pain near a salivary gland.

A dental examination can pinpoint the area. If the dentist deems the area suspicious, she may take a sample of the tissue for a biopsy and/or request a CT scan or MRI (magnetic resonance imaging) or refer the patient to a physician or oral surgeon who specializes in treating cancer of the head and neck.

Treatment Options and Outlook

The first treatment option for cancer of the salivary gland that has not spread is surgery to remove the tumor and the gland. The surgeon may also remove lymph nodes near the gland to see if the cancer has spread. If it has, the patient may require surgery to remove adjacent tissue, including muscles and nerves. Following surgery, the doctor may order radiation therapy to kill any malignant cells remaining in the area around the tumor. (In some cases, radiation therapy alone may be used to destroy the tumor.)

If the surgery is extensive, the patient may require physical therapy to alleviate difficulties in eating and speaking and/or plastic surgery to reconstruct the area from which the tumor was removed. The adverse effects of radiation therapy include dry mouth, mouth sores, hoarseness, difficulty in swallowing, stiffness in the jaw, change in the ability to taste food, nausea, and fatigue.

Risk Factors and Preventive Measures

Cancer of the salivary glands is more common in men than in women and in people older than 50. Risk factors include tobacco (smoking and/or chewing tobacco) and excess exposure to radiation. Occasionally, there is a family history of the tumor.

See also MAGNETIC RESONANCE IMAGING (MRI); ORAL CANCER; SALIVA.

saliva substitutes/stimulants Nonprescription products and prescription drugs used to moisten the mouth or to stimulate the secretion of saliva for people suffering from XEROSTOMIA ("dry mouth").

Nonprescription Products

Artificial saliva Over-the-counter (OTC) artificial saliva products are formulated as liquids or gels similar in chemical composition and physical properties to natural saliva. Unlike natural saliva, these liquids do not remineralize teeth nor do they stimulate the production of saliva from the salivary glands. Lozenges or simple nonmedicinal hard candies may both moisten and stimulate saliva production.

A typical artificial saliva liquid, spray, or gel contains:

- liquid, commonly distilled water
- thickeners, such as glycerin and carboxymethylcellose or starch to make the product feel natural in the mouth
- minerals such as calcium that are found naturally in saliva (the minerals in natural saliva continually strengthen the surface of the teeth; there is no proof that the minerals in artificial saliva behave the same way)
- flavoring agents and sweeteners to make the product taste good
- emulsifiers, such as phosphates to ensure that the ingredients in the products do not separate out into the solution
- preservatives—commonly one of a group of chemicals called parabens—to protect the product from microbial contamination

Adverse reactions to artificial saliva products appear to be rare, but some patients may be sensitive to one or more ingredients in a specific product leading to allergic reactions such as rash, hives, or itching. Swelling of the mouth, face, lips, or tongue, or difficulty breathing/tightness in the chest, require immediate medical attention. Some examples of artificial saliva products are:

- *liquid*: V.A. Oralube
- *sprays*: Entertainer's Secret, Glandosane, Moi-Stir, MouthKote, Optimoist, Salivart, Xero-Lube
- *swabs*: Moi-Stir Oral Swabsticks

Dietary Saliva Stimulant Natural Dry Mouth Relief lozenges contain a patented form of water-free crystals of maltose (ACM), a sugar compound that stimulates saliva production. In two clinical trials, patients taking the lozenges two or three times a day for up to 24 weeks produced more saliva and experienced no significant side effects. This product does not work for patients whose salivary glands have been ablated, for example, by radiation therapy.

Enzymatic Salivary Stimulants Biotène and Oral balance, available over-the-counter, are anti-xerostomia dentifrices that contain three salivary enzymes—lactoperoxidase, glucose oxidase, and lysozyme—specifically formulated to activate intraoral bacterial systems.

Prescription Products

Saliva Stimulants Pilocarpine (Salagen) and cevimeline (Evoxac) are medicines that stimulate secretion from the exocrine glands (salivary glands, sweat glands, mammary glands, stomach, liver, and pancreas). In clinical trials, pilocarpine tablets were significantly more effective than nonprescription saliva substitutes or a placebo (a look-alike pill) in relieving dry mouth due to Sjögren's syndrome or radiation therapy. (Similar trials with cevimeline are not yet complete.)

The side effects of these medicines, which should not be used by patients with glaucoma, may include dry eyes and disturbances in vision; excessive sweating or saliva secretion; runny nose; upset stomach (nausea, diarrhea, constipation); loss of appetite; muscle pain; and vaginal itching or discharge. More serious adverse effects may include breathing difficulties; irregular heartbeat and chest pain; severe gastric upset (nausea and vomiting, bloating); fever or chills; swelling of the hands and/or feet; mouth sores; and jaundice (yellow color of the skin or whites of the eyes).

In addition, pilocarpine and cevimeline may interact with other medicines, including, but not limited to, certain antibiotics, antidepressants, anti-asthmatics, antihypertensives (drugs used to treat high blood pressure), and medications used to treat HIV/AIDS.

Cholagogue A cholagogue is a chemical that stimulates the secretion of the neurotransmitter acetylcholine, a compound that stimulates the transmission of messages between nerves. The secretion of acetylcholine stimulates the secretion of saliva. One cholagogue, anethole trithione, has been used to treat dry mouth, but data regarding its effectiveness remain inconclusive with some studies showing an improvement and others not.

Interferons Interferons are protein and carbohydrate molecules released by body cells in response to triggers such as exposure to an infectious agent. Interferons adjust or modify some cellular functions; for example, in one 12-week study, lozenges containing low doses of human interferon alfa (IFN-a) appeared to stimulate saliva production in patients with Sjögren's syndrome.

scaling In dentistry, the process of removing hardened PLAQUE deposits from teeth during periodontal treatment.

Procedure

The instruments commonly used by the dentist or dental technician to remove calculus (tartar) from the teeth are a hand scaler, a sonic scaler, and an ultrasonic scaler.

A hand scaler is a simple metal rod with a hook-shaped or curved strip used to reach beneath the gum line to physically scrape away CALCULUS (soft or hardened debris).

A sonic scaler is a compressed-air driven instrument whose tip moves at 7,000 or more cycles per second. The sonic scaler is used to remove softer debris from the tooth surface.

An ultrasonic scaler is an instrument powered by an electronic generator, which transmits energy in the form of high-frequency vibrations at a rate of 40,000 or more cycles per second. The ultrasonic scaler is used to remove all types of deposits from various tooth surfaces.

Risks and Complications

The sonic and ultrasonic scalers do not emit heat, but their vibrations do heat the oral tissue. To avoid injury, the tissues are bathed in cool water during scaling with these instruments. Patients with dental sensitivity due to severe gum recession may experience discomfort from the cool water, but not the scaling itself.

Outlook and Lifestyle Modifications

Professional scaling, often recommended to be done once every three months, removes calculus and reduces the risk of infection and bone loss from PERIODONTAL DISEASE for a time immediately after the treatment.

However, to maintain good oral health, a patient with periodontal disease must practice serious home health care, which includes using special brushes and floss to remove debris between the teeth, special tools (usually round-headed wooden toothpicks) to scrape material off the tooth surface, regular brushing (usually with a powered brush), and rinsing regularly with medicated mouthwash. Failure to practice this regimen increases the risk of disease-related bone loss.

schools of dentistry   In the United States, dentists must complete an undergraduate degree commonly characterized by a "pre-dentistry" major that must include courses in basic science with laboratory experience including (but not limited to):

- two semesters of general biology
- two semesters of general chemistry
- two semesters of organic chemistry
- two semesters of general physics

They must then attend a four-year graduate program leading to the D.D.S. (doctor of dental surgery) or D.M.D. (doctor of dental medicine) degree. At some universities with graduate schools of dentistry the program may be shortened to three years' undergraduate work followed by four years' graduate work. Upon completing dental school, the student may choose to specialize in a field of dentistry such as ENDODONTICS, ORAL AND MAXILLOFACIAL SURGERY, ORAL AND MAXILLOFACIAL PATHOLOGY, ORTHODONTIC AND DENTOFACIAL ORTHOPEDICS, PEDIATRIC DENTISTRY, PERIODONTICS, PROSTHODONTICS, or PUBLIC HEALTH DENTISTRY, all of which require additional training.

History of Dental Schools in the United States

The first dental school in the United States (also the world's first dental school) was the Baltimore School of Dentistry, established in 1840. The school, which created the doctor of dental surgery degree, merged with the University of Maryland School of Dentistry in 1923. In 1867, Harvard University set up the Harvard University Dental School, the first school of dentistry associated with a university. Unlike the Baltimore school, Harvard named its dentistry degree *dentariae medicinae doctorase* (D.M.D.). The two degrees, D.D.S. and D.M.D., describe the same professional status; they persist to this day.

By 1900, there were 57 schools of general dentistry in the United States, and schools devoted to dental specialties soon followed.

- The first dental specialty school was the Angle School of Orthodontia, established by EDWARD HARTLEY ANGLE in Saint Louis in 1900.
- The first academic program for nurses specializing in dentistry opened in 1910 at the Ohio College of Dental Surgery in Cincinnati.
- The Fones Clinic for Dental Hygienists, the first school specializing in oral hygiene, opened in Bridgeport, Connecticut, in 1913. Four years later, Irene Newman became the first person to be awarded a license as a dental hygienist.

As the practice of dentistry grew, the composition of the student body at each school became more inclusive. For example:

- In 1866, LUCY BEAMAN HOBBS graduated from the Ohio College of Dental Surgery, becoming the first woman to earn a dental degree in the United States.
- In 1869, Robert Tanner Freeman graduated from Harvard University Dental School, the first African American to earn a dental degree.
- In 1890, Ida Gray (Rollins) graduated from the University of Michigan School of Dentistry, becoming the first African-American woman to earn a dental degree.

In 2004, based on the AMERICAN DENTAL ASSOCIATION'S 2002/2003 Survey of Advanced Dental Education, the American Dental Education Association (ADEA) listed:

- More than 50 dental schools in the United States, the District of Columbia, and Puerto Rico, with 17,800 students seeking D.D.S./D.M.D. degrees and an annual average of approximately 4,400 newly graduated dentists
- 727 school- and hospital-based dental resident programs accommodating 5,257 dental residents
- 266 dental hygiene programs enrolling 12,826 dental hygiene students

- 259 dental assisting programs serving 5,707 dental assistant students
- 25 dental laboratory technology programs enrolling 754 dental laboratory students

ADEA projects that in the year 2020 there will be approximately 54 practicing dentists for every 100,000 people in the United States, down from the 1999 high of 60.4 dentists per 100,000 Americans. However, the distribution of dental services remains uneven through the country, with more than 41 million people living in areas with an inadequate number of dental professionals. In December 2003, the federal Bureau of Health Professions' National Center for Health Workforce Analysis estimated that it would require an additional 8,600 dentists to bring the ratio of dentists to patients to an acceptable level of one dentist per 3,000 patients across the United States.

Accredited Schools of Dentistry

In the United States, schools of dentistry are accredited by the Commission on Dental Accreditation (CODA), a peer-review group that inspects and attests to the academic and professional standards of each school. CODA, which operates under the aegis of the American Dental Association, includes representatives of the dental professional, educational, and licensing communities, as well as members of the public. Appendix V lists the currently accredited schools of dentistry in the United States, District of Columbia, and Puerto Rico.

sealant   A dental sealant is a plastic resin the dentist applies to the chewing surfaces of the teeth in the back of the mouth. The resin bonds to the irregular surface of the tooth, reducing the risk of cavities and other defects by protecting the enamel from acidic substances such as food and the bacteria in PLAQUE.

Procedure

Applying dental sealant is a four-step procedure. First the dentist or dental assistant cleans the teeth to which the sealant will be applied. Step two is to roughen the tooth's enamel surface with a very weak acid, creating very small craters and crevices that enable the sealant to hold more firmly. The third step is simply to paint the sealant onto the enamel surface. Finally, the dentist may use a special high-intensity light to cure (harden and set) the sealant.

Risks and Complications

Some older dental sealants contain bisphenol A (BPA), a hard plastic used in some food containers such as baby bottles and the lining of some food cans. BPA has some estrogenlike effects. Some studies show that it may increase the risk of diabetes and heart disease and may be a potential carcinogen. However, the National Institute of Environmental Health says most modern dental sealants are free of BPA.

Outlook and Lifestyle Modifications

Sealants reduce the risk of decay. The protection appears to last for several years and can be reapplied as needed. In 2005, in THE SURVEILLANCE FOR DENTAL CARIES, DENTAL SEALANTS, TOOTH RETENTION, EDENTULISM, AND ENAMEL FLUOROSIS, UNITED STATES, 1988–1994 AND 1999–2002, a joint project of the National Center for Health Statistics and the Centers for Disease Control (NCHS/CDC), the U.S. Surgeon General noted with approval that the use of dental sealants among Americans age 6–19 years had risen from 19 percent in 1988–94 to 32 percent in 1999–2002 and strongly advocated wide use of the protective coating.

Sjögren's syndrome A chronic, inflammatory autoimmune disease, similar to arthritis or lupus, in which the body attacks its own tissues. In Sjögren's, the body attacks moisture-producing glands including the salivary glands, resulting in an insufficient amount of SALIVA to moisten the mouth. The condition is named after Henrik Sjögren, the Swedish ophthalmologist who first identified it. Primary Sjögren's syndrome is a condition that exists on its own; secondary Sjögren's syndrome develops in conjunction with another autoimmune disorder such as lupus.

Symptoms and Diagnostic Path

The oral and dental symptoms of Sjögren's syndrome are:

- extreme dryness of the mouth and throat that make it difficult to chew and swallow and may diminish the sense of taste; hoarseness and cough
- increased risk of dental CAVITIES due to an insufficient amount of mineral-rich SALIVA to replenish the surface of the teeth
- enlarged and/or infected parotid salivary glands, found at the angle of the JAW
- stiffness and pain in the jaw muscles and joints

Sjögren's syndrome is identified by its symptoms. The diagnosis is confirmed by blood tests that show the presence of antibodies called anti-RO/anti-SSA or anti-La/anti-SSB, a reaction to the attack by the immune system on the tissue. A second confirming test is a biopsy of the inside of the lip showing inflammation in the salivary glands.

Treatment Options and Outlook

There is no cure for Sjögren's syndrome. Treatment for oral symptoms includes mild pain relievers, saliva substitutes, special dentifrices and mouthwashes to relieve dryness and protect the tissues of the mouth, and good oral hygiene to reduce the risk of infection.

Risk Factors and Preventive Measures

Of the estimated 4 million Americans with Sjögren's syndrome, more than 90 percent are women who develop the condition in their late 40s.

The cause of Sjögren's has not been identified. Some researchers suggest that a viral or bacterial infection may trigger the immune system attack on the glands. Because Sjögren's may affect more than one member of a family, others believe there may be a genetic susceptibility.

See also IMMUNE SYSTEM.

smile See FACIAL LANDMARKS; LIPS; MOUTH.

socket See ALVEOLUS.

solution A liquid in which one compound is dissolved in another. For example, a saline solution, which may be used to rinse out the mouth during a dental procedure, is salt dissolved in water. Some other solutions used in dentistry are:

- *cleansing solution:* a liquid used to remove food particles from DENTURES by soaking the dentures rather than using brushes that might scratch

- *disclosing solution:* a liquid containing a dye that clings to and reveals PLAQUE and other debris on teeth so that the patient can remove them

- *hardening solution:* a liquid used to prevent the loss of moisture from a dental impression so that the impression retains its shape

- *parenteral solution:* a sterile liquid used in injections

- *pickling solution:* a liquid used to remove impurities from a dental casting (a piece of metal, such as a gold CROWN, formed in a mold)

- *sclerosing solution:* a liquid that mildly inflames and swells tissues to stop minor bleeding

special-needs patients A special-needs patient is one whose general health affects his dental health or the treatment he receives. Some health conditions lower a patient's immunity, increasing the risk of infection and requiring the dentist to adopt special procedures such as prescribing antibiotics before treatment or suggesting a soft toothbrush to avoid irritating and/or inflaming the gums. Other health conditions may make a patient sensitive to drugs used during dental treatment or produce symptoms such as mouth sores that are likely to be identified first by the dentist. There are many such conditions that affect dental health.

Acromegaly is a condition characterized by continuing abnormal growth of the head, face, hands, and feet due to the body's oversecretion of the pituitary growth hormone somatotropin. The complications of acromegaly (from the Greek *akron,* meaning "extreme," and *megas,* meaning "large") most likely to affect dental treatment are high blood pressure and problems with the heart muscle.

Addison's disease is an abnormality of the adrenal glands characterized by increasing weakness and fatigue, along with the loss of appetite, weight loss, and gastric upset (nausea and vomiting). Because an early sign of Addison's disease is the appearance of blue-black or dark brown pigmented spots on the mucous membrane surface of the inside of the cheeks, lips, or, less commonly, the gums, this condition may be spotted first by the patient's dentist.

Atrial fibrillation is an abnormal rhythm in the contraction of the chambers of the heart that may leave some blood pooled in the heart. While pooled, the blood may form a clot. When this clot is finally ejected out into the bloodstream, it poses a risk of stroke. To reduce this risk, patients with atrial fibrillation are often given the anticoagulant (blood thinner) warfarin (Coumadin). This drug prolongs the time it takes for blood to clot, so patients using warfarin must check with their physicians to decide when or whether to stop taking the anticoagulant for a period of time before and after a procedure such as dental surgery or SCALING that causes bleeding.

Bleeding disorders such as *hemophilia* are inherited conditions that interfere with the normal ability of blood to clot. Before scheduling or proceeding with dental surgery on a patient with a bleeding disorder, the dentist will check with the patient's hematologist (a physician specializing in blood conditions) to ascertain the patient's ability to deal with the surgery.

Cancer patients may be given treatments that reduce the ability of the IMMUNE SYSTEM to fight infection. As a result, dental professionals and cancer specialists recommend that cancer patients:

• schedule a dental exam and cleaning before cancer treatment begins

• practice good dental hygiene to reduce the risk of infection

• plan regular checkups throughout the treatment period

• tell the dentist about any incidents of dental bleeding, soreness, or infection to both dentist and oncologist (the physician treating the cancer)

• discuss any dental procedures with the oncologist before proceeding

Cardiovascular disease increases a patient's risk of a forming a blood clot that might block an artery and cause a heart attack or stroke. Patients with cardiovascular disease are often given daily doses of aspirin, an anticoagulant that prolongs the time it takes blood to clot. Patients on aspirin therapy must check with their physicians to decide when or whether to stop taking the anticoagulant for a period of time before and after dental surgery, scaling, or any other procedure that causes bleeding.

Crohn's disease is a chronic disorder that causes inflammation of the intestinal tract, most commonly in the small intestine. However, Crohn's may affect any part of the gastrointestinal tube, from the mouth to the anus. One symptom, lesions on the mucous membrane lining of the mouth, are visible during a dental exam.

Developmental disability may increase a patient's anxiety regarding dental treatment, as well as his/her physical reaction to various medications, specifically anesthesia.

Diabetes mellitus increases the risk of infection; it is considered a major risk factor for chronic PERIODONTAL DISEASE, but a diabetic patient who controls his condition can reduce his risk by half or more. Insofar as dental treatment is concerned, a patient with diabetes must schedule his dental appointments at times that enable him to avoid hypoglycemia (low blood sugar) and maintain the proper insulin regimen. If the dental work includes a procedure that makes it hard for him to eat for some time afterward, he should confer with his physician in advance to readjust his insulin dosage as required. *Note*: Many cases of diabetes go undiagnosed. A dental patient with aggressive periodontal disease that does not respond rapidly to treatment may be referred to his physician to be evaluated for diabetes.

HIV/AIDS reduces the patient's ability to fight off infection, requiring stringent adherence to infection-control measures to protect the patient and reduce the risk of transmitting the infection to dental personnel.

Thyroid disorders make a patient sensitive to medicines used in dentistry. Patients with hyperthyroidism (overproduction of thyroid hormones) may be sensitive to vasoconstrictors (drugs that constrict blood vessels) found in local anesthetics. In extreme cases, exposure to these chemicals may worsen the symptoms of the thyroid disorder leading to fever, central nervous system problems (agitation, confusion), gastrointestinal reactions (vomiting, diarrhea), irregular heartbeat, and congestive heart failure. Patients with hypothyroidism (underproduction of thyroid hormones) may be sensitive to sedatives and narcotics. Before proceeding with treatment, the dentist should make sure that the patient's medication and condition have not changed.

See also ANTIBIOTIC PROPHYLAXIS; HERPES, ORAL; INFECTION CONTROL; ORAL CANCER; STOMATITIS.

specialties, dental See AMERICAN DENTAL ASSOCIATION; DENTISTRY; ENDODONTICS; ORAL AND MAXILLOFACIAL PATHOLOGY; ORAL AND MAXILLOFACIAL RADIOLOGY; ORAL AND MAXILLOFACIAL SURGERY; ORTHODONTICS AND DENTOFACIAL ORTHOPEDICS; PEDIATRIC DENTISTRY; PERIODONTICS; PROSTHODONTICS.

splint A rigid support; in dentistry, an appliance made of metal, plastic, or a resin compound similar to that used to fill cavities that provides temporary or permanent support for a tooth knocked out and replanted or a fractured tooth or a tooth loosened by extensive loss of jawbone due to PERIODONTAL DISEASE. Splints may also be used to tie together parts of a denture.

Classifying Dental Splints as Temporary or Permanent

One way to characterize dental splints is by the length of time they remain in the mouth. A fixed splint, which may include a replacement tooth, is designed to remain permanently in place. A provisional splint provides temporary support. For example, a cast bar splint (a.k.a. a Friedman splint), a continuous clasp splint, and a crib splint are used to hold one or more teeth steady during the period when the dentist is preparing a permanent appliance.

Classifying Dental Splints by Site and Function

Dental splints may be named for the place on the teeth to which they are attached. For example, an abutment splint unites two adjacent teeth. A cap splint covers the top of the tooth. A cross arch bar splint links teeth on one side of the dental arch (the curve formed by the teeth in the jaw) to the other. A labial splint (from the Latin *labium*, meaning "lip") sits on the side of the teeth facing the lips. A lingual splint (from the Latin *lingua*, meaning "tongue") sits on the side of the teeth facing the tongue. An interdental splint is wired to the inside and/or outside of teeth on the upper and lower jaw to keep the jaw rigid after an injury or surgery.

Dental splints are also described by their function. For example, a bite-guard splint covers the occlusive (biting) surface of the teeth so as to reduce the effects of tooth-grinding.

stages of oral cancer, staging See ORAL CANCER.

sterilization, dental instruments See INFECTION CONTROL.

stomatitis From the Greek *stoma*, meaning "mouth," and *itis*, meaning "inflammation." Mouth sores; any inflammation of the soft tissues in the mouth (cheeks, gums, LIPS, palate, TONGUE) due to a bacterial, fungal, or viral infection; an allergic reaction; a physical irritation due to a food or drug (including a burn caused by accidentally taking a mouthful of a very hot food); a chronic condition such as leukemia; or radiation treatment to the head or neck. Inflammation may also result from irritation or damage due to an injury from badly fitted dentures, an orthodontic appliance, a hard TOOTHBRUSH, a chipped tooth, or a sharp-edged food such as a broken hard candy. In rare cases, mouth sores may be a symptom of exposure to poisonous heavy metals, such as mercury or lead.

Symptoms and Diagnostic Path

The general symptoms of stomatitis due to an injury or bacterial infection are redness, swelling, pain, and in some cases accompanied by bad breath.

A viral infection such as an APHTHOUS ULCER (canker sore) or a HERPES lesion (cold sore) usually produces a characteristic small, whitish sore. Oral THRUSH, a fungal infection due to the *Candida albicans* organism, causes slightly raised but rarely painful small yellow, cream, white, or even bluish patches on the tongue, gums, or inside surface of the cheeks.

Identifying the cause of the mouth sores may be as simple as noting an incident of radiation treatment on the patient's chart or locating a rough spot on a dental appliance. Diagnosing a bacterial, fungal, or viral stomatitis may require blood tests, a biopsy of scrapings from the affected area, and culturing to isolate the specific infectious agent.

Treatment Options and Outlook

The treatment for mouth sores varies depending on the cause. A rinse or topical anesthetic gel, or a coating of an alkaline product such as Kaopectate, or a paste of baking soda and water may neutralize the acidity and relieve discomfort.

Bacterial Stomatitis A mouth sore due to an infection, either after an injury or arising from periodontal disease, is treated with the appropriate antibiotic. NOMA (a.k.a. noma stomatitis, gangrenous stomatitis, or cancrum oris) is a severe form of bacterial infection most commonly found among very young (age two to five years), malnourished children living in areas where the sanitation is poor. The infection begins as a small ulcer on the gum tissue and quickly moves on to damage and eventually destroy tissue inside the cheek and lips. If left untreated, noma may cause massive necrosis (death) of facial bones and soft tissue, and then either spontaneously disappear or, conversely, spread to the face and become potentially lethal. Antibiotics and a nutritionally adequate diet can effectively halt the infection; plastic surgery may be required to cut away the damaged tissue and perhaps to rebuild bones.

Fungal Stomatitis Otherwise healthy adults with mild cases of thrush may be able to control the infection simply with capsules or unsweetened yogurt containing acidophilus bacteria.

More serious cases are treated with lozenges, liquids, or gels containing the fungicide nystatin (Mycostatin); an infection that spreads from the mouth to other parts of the body may require systemic antifungal medicines.

Viral Infection A single aphthous ulcer usually heals fairly quickly on its own; a cluster of the sores may be treated with tetracycline antibiotics to prevent infection or corticosteroids to reduce swelling and pain. Some dentists also use a carbon dioxide laser to reduce pain and inflammation and speed healing. A single herpes infection on the lips or in the mouth is treated with prescription or nonprescription antiviral medicine; recurrent attacks may be controlled, but not eliminated, with systemic antiviral medicines such as a cyclovir (Zovirax).

Risk Factors and Preventive Measures

To reduce the risk of mouth sores, the patient must avoid the common triggers such as poorly fitting dentures, sharp edges on braces, or chipped teeth, all of which can be ameliorated by proper dental care. Avoiding accidents such as hitting the inside of the mouth with the toothbrush requires the patient's attention to detail, as does using certain products such as high-alcohol MOUTHWASH strictly according to the directions, and avoiding cosmetics, drugs, or foods to which the patient has experienced allergic reactions. Good oral hygiene, regular checkups, and adequate nutrition may reduce the risk of bacterial, fungal, and viral infections.

See also DENTURES.

stress, emotional See BRUXISM; PERIODONTAL DISEASE.

sulcus Groove; an indentation on the surface of the brain such as the central sulcus separating the frontal lobe of the brain from the parietal lobe immediately behind it, or a groove on a mucous membrane such as the terminal sulcus separating the front of the tongue from the back of the tongue. Other examples are the alveolo-lingual sulcus, the groove in the space between the jawbone and the tongue, and a groove on a tooth surface such as the occlusal sulcus, the indentation on the top of a tooth.

Each tooth is circled by a gingival sulcus, a groove in the gum tissue normally less than 3 millimeters/0.1 inch deep where PERIODONTAL DISEASE occurs. Repeated episodes of inflammation or infection in this area can destroy the tissue holding the gum to the tooth and jawbone, eventually creating a deep depression called a pocket. Note: The implant gingival sulcus is the groove in the gum around an implant.

See IMPLANTOLOGY.

Surgeon General   The U.S. Surgeon General is the country's chief medical officer and educator. He or she is a member of the U.S. Department of Health and Human Services appointed by the president of the United States to oversee the operations of the U.S. Public Health Service. From time to time, the Surgeon General has released reports on various health issues, perhaps the most famous being those relating the health consequences of tobacco use beginning in 1964 with *Smoking and Health: Report of the Advisory Committee of the Surgeon General of the Public Health Service* and continuing through 2006 with *The Health Consequences of Involuntary Exposure to Tobacco Smoke: A Report of the Surgeon General.*

In May 2000, then–Surgeon General David Satcher released *Oral Health in America,* the first-ever Surgeon General report on the relationship between oral health and overall good health. The report identified a "silent epidemic" of dental and oral conditions such as tooth DECAY, PERIODONTAL DISEASE, mouth sores, oral birth defects, chronic facial pain, and ORAL CANCER that "may interfere with vital functions such as breathing, eating, swallowing, and speaking. The burden of disease restricts activities in school, work, and home, and often significantly diminishes the quality of life." A follow-up "National Call to Action to Promote Oral Health" (2003) proposed ways to remedy defects in the state of oral health in the United States. In 2005, a third report—*The Surveillance for Dental Caries, Dental Sealants, Tooth Retention, Edentulism, and Enamel Fluorosis, United States, 1988–1994 and 1999–2002*—laid out statistics on dental and oral health drawn from the National Health and Nutrition Examination Surveys, conducted by the National Center for Health Statistics of the Centers for Disease Control and Prevention. Together, these three documents provide an accurate picture of dental and oral health in the United States at the beginning of the 21st century.

See *ORAL HEALTH IN AMERICA: A REPORT OF THE SURGEON GENERAL;* NATIONAL CALL TO ACTION TO PROMOTE ORAL HEALTH; *THE SURVEILLANCE FOR DENTAL CARIES, DENTAL SEALANTS, TOOTH RETENTION, EDENTULISM, AND ENAMEL FLUOROSIS, UNITED STATES, 1988–1994 AND 1999–2002.*

The Surveillance for Dental Caries, Dental Sealants, Tooth Retention, Edentulism, and Enamel Fluorosis, United States, 1988–1994 and 1999–2002   From time to time, the U.S. Centers for Disease Control and Prevention issues surveillance summaries, reports containing data gathered from the National Health and Nutrition Examination Survey (NHANES), an ongoing sampling of medical information about Americans older than two months who are not living in institutions such as nursing homes. Note: Because children younger than two rarely have all their primary teeth, this surveillance summary for dental health and practices, released in August 2005, contains information applicable to Americans older than two years.

Results of the Surveillance Summary (2005)

Comparing the two periods (1988–94 and 1999–2002) the NHANES data shows four clear trends in dental information for American older than two years:

- No change in the percentage (41) of children aged 2–11 with cavities in their primary teeth.
- Up to 10 percent reduction (down from 52 percent in 1988–94 to 42 percent in 1999–2002) in the incidence of cavities in permanent teeth among Americans aged 6–19 years; and a 3.3 percent reduction among all adults older than 20, down from 94.6 percent in 1988–94 to 91.3 percent in 1999–2004.
- Among adults older than 20 who had not lost all their teeth, slightly more than one-fifth had untreated tooth decay. The incidence was higher among men than among women and higher among those aged 20 to 39 than among other age groups.
- An increase of 13 percent in the use of dental sealants among Americans aged 6–19 years, from 19 percent in 1988–94 to 32 percent in 1999–2002.
- A reduction of 6 percent in the number of Americans older than 60 years who had lost all their natural teeth, down from 14 percent in 1988–94 to 8 percent in 1999–2002.
- In 1999–2002, 23 percent of Americans aged 6–39 years had enamel fluorosis (discoloration of the teeth due to exposure to fluoride), an increase apparent in people born after the 1980s that is presumed due to the increased availability of fluoridated water.

Recommendations for Public Health Action

Based on the data in this surveillance summary, the Centers for Disease Control and Prevention issued a number of recommendations.

- First, because dental services leading to good dental health are not currently equally available to all socioeconomic groups in the United States, the report recommends improving access to dental professionals for all Americans. For example, among all Americans older than 20 years who still had their natural teeth, the incidence of untreated tooth decay was higher among Mexican-Americans (35.9 percent) and non-Hispanic black Americans (41.3 percent) than among non-Hispanic white Americans (18.4 percent). The incidence of untreated decay among adults was up to 2.5 times higher among Americans with low-income levels versus those with incomes twice the poverty level, and those with less than a high school education versus those who had graduated from high school.
- Second, the report notes the necessity for research to specifically study why the percentage of children with cavities in primary teeth has not declined.
- Third, the report notes that the number of older Americans is growing and urges an increase in preventive individual, community-based, and clinical practices to reduce the age-related loss of natural teeth.
- Fourth, the report urges an increase in the number of public health programs to promote oral health (i.e., the use of dental sealants and quit-smoking regimens) and urges that these programs be set up so as to make them equally available across income and socioeconomic lines.
- Fifth, the report suggests a need for increased information to monitor the exposure to fluoride from various sources including, but not limited to, fluoridated water supplies.

This is a précis of the CDC report. The entire report is available online at www.cdc.gov/MMWR/preview/mmwrhtml/ss5403a1.htme dental.

suture   Stitch; fine material (thread, WIRE) used to join tissues or close the edges of a surgical incision or a wound; for example, after periodontal surgery.

Sutures are usually described in one of five ways: the suture material (natural or synthetic), the suture's construction (monofilament or multifilament), the suture's interaction with the body (absorbable or nonabsorbable), the size of the thread, and the suture's placement (where it sits in the mouth) and style (how the thread is inserted and anchored).

Suture Material

The natural material most commonly used in dental sutures is silk. Other natural materials used in sutures are cotton fibers and sterilized "gut," a twisted, threadlike absorbable wound closure, originally derived from catgut but now made from beef (bovine gut suture) or sheep (ovine gut suture) intestinal connective tissue. A thin iron-chromium-nickel-molybdenum alloy wire suture may be used to immobilize a fractured JAW.

The synthetic materials commonly used to repair the soft tissue in the mouth after dental surgery are polymers, substances composed of long chains of molecules.

Suture Construction

Sutures may be monofilament (a single strand) or multifilament/polyfilament (several strands braided or twisted together). Monofilament sutures are easier to tie, pass more easily through tissue, and are less likely to collect bacteria once in place. Multifilament sutures are more flexible, less likely to break or crimp, and stronger once in place.

Both natural and synthetic monofilament and multifilament sutures may be coated with substances that make them easier to handle, improve their ability to pass smoothly through body tissue so as to avoid excess injury, to reduce the risk of reaction with body tissues, and to maintain the suture's strength by slowing absorption or dissolution. Some sutures are colored with dye to make them more visible to the surgeon.

Suture Interaction with the Body

Absorbable sutures are dissolved by body fluids; nonabsorbable sutures must be removed by the surgeon. The sutures most commonly used in dental surgery are made of Dexon and Vicryl. Dexon (polycyclic acid), the first absorbable synthetic suture material, was introduced in 1983. Vicryl (polyglactin 910) was introduced in 1985.

Nonabsorbable sutures (silk, cotton, plastic, wire) on a body surface are removed as soon as the incision has healed sufficiently to remain closed on its own, usually within a week after surgery. Note: Although silk is commonly classified as a nonabsorbable material for dental purposes, if it is left inside the body after general surgery it is usually degraded by enzymes over a period of perhaps two years. Cotton and plastic suture left inside the body are eventually covered and encased in connective tissue or bone tissue when used to stabilize bone.

In the summer of 2007, researchers at the University of Texas Southwestern Medical

COMMON DENTAL SUTURES

Suture	Description
Blanket	A continuous suture that loops each stitch over the one before; also known as a continuous lock stitch
Continuous	A single thread used to make repeated loops along a line in the gum with a knot at the beginning and the end; also known as a running suture
Crisscross	An X-shaped stitch formed by running a thread from one side of the gum diagonally across to the other side and back again to close a gap in the gum left by a missing tooth
Interrupted	A line of individual sutures, each tied with a knot
Mattress	A continuous suture that goes back and forth though the same tissue (such as the gum) but at different levels
Single interrupted	A single loop tying one side of the gum to the other
Suspension	A stitch that goes around a tooth to anchor a flap on the side of the gum next to the tongue or cheek

Center (Dallas) reported in the *Archives of Facial Plastic Surgery* that using hydrogen peroxide to clean wounds closed with absorbable and gut sutures could weaken the suture material. The hydrogen peroxide did not affect nonabsorbable sutures; cleaning the wound with distilled water was safe for both absorbable and nonabsorbable sutures.

Suture Size

The U.S. Pharmacopoeia (an official list of drugs published each year by the United States Pharmacopoeia Convention) has established standard sizes for sutures as measured by the diameter of the suture. Currently, standard sutures range in size from 3-0 to 4-0 (the largest) down to 12-0 (the finest). For comparison, a 0 suture made of any material other than catgut is 0.350–399 mm in diameter; a 6-0 suture made of any material other than catgut is 0.070–0.099 mm in diameter. Sutures smaller than 7-0 are visible only under a microscope. As a general rule, the sutures most commonly used in surgery inside the mouth are sizes 3-0 and 4-0.

Suture Placement and Style

Dental sutures may be described by their location near or next to a tooth or part of the jaw. For example, a circumferential suture is one that loops entirely around a tooth; an interdental suture passes between two teeth to join opposing sides of the gum; and an intermaxillary suture, also known as a median palatine suture, runs from one side of the upper jaw (maxilla) to the other.

Finally, dentists characterize their sutures by style, that is, the way the suture is inserted so as to hold the open edges (flaps) of tissue together. The table shows a selected list of dental sutures listed by style.

tartar See CALCULUS.

taste, sense of The sense of taste is the ability to respond to molecules in food and drink that carry flavor messages.

The Chemistry of Taste

The sense of taste is a chemical process conducted by specialized sensory organs called taste buds located in small protuberances on the TONGUE. Each taste bud contains a microvillus, a thread-like receptor that reacts to chemicals in food and drink, delivering a message via nerves to the brain. The nerves that deliver taste messages to the brain are the facial nerve, which serves the front two-thirds of the tongue, and the glosso-pharyngeal nerve, which serves the back third of the tongue. The brain translates messages carried from the taste buds via the facial and glosso-pharyngeal nerves as flavors: sweet, sour, bitter, salty, and umami (a rich flavor most commonly associated with soy products). A second set of sensory messages related to taste is delivered via nerve endings on the mucous membrane lining of the nose, mouth, and throat. These nerve endings transmit sensations such as the "cool" sensation of mint and the "bite" of hot peppers.

Originally, researchers assumed that specific taste buds delivered specific messages related to one or another of the five flavors. Today, the prevailing theory is that the taste buds work together to create patterns the brain recognizes as one of the flavors, a process described in scientific terms as the "across fiber pattern theory of gustatory neural coding."

Factors that Influence the Sense of Taste

Age, illness, and medicine may impact the sense of taste, producing partial or total ageusia (the medical term for "loss of taste"). Food interactions may cause "flavor confusion," that is, interpreting a sour flavor as bitter, a sweet flavor as salty, or vice versa.

Age and the Sense of Taste With increasing age, the sense of taste becomes less acute because taste buds that are lost as a person grows older are not replaced. One solution to this problem is to season food more aggressively.

Illness and the Sense of Taste Several dental and medical conditions or treatments may affect the sense of taste. For example:

- Poor oral hygiene or an episode of PERIODON-TAL DISEASE may alter the transmission of messages from the oral nerves.

- A bacterial or viral infection of the upper respiratory tract or a bacterial, viral, or fungal infection of the mouth may produce secretions that coat the tongue and block the taste buds.

- An injury, radiation therapy to the mouth, nose, or throat, or a nutritional deficiency (i.e., a niacin deficiency) may damage nerves that transmit flavor messages.

- An injury or illness of the brain such as a tumor or a vascular incident (stroke) may interfere with the ability to interpret flavor messages, as may any disease of the central nervous system such as Parkinson's disease.

Medical Drugs and the Sense of Taste Some medical drugs may reduce the ability to taste food. These drugs include (but are not limited to) some anti-infective agents (antibiotics and anti-fungal products), cancer chemotherapy agents, psychotropic medications, and drugs used to treat rheumatoid arthritis and thyroid conditions.

Food Interactions and the Sense of Taste   Some food combinations reduce the ability to interpret flavor signals correctly. For example, alcohol beverages commonly deliver an acidic flavor sensation, but tasting cheese before the beer, wine, or spirits causes fat molecules in the cheese to coat receptor cells on the tongue, thus reducing the ability of the acidic flavor cells in the beverage to link up with the receptor cells. A similar phenomenon occurs when one eats a globe artichoke. The flesh of the artichoke heart contains cynarin, a sweet-tasting chemical that dissolves in water-based liquid such as saliva so that any food eaten immediately after the artichoke will taste sweet.

teeth   See TOOTH.

teething   The eruption of the primary (first) teeth through the gums, usually when a child is between three and 12 months of age. In most cases, the lower front teeth are the first to appear, followed in a month or two by the top front teeth.

Symptoms and Diagnostic Path

The signs that a baby is teething may including an increase in fussiness and a refusal to eat or drink due to the discomfort of swollen gums. Drooling is common once the teeth actually begin to break through the gum.

Treatment Options and Outlook

Classic remedies such as a teething ring or gently rubbing the baby's gums with a clean finger may help relieve the discomfort of a swollen gum. If the discomfort is severe, the pediatrician may recommend a mild pain reliever such as Tylenol. *Caution:* Never give a baby aspirin without consulting a doctor; in young children, all salicylates, including aspirin (acetylsalicylic acid) have been associated with a seriously increased risk of Reye's syndrome, a potentially fatal condition.

Teething gels or powders should not be used without consulting a doctor. The gels, which contain local anesthetics to numb the baby's gums, may be harmful if swallowed or used to excess, and the powder may cause a baby to accidentally inhale particles.

Risk Factors and Preventive Measures

There are no preventive measures and no risk factors other than being an infant.

template   A pattern; in dentistry, a mold or IMPRESSION that is an accurate replica of the shape of a part of the mouth. There are many different types of templates.

- An *occlusal template* is a mold made from WAX impressions of the movement of the teeth against each other. This template shows the dentist how the jaws move and where the teeth do and do not meet correctly.

- An *orthodontics template* is a tracing made from a cephalometric radiograph (an X-ray taken with a camera that rotates around the head to provide a full circle picture). This template can be used to compare the patient's facial and dental characteristics against a norm established for a specific age and gender when planning orthodontic treatment.

- A *prosthetic template* is a plate used to set teeth in dentures.

- A *surgical template* is a transparent plastic base that mimics the underside of an immediate denture (a temporary denture put into the mouth immediately after one or more teeth are removed). It is used as a guide in shaping the tissue and bone of the jaw so that the denture fits well.

- A *wax template* is an impression showing how the teeth meet when closed. This template may be used in planning a variety of corrective treatments from simply filing down a slightly-too-long tooth to complicated orthodontic corrections.

See also IMPRESSION, DENTAL.

temporomandibular disorder   The temporomandibular joint is a ball-in-socket joint (cartilage) that connects the lower jaw to the flat temporal BONE, the part of the skull that forms the side of the face. The movement of the ball (the condyle) at the back on each side of the lower jaw in the socket (fossa) on each side of the skull enables the lower jaw to move up and down and side to side.

Temporomandibular disorder (TMD) is a term commonly used to describe a temporary or persistent pain in the joint arising from:

- an injury to the JAW, the joint, or the muscles that move the joint, including dislocation of the joint
- persistent BRUXISM—grinding or clenching the teeth—usually resulting from emotional stress
- arthritis in the joint

Symptoms and Diagnostic Path

The common symptoms of TMD include (but are not limited to):

- pain or tenderness in the area around the joint, sometimes extending as far as the ear when the patient chews or opens her mouth wide
- headache, or earache with no identifiable cause such as an infection
- a feeling of being locked in position when the jaws are open wide or closed tight
- a click, grating, popping or other unusual sound whenever the joint moves

To rule out other conditions some of whose symptoms may be similar—for example, migraine headaches or an ear infection—the dentist will examine the affected joint and surrounding muscles manually while observing how the patient moves the jaw, and may request imaging studies such as X-rays to check for any structural abnormality in the joint or surrounding bone.

Treatment Options and Outlook

The treatments for TMD vary with the cause and severity of the problem. However, they can usually be grouped into one of three categories: Simple self-care treatments; conservative, reversible treatments; and invasive and/or irreversible treatments.

Simple Self-Care Treatments for TMD   Simple stratagems such as avoiding hard or chewy foods, or applying heat or cold packs to the joint, or avoiding extreme jaw movements such as opening wide to yawn may relieve the discomfort of temporary or mild TMD. For mild short-term discomfort, dentists usually prescribe over-the-counter pain relievers such as acetaminophen (Tylenol) or ibuprofen (Advil).

Conservative, Reversible Treatments for TMD   Wearing a MOUTH GUARD that prevents clenched teeth from grinding against each other may temporarily relieve TMD arising from bruxism. Relaxation techniques such as BIOFEEDBACK, as well as hypnotism or psychotherapy, may help alleviate stress that leads to bruxism. Physical therapy exercises to stretch and relax the muscles around the temporomandibular joint may also be useful.

Invasive and/or Irreversible Treatments for TMD   This class of remedies includes various therapeutic injections, arthroscopy, and joint replacement.

- *Therapeutic injections* As with other forms of arthritis, some dentists recommend steroid injections to relieve pain in an arthritic temporomandibular joint. Another injectable treatment is Synvisc, a synthetic product similar to synovial fluid, which is a lubricant found naturally in joints.
- *Arthroscopy* A surgery performed under general anesthesia during which the surgeon makes

a small incision in front of the ear to insert a thin tube; through this tube the doctor passes a light and camera that display the inside of the joint on a video screen. A second tube through which the doctor passes surgical instruments is inserted to facilitate removal of inflamed tissue or realignment of the components of the joint so that it moves more smoothly.

- *Joint replacement surgery* The U.S. Food and Drug Administration (FDA) has approved several devices for replacing the temporomandibular joint when reconstructing the jawbone for patients who have severe arthritis or degenerative disease of the joint, previous multiple surgeries, severe fractures, tumors, or severe developmental abnormalities such as birth defects that cannot be treated by other means. However, as of this writing the FDA does not recommend these devices for use as partial temporomandibular joint (TMJ) replacements or for any patient who has an active or chronic infection or a disease that increases the likelihood of infection; who has insufficient bone to support the device or is skeletally immature; who has an allergy or a previous reaction to any of the materials used in the replacement joint; or who is unable to follow instructions after the surgery. The FDA is currently conducting long-term studies on the safety and effectiveness of these replacement joints.

Risk Factors and Preventive Measures

TMD is most common among people aged 20 to 40, and the most common risk factor in this, and any other group, is stress. Therefore, any technique that reduces stress may help prevent or reduce the severity of TMD.

thermal sensitivity   A temporary sensitivity to heat or cold, most commonly to hot or cold foods but also to hot or cold air breathed in through the mouth.

Symptoms and Diagnostic Path

Immediate sensation of pain upon exposure to hot or cold food or air. The most likely causes for this sensitivity are recent dental work that has temporarily inflamed the tissues around a tooth, a cavity, a filling that has come loose, or a chip or fracture in the tooth that allows hot or cold food or air to reach the nerve inside the tooth. Gum recession that has left the surface of the root of the tooth exposed can also cause thermal sensitivity.

Treatment Options and Outlook

The treatment for sensitivity to heat and cold depends on the cause.

- Sensitivity due to a cavity or a loose filling is remedied by filling the cavity or replacing the filling.

- Sensitivity due to a fractured tooth requires endoscopic treatment during which the dentist rebuilds the tooth or, if that is not possible, extracts the fractured tooth and replaces it with a false tooth or—most likely with a back tooth—leaves the space open.

- Sensitivity due to gum recession is usually treated by brushing with toothpaste designed specifically to reduce sensation on the tooth surface.

Risk Factors and Preventive Measures

Regular dental and periodontal checkups as well as good ORAL HYGIENE may reduce the risk of some causes of thermal sensitivity.

See also DECAY; PERIODONTAL DISEASE.

3-D conformal radiotherapy (3DCRT)   See RADIATION THERAPY.

thrush   Candidiasis, oral; a fungal (*Candida*) infection of the tongue and membrane lining of the mouth. The thrush organism lives naturally in the mouth and is ordinarily kept in check by other naturally resident organisms. When the IMMUNE SYSTEM is weakened, the infection may flare up.

Symptoms and Diagnostic Path

The signs of a thrush infection are soft white spots on the tongue or lining of the mouth.

Under the white surface, the tissue is red and may bleed. In people with weakened immune systems, such as those who are getting chemotherapy for cancer or who are HIV positive, the fungal infection may spread to the throat and, in rare cases, throughout the body.

A biopsy or culture of a small tissue sample can confirm the presence of *Candida* organisms and thus a diagnosis of a thrush infection.

Treatment Options and Outlook

In infants, thrush often resolves spontaneously; to prevent recurrence, parents are advised to sterilize bottle nipples and pacifiers.

The simplest treatment for thrush in an otherwise healthy adult is simply to practice good oral hygiene and allow the illness to run its course naturally. A second simple treatment is antifungal MOUTHWASH or antifungal lozenges. If these fail to clear the infection, or if it begins to spread, or if the patient has a compromised immune system, the doctor/dentist may prescribe systemic antifungal medication such as ketoconazole (Nizoral) or fluconazole (Diflucan).

As with any infection, the effectiveness of treatment for thrush depends to a large degree on the overall health of the patient's immune system. The stronger the immune system is, the better the predicted outcome.

Risk Factors and Preventive Measures

The primary risk factor for thrush is a weakened immune system. Those at highest risk are the very young and the very old; patients in generally poor health; patients whose immune responses are reduced by HIV/AIDS, cancer chemotherapy, or medications to suppress the immune system after an organ transplant; and persons with diabetes.

For persons who experience frequent thrush infections, prevention may include regular antifungal medication. Safe sex practice can prevent the spread of thrush from one person to another.

thumb sucking Sucking is a natural reflex that not only enables infants to feed but also provides them with information about their own bodies and lends older children with a sense of comfort and security.

Most children stop thumb sucking (or sucking on pacifiers) by the time they are two to four years old. Thumb sucking that continues after this age may affect the alignment of the permanent teeth, commonly requiring orthodontic treatment to reposition the teeth.

Symptoms and Diagnostic Path

Thumb sucking that continues after the primary teeth appear may alter the alignment of the teeth, a situation clearly visible to the child's parent or her dentist. Children who simply put their thumbs in their mouths and do not suck strongly are less likely to alter the alignment of their teeth than are children who suck vigorously enough to produce a pop sound when the thumb comes out of the mouth.

Treatment Options and Outlook

Punishing a young child for sucking behavior or attempting to force him to stop may interfere with sleep patterns or other development. Praising the child or rewarding him for not sucking the thumb or a pacifier appear to be more effective, especially if the child seems to suck his thumb more frequently during stressful situations, such as being separated from a parent. Older children may respond to an offer to participate in choosing the way to stop sucking or to a dentist's explanation of the effects of thumb sucking on the teeth.

In any event, most children give up sucking behavior naturally around the time they begin school or when the first permanent teeth erupt around age six.

Risk Factors and Preventive Measures

Thumb sucking is normal. Thumb sucking among older children may be a reaction to stress; alleviating the stress may reduce the behavior.

tic douloureux See TRIGEMINAL NEURALGIA.

tobacco Tobacco products—chewing tobacco as well as smoking tobacco—are a significant risk factor for dental problems and disorders of the mouth including (but not limited to):

- ORAL CANCER
- PERIODONTAL DISEASE with consequent gum recession and bone loss leading to an increased risk of CAVITIES on the exposed tooth roots and tooth loss resulting from the loss of supporting jawbone; according to the U.S. Centers for Disease Control and Prevention (CDC), nearly half of all daily cigarette, cigar, and pipe smokers have lost all their teeth by age 65 versus less than 20 percent of people who have never smoked
- slowed healing after dental surgery such as an extraction
- increased risk of failure of dental treatment such as implants
- mouth sores
- stained teeth
- bad breath
- disorders of the sense of taste

All tobacco, whether smoked or chewed, contains a variety of known carcinogens. The National Cancer Institute has identified at least 60 such chemicals in tobacco smoke and nearly 30 such chemicals in smokeless tobacco, a product associated with koilocytosis, a precancerous change in cells in the mucous membrane lining of the mouth. Not inhaling the smoke or swallowing the "juice" from chewing tobacco does not reduce the risk of oral exposure to these toxins, nor does the water in a hookah filter out the chemicals.

In addition, the heat from a cigarette, cigar, or pipe is irritating to the oral tissues, and the nicotine in tobacco constricts blood vessels, disrupting the even flow of oxygen- and nutrient-rich blood to oral tissues.

See EXTRACTION; IMPLANTOLOGY.

tongue The tongue is a organ composed of striated (voluntary) MUSCLE covered with mucous MEMBRANE dotted with small protuberances called papillae and taste buds. The front of the tongue, known as the oral tongue, is attached to the floor of the mouth by a fold of tissue called the lingual frenulum (from the Latin word *lingua*, meaning "tongue" and *frenum*, meaning "fold"). The back of the tongue (the part that curves down into the throat) is called the base.

The Role of the Tongue
The tongue plays an important role in the digestive system. First, it contains the taste buds, organs that transmit signals regarding flavor and texture. Second, the tongue pushes food to the back of the mouth, directing it into the esophagus (throat), the tube that leads to the stomach. Finally, the tongue is vital for speech; its position and movement in the mouth produce specific sounds.

Health Conditions of the Tongue
Like other organs in the body, the tongue is subject to a multiplicity of disorders, including birth defects and specific diseases. In addition, the condition of the tongue often provides a clue to other bodily conditions.

Birth Defects or Other Defects of the Tongue These conditions are also known as congenital (present at birth):

- *Aglossia* (from the Greek word *glosso*, meaning "tongue") is a missing tongue.
- *Bifid tongue* is a tongue with a cleft (division) down the middle.
- *Fissured tongue*, also known as a furrowed tongue, is a tongue with wrinkles in the pattern of a leaf coming down from the back of the tongue toward the front. This condition may be present at birth or develop later in life.
- *Lobulated tongue* is a tongue with an extra piece (lobe) rising up from the surface.
- *Tongue tie*, also known as ankyloglossia or short frenulum, is a bunching of tissue around the lingual frenulum that makes it difficult if not impossible to move the tongue freely.

Diseases of the Tongue   The umbrella term for an inflammation of the tongue is glossitis. Geographic glossitis is the loss of tissue from the top of the tongue in several spots. Glossodynia is a burning sensation on the tongue. The most serious disease of the tongue is TONGUE CANCER.

Side Effects of Medication or Nutrient Deficiencies

- *Antibiotic tongue* is a catchall phrase for side effects associated with the use of antibiotic drugs. One common example is hairy tongue, an overgrowth of the papillae.

- *Atrophic glossitis,* also known as bald tongue or smooth tongue, is a shrinkage of the papillae on the tongue surface associated with anemia or a vitamin B deficiency disease such as pellagra.

- *Cobblestone tongue,* an enlargement of the papillae, is associated with a riboflavin (vitamin B_2) deficiency.

- *Magenta tongue* is a reddish/purple coloring due to a riboflavin (vitamin B_2) deficiency.

Disorders of the Tongue Associated with an Infectious Disease or Other Bodily Health Problem

- *Coated tongue* means whitish accumulations on the tongue, a sign of a systemic infection or illness.

- *Glossoplegia* is paralysis of one or both sides of the tongue. *Flat tongue* is paralysis most commonly associated with advanced syphilis, which makes it impossible to curl the tongue.

- *Macroglossia* (an abnormally large tongue) and *thrusting tongue* (the inability to keep the tongue inside the mouth) are most commonly signs of a genetic disorder such as Down syndrome.

- *Strawberry tongue* is a red inflammation associated with scarlet fever.

Care of the Tongue

In the course of a day's eating and drinking, debris such as food particles and microorganisms are likely to accumulate on the tongue. In extreme cases, the pileup of debris may darken the appearance of the tongue, a condition called black tongue or black hairy tongue (*lingua nigra*). It may also contribute to HALITOSIS (bad breath).

To wipe away the smelly, discolored debris, some people brush the tongue with a TOOTHBRUSH or scrape it with a small spoon. A more effective way of cleaning the tongue is to use a specialized tongue cleaner such as a tongue brush or tongue scraper, available in the dental section of most drugstores.

See also NERVES; ORAL HYGIENE; PIERCING, ORAL; TASTE, SENSE OF; TONGUE RECONSTRUCTION.

tongue cancer   A malignant tumor of the tongue, usually occurring on the side of the tongue, commonly discovered during a routine dental or periodontal examination.

Symptoms and Diagnostic Path

About one-third of all cancers of the tongue are diagnosed while the tumor is still localized and has not spread. Almost 50 percent are diagnosed after the cancer has spread to adjacent tissue or to the lymph nodes. Slightly more than 10 percent are diagnosed after the tumor has spread to distant sites in the body, such as the lung.

The early signs of tongue cancer include (but are not limited to):

- a small hard lump
- a hardened thick white or gray-white patch
- an ulcer (a sore with a hard, raised rim and a bleeding center)
- any sore that does not heal within 14 days

The diagnosis of cancer is confirmed by a biopsy of tissue from the affected area.

Treatment Options and Outlook

The primary treatment for cancer of the tongue is removal of the tumor and surrounding tissue, followed, if required, by tongue reconstruction.

INCIDENCE OF TONGUE CANCER BY RACE

Race/Ethnicity	Male	Female
All Races	4.2 per 100,000	1.7 per 100,000
White	4.4 per 100,000	1.7 per 100,000
Black	3.8 per 100,000	1.2 per 100,000
Asian/Pacific Islander	2.1 per 100,000	1.4 per 100,000
American Indian/Alaska Native	1.7 per 100,000	n.a.*
Hispanic	2.2 per 100,000	1.0 per 100,000

The outlook for patients with cancer of the tongue varies with the status of the tumor. National Cancer Institute statistics show that 76 percent of patients diagnosed with localized tumors are likely to survive at least five years. For patients whose cancers are diagnosed after the cancer has spread to adjacent tissues, the five-year survival rate is 53 percent; it drops to 29 percent for those whose tumors have spread to other parts of the body at the time of diagnosis.

Risk Factors and Preventive Measures

The clearest risk factors for most oral cancers, including cancer of the tongue, are the use of tobacco and alcoholic beverages. The risk rises significantly among those who both smoke and drink.

Gender, age, and ethnicity may also be risk factors. First, nearly twice as many men as women develop tongue cancer. Second, the risk rises with age. Statistics from the National Cancer Institute show that fewer than one-tenth of 1 percent of all cases of cancer of the tongue diagnosed between 2001 and 2005 were in people younger than 20, 9 percent occurred in people aged 20 to 44, 50 percent were diagnosed in people aged 45 to 64, and 41 percent in people older than 65. Finally, the following tables show discrepancies among various ethnic groups, although there is some question as to whether different socially acceptable behaviors are the true risk multipliers here. In other words, do more men than women and more American whites than Americans of Hispanic descent smoke and drink?

Statistics aside, the simplest preventive measures are to avoid tobacco and drink only in moderation or not at all, and have regular dental checkups.

DEATH RATES OF TONGUE CANCER BY RACE

Race/Ethnicity	Male	Female
All Races	0.9 per 100,000	0.4 per 100,000
White	0.9 per 100,000	0.4 per 100,000
Black	1.2 per 100,000	0.3 per 100,000
Asian/Pacific Islander	0.5 per 100,000	0.3 per 100,000
American Indian/Alaska Native	n.a.*	n.a*
Hispanic	0.6 per 100,000	0.2 per 100,000

*n.a.—not available

Source: National Cancer Institute, "Surveillance Epidemiology and End Results," *Cancer Statistics Review, 1975–2006* (April 15, 2009), seer.cancer.gov/statfacts/html/tongue.html.

tongue reconstruction Surgery to reconstruct all or part of the TONGUE after removal of a malignant tumor.

Procedure

Tongue reconstruction surgery is performed under general anesthesia. Once the patient is sedated, the surgeon lifts a piece of tissue from another part of the body to rebuild the tongue.

To replace the front part of the tongue, the surgeon may use tissue from the forearm. To replace a large defect or a complete tongue, the surgeon may use:

- skin and underlying tissue from the forearm
- skin and underlying tissue from the side of the thigh
- skin and the underlying muscle from the *latissimus dorsi,* the flat muscle on the side of the trunk behind the arm
- skin and the underlying muscle from the *rectus abdominis,* a.k.a. "abs," the muscle that runs up and down the front of the abdomen

In 2007, a team of surgeons from the National Cancer Center Hospital East, in Chiba, Japan, published a report in the *Journal of Plastic, Reconstructive and Aesthetic Surgery* noting that for very thin patients with little body fat, the *rectus abdominis* flap should have two pieces of skin to bulk up the transplant.

Once the tissue has been harvested, the surgeon moves it into place in the mouth, attaches nerves and blood vessels from the transplanted tissue to the remaining tongue tissue, folds the transplant tissue into the shape of a tongue, and SUTURES it in place. If the surgeon has used tissue from the forearm or the thigh, the last step in the procedure may be a skin GRAFT to cover the wound in the arm or leg.

Risks and Complications

As with any major surgery, tongue reconstruction carries the risk of a reaction to the anesthesia, as well as swelling, bleeding, pain, and the risk of infection, both on the tongue and at the donor site (the site from which the transplant tissue was taken).

The most serious complication, however, would be the failure for the new tongue to prevent food from falling into the trachea, from which point it might be aspirated (drawn into) the lungs.

Outlook and Lifestyle Modification

Successful tongue reconstruction should restore the patient's ability to swallow and speak. Several studies have shown that more than half of all patients who undergo tongue reconstruction are able to take food by mouth, although often with some difficulty. Speech therapy can be useful in teaching the patient to speak clearly after surgery, but the therapy is more likely to succeed for a patient whose reconstruction involved the back (base) of the tongue rather than the front of the tongue.

See also ORAL CANCER; TONGUE; TONGUE CANCER.

tooth A hard, bonelike structure anchored in an ALVEOLUS (socket) in the upper or lower JAW; the body part used for chewing food.

Formation of the Teeth

Odontogenesis (from the Greek words *odontis* or *dont-,* meaning "tooth," and *genesis,* meaning "origin") is the sequence of events that produces a tooth.

The development of the teeth begins about six weeks into a pregnancy. The fetus develops a ridge called the labiodental lamina (from the Latin words *labio,* meaning "lip," and *lamina,* meaning "plate"), the precursor of the oral cavity. Eventually, a thickened U-shape ridge called the dental lamina appears, and soon 10 dental buds arise inside the dental lamina. The dental buds, five on what will be the top jaw and five on the bottom, are also known as enamel organs or dental organs. The buds become a kind of mold called the dental bell in which the teeth begin to develop, and by the fourth month of pregnancy, the hardened primary ("baby") teeth have formed inside the gum. (In rare cases, a child will be born with one or more *natal teeth,* teeth that have erupted prematurely through the gum before birth.)

Occasionally, something goes amiss in the development of the teeth, leading to a variety of developmental disorders. The most common are missing teeth (ANODONTIA), extra teeth, FUSED TEETH, impacted teeth (teeth that are positioned so that they cannot erupt through the gum), and disorders of tooth shape.

The Structure of a Tooth

A tooth is a multilayer structure divided into two basic sections: the crown (the top of the tooth above the natural gum) and the root (the part of the tooth below the natural gum line). The place where the crown and the root meet is called the neck.

- The surface of the crown is made of ENAMEL, a hard calcified tissue composed primarily of calcium crystals.
- Beneath the enamel is a second layer of hard tissue called DENTIN.
- The dentin forms the walls of the PULP chamber, the hollow interior of the tooth.
- The pulp chamber is filled with pulp, a soft tissue that contains blood vessels that nourish the tooth, lymph vessels that carry away waste, and nerves that transmit sensory messages such as heat, cold, and pain.
- The root of the tooth is covered with CEMENTUM rather than enamel. Otherwise, the structure of the root is similar to the crown: a hard outer layer of cementum over a layer of dentin with the root canal (the continuation of the pulp chamber) inside.
- The root (or roots) is covered with the periodontal ligament, connective tissue that holds the tooth in its alveolus (socket).
- At the bottom tip of the root is an opening through which the tooth's blood vessels, lymph vessels and nerves pass into the socket and jawbone.

Naming the Teeth

The collective name for the first teeth to erupt through the gum when a baby teethes is primary teeth, also known as baby teeth or deciduous teeth (from the Latin verb *decidere,* meaning "to fall off"). The secondary, or succedaneous, teeth (from the Latin word *succedere,* meaning "to follow") are the 32 permanent adult teeth that begin to erupt through the gum about age six and continue to develop and erupt well into a person's late teens.

- *Central.* One of the two upper and two lower center teeth. The central is also known as an incisor (a cutting tooth).
- *Lateral.* The tooth right next to the central. Like the central tooth, the lateral is also known as an incisor.
- *Cuspid.* The single cusp (tip) tooth next to the laterals. An alternate name for the cuspid is a canine tooth.
- *First Bicuspid.* The two-cusp tooth right behind the cuspids.
- *Second Bicuspid.* The two-cusp tooth behind the first bicuspids.
- *First Molar.* The four-cusp tooth right behind the second bicuspid. The first molar is also known as a six-year molar because it is likely to erupt when a child is six years old.
- *Second Molar.* The four-cusp tooth behind the first molar. Another name for the second molar is a 12-year molar, because this tooth is likely to erupt when a person is 12 years of age.
- *Third Molar.* The four-cusp tooth behind the second molar. The third molar is also known as a wisdom tooth because it erupts last, presumably at an age when a person has acquired wisdom.

Positioning the Teeth

As a group the teeth in the front of the mouth are known as the anterior teeth; those in the back are known as the posterior teeth.

Numbering the Teeth

There are three basic systems for numbering the individual teeth: the Palmer's notation, numerical notation, and universal numerical notation.

Palmer's Notation This system, originally known as the Zsigmondy system, divides the mouth into four sections called quadrants: Upper left, upper right, lower left, and lower right. Dentists then use the system to link the name of each tooth to the quadrant in which the tooth is located. For example, the central tooth on the left side of the upper jaw is called the upper left central.

Numerical Notation for Teeth The system names the central tooth #1 and goes back from

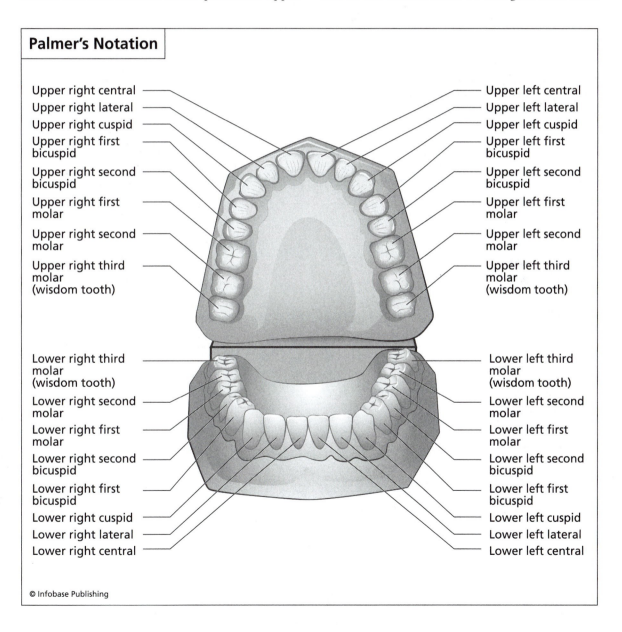

Palmer's Notation

Upper right central
Upper right lateral
Upper right cuspid
Upper right first bicuspid
Upper right second bicuspid
Upper right first molar
Upper right second molar
Upper right third molar (wisdom tooth)

Upper left central
Upper left lateral
Upper left cuspid
Upper left first bicuspid
Upper left second bicuspid
Upper left first molar
Upper left second molar
Upper left third molar (wisdom tooth)

Lower right third molar (wisdom tooth)
Lower right second molar
Lower right first molar
Lower right second bicuspid
Lower right first bicuspid
Lower right cuspid
Lower right lateral
Lower right central

Lower left third molar (wisdom tooth)
Lower left second molar
Lower left first molar
Lower left second bicuspid
Lower left first bicuspid
Lower left cuspid
Lower left lateral
Lower left central

© Infobase Publishing

there. The lateral becomes #2; the cuspid, #3; the first bicuspid, #4; the second bicuspid, #5; the first molar, #6; the second molar, #7; and the third molar, #8. To identify an individual tooth, the number is simply located in its quadrant. For example, the central tooth on the right side of the upper jaw is the upper right #1.

Universal Numerical Notation Where Numerical notation numbers teeth starting at the front in each quadrant, universal numerical notation begins at the back and treats the entire set of teeth as one continuous system. The upper right third molar is #1, the upper right second molar is #2, and so on across the upper jaw from right to left and then down across the lower jaw from left to right until #32, the total number of permanent teeth if all the molars erupt successfully.

The Eruption of the Teeth

The first primary tooth to erupt through the gum (see TEETHING) is almost always one of

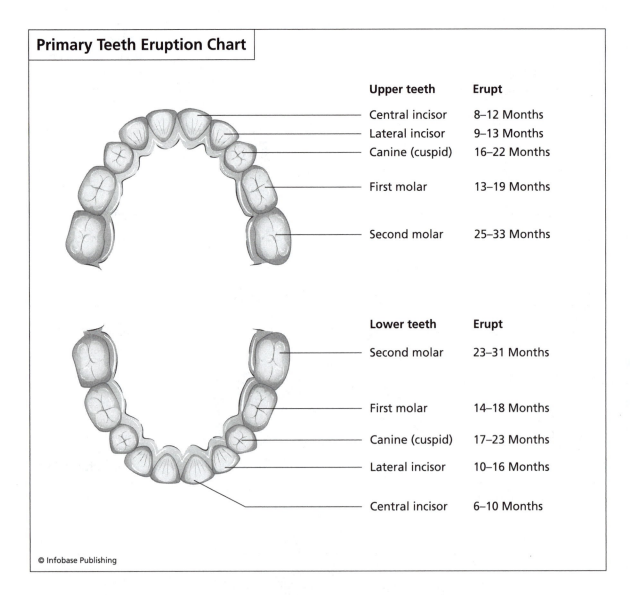

Primary Teeth Eruption Chart

Upper teeth	Erupt
Central incisor	8–12 Months
Lateral incisor	9–13 Months
Canine (cuspid)	16–22 Months
First molar	13–19 Months
Second molar	25–33 Months

Lower teeth	Erupt
Second molar	23–31 Months
First molar	14–18 Months
Canine (cuspid)	17–23 Months
Lateral incisor	10–16 Months
Central incisor	6–10 Months

© Infobase Publishing

Permanent Teeth Eruption Chart

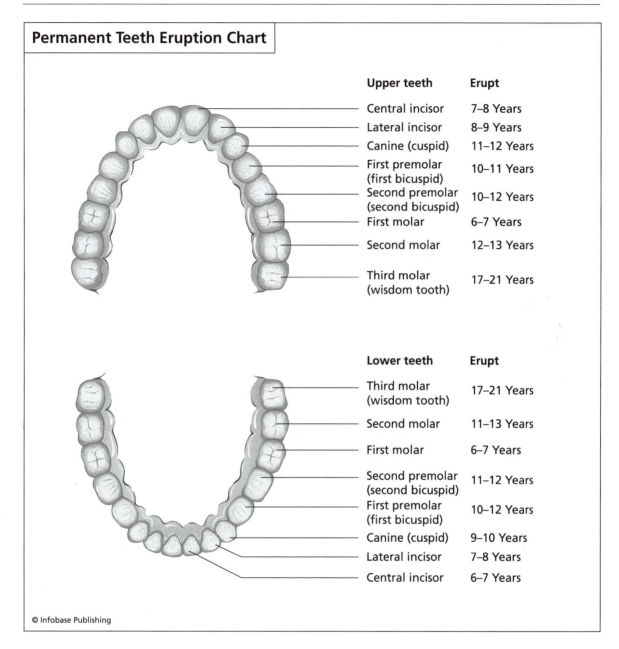

Upper teeth	Erupt
Central incisor	7–8 Years
Lateral incisor	8–9 Years
Canine (cuspid)	11–12 Years
First premolar (first bicuspid)	10–11 Years
Second premolar (second bicuspid)	10–12 Years
First molar	6–7 Years
Second molar	12–13 Years
Third molar (wisdom tooth)	17–21 Years

Lower teeth	Erupt
Third molar (wisdom tooth)	17–21 Years
Second molar	11–13 Years
First molar	6–7 Years
Second premolar (second bicuspid)	11–12 Years
First premolar (first bicuspid)	10–12 Years
Canine (cuspid)	9–10 Years
Lateral incisor	7–8 Years
Central incisor	6–7 Years

the middle front teeth on the lower jaw, which normally appear about two months before the teeth on the upper jaw. The usual sequence after that is the appearance of the incisor next to the bottom central tooth, followed by the lateral incisors, the cuspids, and the molars. At about age six, a child begins to lose his or her primary teeth, starting once again with the central teeth. The following charts show the normal pattern of tooth eruption.

toothbrush A bristled tool for cleaning the teeth and, sometimes, the tongue.

The Evolution of the Toothbrush

The history of the toothbrush begins with twigs and then winds its way through natural bristles, bone tools, nylon and plastic, to electricity.

The Chewstick The first tooth cleaner was a primitive version of a toothpick, a twig used to pick out debris from the teeth. Other early toothpick-type instruments included the hard, sharp end of a feather, a porcupine quill, or even a sliver of bone. By 3500 B.C.E., the Babylonians and their contemporaries across the populated world were cleaning their teeth with chewsticks, long twigs chewed at one end and rubbed against the teeth. Most commonly, the twigs were taken from trees whose leaves and branches contained fragrant oils that served to freshen the mouth and breath.

The Bristled Brush Sometime after 1498, the Chinese invented the first bristle toothbrush with stiff hairs pulled from the backs of wild hogs and anchored to handles made of bone or bamboo. French dentists are said to have been the first in Europe to promote the use of bristled brushes starting around 1600, but it was not until 1780 that William Addis of Clerkenwald, England, created the first British toothbrush with handles of cattle bone and natural hog bristles. As their reputation spread, the Addis brushes quickly became popular on the Continent as well.

In 1844, across the Atlantic in the United States, New York physician and dentist Meyer (Myer) L. Rhein handcrafted and patented a toothbrush with three rows of serrated bristles. Thirteen years later, in 1857, H. N. Wadsworth obtained U.S. patent No. 18,653 for a toothbrush with a bone handle and Siberian boar bristles. In 1885, Meyer Rhein joined with the Florence Manufacturing Company of Massachusetts to produce and market the Pro-phy-lac-tic brush. (Florence was also the first company to sell toothbrushes packaged in boxes.)

The next major step in bristled brushes was the switch from natural boar bristles to nylon. In 1938, one year after nylon was invented by Wallace H. Carothers of the DuPont Laboratories, the synthetic material was used to make toothbrushes, starting with "Dr. West's Miracle Toothbrush." Since then, the developments in toothbrushes have been both cosmetic and ergonomic and have included attractive colors and designs, different sized handles to fit different sized hands, different sized heads (bristles) to fit different sized mouths, and different bristle strengths (hard, medium, soft) and hardness to match individual needs.

The Electric Toothbrush. The first electric toothbrush, introduced about 1939 in Switzerland, was engineered simply to move back and forth as though someone were brushing with a plain toothbrush. The brush did not sell well and was quickly withdrawn from the market.

In 1955, American dental inventor Phillippe Guy E. Wood founded Broxo, a small business whose intent was to develop an effective electric toothbrush. In 1959, Wood's entry, the Broxodont, was introduced by Squibb (now Bristol Meyers Squibb); the brush went on sale one year later.

In 1961, General Electric introduced the first cordless rechargeable electric toothbrush. In 1987, Interplak began to market the first electric toothbrush with a rotary action, cleaning in circles rather than in straight lines. In 1983, Koninklijke Philips Electronics N.V. introduced Sonicare, the first sonic toothbrush. This was another major advance: The brush head on basic electric toothbrushes vibrates at 2,500 to 7,500 strokes per minute. By comparison, the brush head on the Sonicare generation of electric brushes vibrates at more than 30,000 strokes per minute.

A 2005 study by the Cochrane Collaboration, an international, nonprofit, independent organization that produces and disseminates systematic reviews of health-care interventions and promotes the search for evidence in the form of clinical trials and other studies of interventions, concluded that the rotary head electric brush had no benefit over manual brushing insofar as decay is concerned. However, the study also concluded that electric brushes are valuable for people with hand and wrist conditions that make it difficult to hold and move a manual brush.

Using the Toothbrush

Regular brushing, at least twice a day, is considered an integral part of an ORAL HYGIENE regimen. Brushing cleans the teeth and reduces the risk of PERIODONTAL DISEASE by removing bacterial debris that can harden into dental CALCULUS.

Recommended technique The brushing technique most commonly taught in dental schools is called the modified Bass technique created by microbiologist CHARLES CASSIDY BASS.

- To clean the buccal (cheek-side) and lingual (tongue-side) surfaces of the teeth, position the brush head at a 45-degree angle against the gum and move back and forth in short strokes, one tooth or, at the most, two teeth wide.
- To clean the lingual surface of the front teeth, position the brush head vertically against the surface and move gently up and down.
- To clean the broad occlusal (chewing) surface of the back teeth, position the brush flat against the top of the tooth and, again, move back and forth in short strokes.

Other Brushing Techniques In certain cases, more specific methods for brushing may be required. Examples of the methods are:

- *The Charters method:* The toothbrush is held with the bristles lying against the teeth and pointed toward the top of the tooth, and the brush is moved in a circle to dislodge debris between the teeth.
- *The Collis method:* A curved brush that reaches the top and side of the tooth is used for short strokes to clean the teeth and around the gum line when brushing teeth for a person who is ill or unable to brush himself.

- *The Fones method:* The brush is used in large circles on closed teeth and, when the jaws are open, smaller circles on the tongue- and palate-side surfaces of the teeth.
- *The Hirschfeld method:* The toothbrush is held against the teeth and brushes the tooth and the gum at the same time with very small, circular strokes. The occlusal (biting) surfaces of the teeth are brushed with strong strokes.
- *The Leonard method:* The toothbrush is used for strong up and down strokes against the teeth, a method also known as vertical toothbrushing.
- *The rolling stroke method:* Simple rolling strokes are used over the teeth, often used as an introductory teaching tool for children.
- *The Stillman method:* The toothbrush is held so that the bristles are against both the gum line and the tooth surface, then the brush is vibrated to stimulate the gum and clean the teeth.
- *The sulcal method:* The tips of the bristles are placed into the sulcus (the rim of gum around the base of the visible part of the tooth) and vibrated from side to side to eliminate plaque-forming debris at the gum line.

Caring for the Toothbrush

The toothbrush is a health appliance that requires proper care to keep it clean, safe, and effective.

Toothbrush Care for Healthy People After each use, the brush should be rinsed thoroughly and stored uncovered and exposed to air so that it can dry completely.

If several people store their toothbrushes in the same area, the brushes and brush heads should not touch so as to avoid any contamination from one brush to another.

For maximum effectiveness, the brush should be replaced with a new one every four months or as soon as the bristles begin to bend or split. Some new brush bristles are coated with a dye that fades as the brush ages to indicate when a new brush is needed.

Extra Toothbrush Care for People with Health Problems A person with a transmissible disease (including even so simple an illness as a cold) or a weakened immune system can reduce his risk of transmitting or acquiring an infection by rinsing the brush with a dentist-recommended antibacterial solution before brushing. Afterward, depending on the advice of his dentist, he may

- wash the brush thoroughly with running tap water
- soak the brush in an antibacterial solution
- replace the toothbrush more frequently than every three to four months to decrease the number of bacteria on the bristles
- use throwaway toothbrushes

tooth discoloration Any change in the natural color of the teeth. There are two types of tooth discoloration: Intrinsic discoloration (a change in the color of the interior of the tooth) and extrinsic discoloration (a change in the color of the exterior surface of the tooth). In either case, the color change may appear in primary and/or secondary (permanent) teeth, and it may be local, affecting one or two teeth, or regional, affecting several adjacent teeth.

Intrinsic Tooth Discoloration The list of incidents and materials that produce color changes emanating from inside the tooth includes (but is not limited to):

- *Antibiotics:* Tetracycline antibiotics taken by a pregnant women or by a young child while the teeth are developing may bind to the calcium in developing teeth to cause a yellow discoloration that may darken to gray or reddish brown. Minocycline, a tetracycline derivative used to treat adolescent and adult acne, may stain the surface of the tooth, as may doxycycline, another tetracycline antibiotic.

- *Birth defects:* Birth defects such as AMELOGENESIS IMPERFECTA (AI) interfere with the formation of ENAMEL or DENTIN, leaving the surface of the tooth thin enough to permit the natural yellowish color inside the tooth to show through.

- *Dental compounds and materials:* Compounds such as silver AMALGAM may corrode to leave a gray-black tint inside the tooth that shows through if sufficient amounts of enamel have been removed while filling a CAVITY. Other compounds that may change the color inside the tooth include eugenol (used to relieve a toothache and to reduce irritation from a temporary filling) and materials used to seal a tooth canal.

- *Fluorides:* FLUORIDES are particles of the element fluorine that, like calcium, are incorporated into teeth and bone. Excessive amounts of fluorides, 3–4 times the RDA (4 mg for adult men; 3 mg for adult women) produces dark mottling of the teeth, a condition known as dental fluorosis. Doses twice the RDA cause white spots on the teeth.

- *Infection:* An infection at the root of a developing tooth may interfere with the normal production of enamel, leaving a thinner-than-normal surface. In rare cases, a mother's having rubella (German measles) or another infection such as toxemia of pregnancy may interfere with the child's developing a normal enamel surface. Once the child is born, infectious diseases such as measles, chicken pox, and streptococcal infections may interfere with her developing a normal enamel surface on her secondary (permanent) teeth.

- *Inherited disorders:* A disorder of porphyrin metabolism, such as erythropoietic porphyria, affects the body's ability to metabolize these natural red-to-burgundy compounds in blood. The unmetabolized porphyrins bind to elements, including the calcium in teeth, causing the teeth to turn pink to (in rare cases) dark brown. Other sources of intrinsic discoloration are illnesses such as sickle-cell anemia, or thalassemia, or hemolytic disease of the newborn (HDN) due to Rh factor that leads to hyperbilirubinemia, which is excess bilirubin, a pigment, in blood. The pigment is incorporated into developing teeth to produce a yellow-green tint that shows through the enamel surface.

- *Injury:* Injury to developing teeth produces a thinner enamel surface. Occlusal injury (teeth that meet with great force) and injury to the pulp inside an erupted tooth may cause a hemorrhage leading to the deposit of dark particles under the surface.

- *Nutritional deficiency:* Calcium, phosphorus, and vitamins C and D are required for the development of healthy bones and teeth. A deficiency of any of these nutrients may lead to a thinner-than-normal enamel surface, allowing discoloration on the interior of the tooth to show through.

- *Salivary problems:* An adequate supply of saliva is essential for removing debris from the mouth. If the production of saliva diminishes due to infection or obstruction of the salivary glands; a systemic disease (such as SJÖGREN'S SYNDROME); radiation therapy or chemotherapy for cancer of the head and neck; or medications such as antihistamines, the debris is not washed away and staining increases.

Extrinsic Tooth Discoloration In 1997, Salim Nathoo, a dentist and biochemist, described three basic types of discoloration occurring on the surface of the tooth. The descriptions, known collectively as the Nathoo Classification System of Extrinsic Dental Stains, are:

- *Nathoo type 1 (N1):* The chromogen (coloring agent) attaches to the surface of the tooth, producing an immediate stain. Examples of this type of material include foods such as tea, coffee, and wine; chromogenic (color-produc-

ing) bacteria that bind to metals or change hue when exposed to sunlight; and metals such as iron, manganese, silver (black stains), mercury, and lead dust (blue-green), chromic acid fumes (orange), and iodine (brown).

- *Nathoo type 2 (N2):* The coloring agent causes stains after binding to the tooth. Examples include food stains that darken with time.

- *Nathoo type 3 (N3):* After binding to the tooth, a previously colorless material goes through a chemical reaction that produces a colored stain. Examples of this type of material include carbohydrate-rich foods (e.g., apples, potatoes), fluorides, and chlorhexidine, an antiseptic used in mouthwashes.

Symptoms and Diagnostic Path
Discolored teeth are clearly visible. Establishing the cause of the discoloration, however, requires a thorough review of the patient's general health, her dental health and previous dental treatments, her exposure to various environmental factors such as metals, her oral hygiene regimen, and her dietary habits.

Treatment Options and Outlook
The treatment of discolored teeth varies with the cause of the stain, the type of stain, and the severity of the discoloration. These techniques are usually successful in either removing stains or improving the appearance of previously stained teeth.

Changes in Diet or Other Habits For example, if excess amounts of coffee, tea, or another food, or tobacco, are staining the teeth, the patient is advised to change her habits to reduce the risk of stains.

Cleaning Techniques At home, the patient is advised to brush the teeth twice a day or after each meal to remove food and bacterial debris. Professional dental cleaning methods such as polishing or bleaching the teeth can remove both intrinsic and extrinsic stains. These methods may thin the enamel or make the teeth more sensitive, so they are not used repeatedly.

Restorations Dental VENEERS and CROWNS make the surface of badly stained teeth more attractive. Discoloration due to extensive CAVITIES and/or genetic defects may require extracting the affected tooth or teeth and replacing them with DENTURES or implants.

Risk Factors and Preventive Measures

There is no effective prevention for tooth discoloration due to a genetic, inherited, or infectious medical condition. However, the most common cause of extrinsic stains or intrinsic stains such as those resulting from dental cavities is poor oral hygiene, including the failure to use stain-removing toothpastes and powders, along with a lack of regular dental care.

tooth grinding   See BRUXISM.

tooth loss   See DECAY; DENTURES; IMPLANTOLOGY; PERIODONTAL DISEASE; TOBACCO.

tooth mobility   See PERIODONTAL DISEASE.

toothpaste   See DENTIFRICE.

tooth whitening   See WHITENING.

tooth transplant   Autogenous tooth transplantation (from the Greek words *autos,* meaning "self," and *genesis,* meaning "birth"); auto transplantation. A procedure during which one tooth in the patient's mouth is moved from its original (donor) site to another (recipient) site; implanting one of the patient's own teeth eliminates the major transplantation risk: rejection of the transplanted organ/tissue.

A tooth transplant is performed to replace a missing tooth, either a tooth lost to decay, injury, or periodontal disease, or a tooth that is missing or misshapen due to a genetic or developmental defect.

Procedure

The first steps in a tooth transplant are to ascertain that the patient is healthy; that both the donor site and the recipient site are free of inflammation or infection; that the bone structure at the recipient site can support an implanted tooth; and the tissue sheath surrounding the root of the tooth to be implanted is healthy enough and undeveloped enough to grow into place at the new site. In addition, the dentist or oral surgeon takes a series of X-rays to provide guidance for inserting the transplanted tooth into its new site.

Once the patient and her tooth are approved for surgery, the procedure is performed under local anesthesia plus general anesthesia. The patient is sedated. The misshapen or damaged tooth to be replaced is removed from its socket and the socket is prepared to receive the new tooth. The donor tooth is removed from its socket and the wound closed. The tooth is positioned in its new socket and the wound closed.

Risks and Complications

As with any surgery, the patient may experience slight bleeding, pain, and swelling for a few days; to alleviate discomfort, she will be advised to stick to a soft diet and avoid chewing on the site of the transplant. If bleeding, pain, or swelling worsens, the patient should contact the dentist. The most serious complication of a transplant would be failure of the tooth to implant and thrive in its new site.

Outlook and Lifestyle Modifications

A successful tooth transplant provides a functioning tooth surrounded by healthy gum and bone.

trigeminal neuralgia   Also known as *tic douloureaux,* this is a painful disorder of the trigeminal nerve. The trigeminal nerve sends motor messages to the muscles of the jaws that make it possible to chew and sends sensory messages such as the awareness of pain and temperature to the face, jaws, and teeth. Although some cases of trigeminal neuralgia are linked to an illness of the central nervous system such as multiple sclerosis, most patients with this condition show no identifiable underlying cause.

Symptoms and Diagnostic Path

The pain of trigeminal neuralgia is sharp, stabbing, and unpredictable. In some cases, it is sufficiently severe as to require hospitalization for pain control medication.

The hallmark of trigeminal neuralgia pain is that it may be triggered by simple daily events such as eating, brushing the teeth, washing the face, or simply experiencing a breeze or the wind against the face. The sensation usually affects one side of the face, along the cheek, nose, upper lip, jaw, and teeth. Less commonly, pain may occur along the lower cheek, lip, and jaw. To avoid the pain, some patients avoid eating and drinking as much as possible; as a result they may suffer from weight loss or dehydration. Between acute attacks, some patients are pain-free; others experience a continuing but not disabling ache.

A conclusive diagnosis of trigeminal neuralgia requires the physician to rule out other possible causes of the pain such as TEMPOROMANDIBULAR DISORDER (TMD), migraine headaches, a sinus infection, or a disease of the facial bones or the bones of the skull.

Treatment Options and Outlook

The basic treatments for trigeminal neuralgia are either medical—(drugs)—or surgical.

Medical Treatment for Trigeminal Neuralgia
There are three common medical treatments for trigeminal neuralgia:

- *Antiseizure drugs.* Medicine such as baclofen (Lioresal), carbamazepine (Tegretol), and phe-

nytoin (Dilantin) reduce excess nerve activity, thus reducing pain messages.
- *Nerve block.* Doctors specializing in pain relief may use an injection or a series of injections of ANESTHETICS to block sensation in a region of the face.
- *Anesthetic injection into the skull.* Guided by X-ray images, the doctor may use a fine needle to inject anesthetic into the nerve that is triggering the pain.

Surgical Treatment for Trigeminal Neuralgia
If the cause of the trigeminal neuralgia is determined to be pressure exerted by an artery in the brain against the nerve, the neurosurgeon may decide to perform vascular surgery to move the artery away from the nerve.

Risk Factors and Preventive Measures

Some experts suggest that abnormal blood vessels or damage to the trigeminal nerve may lead to trigeminal neuralgia, but there is as yet no conclusive proof for any cause and no identifiable risk factors.

Tweed, Charles H. (1875–1970) American orthodontist who worked closely with EDWARD HARTLEY ANGLE. In 1932, when he published his first article in *The Angle Orthodontist,* the journal published by the Angle School of Orthodontics, in California, Tweed shared Angle's disdain for extraction as an orthodontic tool. However, as time went on, Tweed collected the records of more than 100 patients who were first treated without extraction and then treated after extraction.

The data convinced him that carefully planned extraction made it possible to make a patient look better and improve the stability of the teeth, which often move back once orthodontic treatment is done. As a result, Tweed created the Tweed Facial Triangle, a pattern formed by teeth and jaws, and most importantly, the degree of protrusion or recession of the teeth in relation to the upper and lower jawbones. This diagnostic tool is used in planning orthodontic treatment, as well as in planning plastic surgery or cosmetic dental surgery to create a more pleasing appearance.

To honor Tweed's mastery of his profession, in 1947 a group of his peers proposed the founding of the Charles H. Tweed Foundation for Orthodontic Research. Today, the Charles H. Tweed International Foundation for Orthodontic Research and Education in Tucson, Arizona, and its journal, *The Tweed Profile*, remain a center for continuing education and international study of orthodontics.

See NERVES; ORTHODONTIC BRACES; ORTHODONTICS AND DENTOFACIAL ORTHOPEDICS.

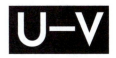

ugly duckling stage See MALOCCLUSION.

ulcer See APHTHOUS ULCER; HERPES, ORAL.

ultrasonic See PERIDONTAL DISEASE; SCALING.

underbite See MALOCCLUSION.

universal precautions See INFECTION CONTROL.

varnish See FLUORIDE; SEALANT.

vasoconstrictor A medicine, a chemical, or a physical factor such as exposure to extreme cold that causes blood vessels to constrict. Conversely, a vasodilator is a medicine, chemical, or physical factor such as exposure to extreme warmth that causes blood vessels to expand.

In dentistry, a vasoconstrictor such as epineph-rine (a hormone secreted by the adrenal glands) or levonordefrin (Nordefrin) is often added to injectable ANESTHETICS to constrict the blood vessels. This increases the anesthetic effect by holding the anesthetic longer at the site, reduces bleeding during the procedure, and reduces the incidence of sensitivity reactions because less anesthetic flows into the bloodstream.

About one person in seven is sensitive to normal doses of any medical drug; some of these sensitive people are hyperreactive, which means their reaction to the drug is more severe. For example, the most common side effect of a vasoconstrictor is a fast heartbeat. A hyperreac-tive person may experience a sudden drop in blood pressure that causes him to faint, or his skin may redden and he may begin to perspire heavily.

Anesthetics with added vasoconstrictors may also be contraindicated for people with heart dis-ease or blood vessel disorders, or who have had a bad reaction to the combination in the past. Taking certain drugs such as tricyclic antidepres-sants—for example, amitriptyline (Elavil) and doxepin (Adapin)—is a definite contraindication because these drugs may interact with the vaso-constrictor to cause dangerously high blood pres-sure. As in similar situations, patients with risk factors should consult their own doctors before a dental procedure.

vasodilator See VASOCONSTRICTOR.

veneer Thin piece of dental porcelain or com-posite resin custom made to cover the front sur-face of a tooth so as to improve the appearance of chipped, discolored, misaligned, misshapen, or unevenly spaced teeth.

Porcelain veneers are more stain-resistant than resin veneers. They are also easier to color-match to natural teeth and they reflect light more like natural teeth than do the resin veneers. On the other hand, porcelain veneers are more expensive. When applying them, the dentist must remove more of the dental enamel than with resin veneers, and chipped porcelain is more difficult to repair than is chipped or bro-ken resin.

Procedure

Preparing and attaching dental veneers may be a two-visit procedure.

If the veneer requires, on the first visit, the dentist prepares the tooth by grinding away about an eighth of a millimeter of dental enamel, the hard surface of the tooth, from the front of the tooth. He then makes a model or impression of the tooth. Depending on the condition of the teeth, this may require local anesthetic. The model is sent to a dental laboratory, which manufactures the veneer and returns it to the dentist, who approves the fit and color, both of which can be adjusted before the veneer is fixed on the tooth. If the ground teeth are unsightly, the dentist may apply a temporary layer of plastic resin.

On the second visit, the dentist cleans and polishes the tooth surface, then etches it with a weak acid solution to provide a firm footing for the veneer. The dentist applies a cement to the back of the veneer, sets the veneer in place, and uses a high-intensity light or a LASER to "cure" (dry and harden) the cement that will hold the veneer in place. Finally, the dentist removes excess cement, and makes adjustments as necessary so as to insure that the teeth meet properly, and schedules a third visit to check the placement and reaction to the veneer.

Risks and Complications

As with any dental procedure, for a few days after the veneers are attached the teeth may be sensitive to heat and cold or the pressure of biting and chewing. If the sensitivity continues, however, the dentist should be consulted.

Veneers may not be a good choice for people whose teeth have been weakened by DECAY or large dental fillings, or who have active PERIODONTAL DISEASE.

Outlook and Lifestyle Modifications

Typically, porcelain veneers may last five to 10 years; resin veneers less than that. However, exactly how long either type of veneer remains intact depends both on how well the veneer is applied and how well the patient protects them after they are in place. Both are breakable and liable to damage from biting on hard food or ice or chewing on hard objects such as a pen or pencil or BRUXISM (grinding or clenching the teeth).

vestibuloplasty In dentistry, the vestibule is the space between the teeth and gums and the lips and cheeks. The specific areas of the vestibule of the oral cavity are named according to the structures they face. For example, the buccal vestibule is the space between the teeth and the cheek in back of the buccal frenum (the fold of mucous MEMBRANE attaching the JAW to the cheek at the side); the labial vestibule is the space between the jaw and teeth in front of the buccal frenum. (The upper buccal vestibule is on the upper jaw; the lower buccal frenum is on the lower jaw.)

Vestibuloplasty is a surgical procedure that alters a vestibular space to increase the size of the area of the alveolar ridge (the part of the jawbone that holds and supports the teeth) when preparing the mouth for DENTURES so that the dentures have a larger platform on which to sit, thus increasing their ability to remain tight in place. Vestibuloplasty is most commonly performed for children born with CLEFT LIP AND/OR PALATE or for older adults who have lost large amounts of BONE to PERIODONTAL DISEASE.

Procedure

Once the patient is sedated, the surgeon enlarges the alveolar ridge by repositioning the muscles that attach the jaw to LIPS, cheek, and TONGUE. In some cases, the surgeon may GRAFT bone tissue to rebuild the alveolar ridge. Depending on the size of the wound, the surgeon may require grafts of mucous membrane tissue to close it.

Risks and Complications

Bleeding, swelling, and discomfort are common. If these problems suddenly worsen, they may be a sign of infection.

Outlook and Lifestyle Modifications

Successful surgery improves the performance of the dentures, making eating and speaking more comfortable and effective.

vitamins Vitamins are compounds that contain carbon, hydrogen, and oxygen atoms, a combination known as organic chemicals. MINERALS, on the other hand, are elements, substances built of only one type of atom. For example, calcium is made solely of calcium atoms, iron of iron atoms, and so on.

The body uses vitamins to regulate various functions. They are essential for the synthesis of proteins and for building body tissues and structures such as the gums and facial bones. Vitamins also play a vital role in the proper healing of wounds, including surgical wounds, such as an incision made during a periodontal procedure.

To function properly, the human body requires 11 specific vitamins: the fat-soluble vitamins A, D, E, and K, and the water-soluble vitamins C and the B vitamins thiamin (B_1), riboflavin (B_2) vitamin B_6, vitamin B_{12}, niacin, and folate. Two more B vitamins, biotin and pantothenic acid, are believed to be valuable but not vital.

Several of these vitamins are specifically relevant to dental and oral health. For example, vitamin A reduces inflammation such as may occur during an episode of periodontal disease and enhances the production of new cells to repair tissues and reduce scarring. Vitamin D helps the body absorb calcium, the mineral that builds strong teeth and bones. Like vitamin A, vitamin E is an anti-inflammatory; it is also an anticoagulant (or blood thinner). Vitamin K, which is manufactured by microorganisms living naturally in the intestinal tract, produces specialized proteins in blood plasma (the clear fluid in blood), including prothrombin, the protein that clots blood and helps form a scab over an injury, including a surgical incision.

Vitamin C develops and maintains connective tissue such as the tissue anchoring the gum to the teeth. It protects against the deficiency disease scurvy, which destroys connective tissue and loosens teeth from gums. Vitamin C is also important for wound healing. A person who is deficient in vitamin C may experience slow healing of wounds, including those experienced during dental surgery, but there is no evidence that giving vitamin C supplements to patients who are not deficient in vitamin C will speed healing. The foods with the most plentiful supply of vitamin C are fresh fruits and vegetables, specifically citrus fruits.

The B vitamins are vitamin B_1 (thiamin), vitamin B_2 (riboflavin), vitamin B_6 (pyridoxine), vitamin B_{12} (cyanocobalamin), niacin, and folate (folic acid). Vitamins B_1, B_2, and B_6 enable the body to extract nutrients and energy from food. Like vitamin A, vitamin B_2 protects the health of mucous membranes, including the lining of the oral cavity. Vitamin B_{12} makes healthy red blood cells and protects myelin, the fatty material that covers nerves and enables the transmission of electrical impulses ("messages") between nerve cells in the brain, as well as between nerve cells that govern movement in muscles such as the tongue. Niacin increases the flow of oxygen into body tissues to hasten healing—for example, after a dental infection or surgical procedure. Folate, found in various green, leafy vegetables, participates in the synthesis of amino acids used to build new body cells. Biotin is used to make fatty acids and amino acids, and pantothenic acid protects hemoglobin, the protein in red blood cells that carries oxygen throughout the body to all tissues including the teeth and gums.

The Food and Nutrition Board, a subsidiary of the National Research Council, which in turn is part of the National Academy of Sciences in Washington, D.C., has established recommended dietary allowances for vitamins, minerals, and some other nutrients. The recommendations for vitamins are shown in Table 1.

TABLE 1. RECOMMENDED DIETARY ALLOWANCES FOR HEALTHY ADULTS (2006)

Age (Years)	Vitamin A (RE/IU)*	Vitamin D (mcg/IU)	Vitamin E (alpha-TE)**	Vitamin K (mcg)	Vitamin C (mg)
Males					
19–24	900/2970	5/200	15	120	90
25–50	900/2970	5/200	15	120	90
51–70	900/2970	10/400	15	120	90
71+	900/2970	15/600	15	120	90
Females					
19–24	700/2310	5/200	15	90	75
25–50	700/2310	5/200	15	90	75
51–70	700/2310	10/400	15	90	75
71+	700/2310	15/600	15	90	75

Age (Years)	Thiamin (Vitamin B_1)(mg)	Riboflavin (Vitamin B_2)(mg)	Niacin (mcg/NE)	Vitamin B_6 (mg)	Folate (mcg)
Males					
19–24	1.2	1.3	16	1.3	400
25–50	1.2	1.3	16	1.3	400
51–70	1.2	1.3	16	1.7	400
71+	1.2	1.1	16	1.7	400
Females					
19–24	1.1	1.1	14	1.3	400
25–50	1.1	1.1	14	1.3	400
51–70	1.1	1.1	14	1.5	400
71+	1.1	1.1	14	1.5	400

Age (Years)	Vitamin B_{12} (mcg)	Biotin (mcg)	Pantothenic acid (mg)***
Males			
19–24	2.4	30	5
25–50	2.4	30	5
51–70	2.4	30	5
71+	2.4	30	5
Females			
19–24	2.4	30	5
25–50	2.4	30	5
51–70	2.4	30	5
71+	2.4	30	5

*RE stands for retinol equivalents, IU for international units.

**alpha- TE stands for alpha tocopherol equivalents.

***this amount is labeled "Adequate Intake" (AI), not RDA.

waste disposal, waste management See INFECTION CONTROL.

waste products, dental See INFECTION CONTROL.

water, drinking See FLUORIDE.

Waterpik See IRRIGATION.

wax Wax is a soft, natural or synthetic fatty material that melts when heated and hardens when cooled. Common waxes are beeswax, the sticky substance secreted by bees; carnauba wax, derived from the leaves of the Brazilian palm tree *Copernicia prunifera;* and paraffin, a petroleum derivative. Dental wax is a mixture of two or more kinds of wax that generally includes carnauba wax, which melts at a higher temperature than other waxes, thus lending stability to the mix. Dentists use waxes for three basic tasks: to make a pattern for a RESTORATION such as an INLAY; to create an IMPRESSION of the teeth; and to build dental paraphernalia such as the base for a dental impression. Some specific types of dental wax are:

- *Baseplate wax*: This is a hard, pink wax used primarily to make the solid base upon which a denture is built.

- *Bite plate wax:* Also known as bite registration wax, this is a sheet of wax into which a patient bites to create an impression showing the relationship between the upper and lower teeth when the jaws are closed.

- *Boxing wax:* A wax used to heighten the borders of a dental impression when making the base of a dental cast, a model of one or more parts of the inside of the mouth.

- *Casting wax:* This is a mixture of waxes that change shape (expand and contract) less when exposed to heat and cold, a valuable quality for wax used to make molds for metal restorations such as an inlay.

- *Fluid wax:* This wax, which can be molded at room temperature, is used to make a model of the teeth that can easily be adjusted.

- *Sticky wax:* This is a very hard mixture of beeswax, paraffin, and resin in shades of orange, red, blue, and purple, used to hold pieces of a broken denture together while it is being repaired.

- *Utility wax:* This is a rope of colorless or red wax that is very soft at room temperature; it is used on an impression tray to keep the impression material from sliding back into the patient's throat.

Wells, Horace (1815–1848) Wells, a dentist practicing in Hartford, Connecticut, was the first person to recognize the fact that nitrous oxide might be an effective surgical anesthetic. Having tested it first on himself by enlisting a colleague to administer the gas and then extract one of Wells's wisdom teeth, he began to use it on his patients. In 1846, his former student, William Morton, persuaded Wells to give a public demonstration of his technique. However, the bag containing the gas was withdrawn too soon from the patient who was not fully anesthetized and thus not free of pain during the extraction. Wells continued to promote the use of nitrous oxide, even traveling to Europe to do so, but by the time he returned to the United States, Morton had done his own successful demonstration of ether anesthesia, eclipsing Wells's efforts and (erroneously) gaining the reputation of having been the first to use dental anesthesia.

whitening Tooth bleaching; cosmetic procedure to remove stains on the surface of the teeth due to environmental factors such as tobacco, coffee, or tea, or to correct color changes arising from alterations to the tooth itself due to:

- exposure to tetracycline antibiotics either in utero or in the first eight years of life

- excessive consumption of FLUORIDE during tooth formation

- death of the PULP (soft tissue inside the tooth)

- genetic influences such as a natural tendency to darker teeth or cavities or a natural heightened response to staining agents

- systemic medical conditions such as jaundice

Procedure

A variety of whitening procedures and products exist.

In-Office Whitening Procedures The two basic in-office techniques for lightening the color of teeth are bleaching and microabrasion. Before beginning any lightening process, the dentist applies protective gel (petroleum jelly) to the patient's gums and inserts a rubber device to protect the interior of the mouth. Before bleaching, he may also use pumice to remove superficial stains or debris from the tooth surface.

Bleaching To bleach vital teeth (teeth with a healthy pulp and nerve inside) the dentist usually begins by etching the tooth (applying a gel that makes the surface more porous). Then, the dentist applies a peroxide gel to the surface of the teeth and uses an argon laser, which emits a blue light, to activate the gel.

To bleach nonvital teeth (teeth from which the pulp and nerve have been removed) the dentist drills a small opening in the back of the tooth, inserts a bleaching paste, and covers the hole with a temporary seal that can be removed to change the bleach paste once a week, as required, until the tooth is the desired color. This procedure, a walking bleach, lightens the tooth from the inside out; several visits to the dentist may be required to renew the bleach solution in order to lighten the tooth properly.

Microabrasion First, the dentist uses a fine abrasive such as pumice to remove stains on the outer surface of the tooth. Then, he applies an acid or acid/abrasive paste to the surface of the tooth. The acid oxidizes and removes stains, dissolves white calcium deposits, and smooths the enamel surface of the tooth so that the tooth reflects light more cleanly.

At-Home Lightening Procedures Over-the-counter products for whitening teeth at home include whitening toothpastes, whitening strips or gels, and tray-based whiteners.

Whitening Toothpastes In addition to the mild abrasives found in all toothpastes and powders, those advertised as whitening products contain stronger polishing (abrasive) agents or bleaching chemicals such as hydrogen peroxide. These products may lighten teeth by about one shade.

Whitening Gels and Gel-Coated Strips The gels are clear, peroxide-based products applied directly to the teeth once or twice a day for two weeks. The peroxide gel-coated strips are also applied twice daily, also for two weeks.

Tray-Based Whitening Kits These products, which are available in drugstores or directly from the dentist, are weaker versions of the in-office tray-based systems used by dental professionals. The consumer fills the tray with the bleach solution and then puts the tray over his teeth for a period of time, once a day or overnight, for a period of several weeks. The bleach in the home kit is a form of peroxide called carbamide peroxide. The concentration of bleach in home-use solutions is about 10 percent carbamide peroxide, the equivalent of a solution that is 3 percent hydrogen peroxide. The concentration of bleach in a professionally applied, in-office whitening solution may be as high as 43 percent hydrogen peroxide.

An alternative to the over-the-counter one-size-fits-all bleaching tray kit is a kit assembled by the dentist with a tray tailored to the patient's mouth and bleaching solution for the patient to apply at home.

Risks and Complications

In-Office Whitening Procedures The strong bleaches used by dentists may in some rare instances injure the gums or damage the surface of a healthy tooth. In addition, the bleach solution for external lightening or a walking bleach may trigger resorption (natural breakdown) of the tooth root; to reduce the risk of serious damage, the patient is usually required to return for periodic checkups.

Etching or microabrasion may thin the enamel, increasing the risk of cavities and making teeth more sensitive to heat and cold.

At-Home Whitening Procedures Repeated use of the peroxide bleach might alter the bacterial content of the mouth, increasing the risk of infection. Repeated use of the bleaching trays, like repeated use of "boil-and-bite" MOUTH GUARDS, might cause teeth to shift or trigger TEMPOROMANDIBULAR DISORDER (TMD). In some instances, the procedure may irritate the gums or make the teeth more sensitive to heat and cold; if this happens, the dentist should evaluate the condition of the patient's mouth.

The effects of bleaching agents on the developing fetus are unknown; it is prudent to avoid these products during pregnancy.

Outlook and Lifestyle Modifications

No whitening procedure produces permanent change in color. In addition, the amount of the change produced by any whitening product depends on several factors, including but not limited to the original color of the tooth and the strength of the bleach product.

At-home Lightening Products Whitening toothpastes, gels, strips, and tray-based products are less expensive than professional treatment in the dentist's office, but all require long-term commitment, none produce permanent change, and all are less effective than the in-office procedures.

In-office Procedures Bleaching a vital tooth may lighten the tooth for several years, after which the tooth is likely to gradually darken again, requiring a second procedure. Teeth with multiple restorations (fillings, VENEERS, caps) or insufficient or cracked ENAMEL may not respond well to bleaching.

Microabrasion does not lighten teeth; it simply removes stains so that the surface of the tooth resumes its natural color.

The primary advantages of in-office over home-based procedures are (1) immediate whitening, (2) no work for patient at home, (3) better color matching, and (4) reduced risk of problems such as irritation of the soft tissue of the gum.

Wilson, curve of See CURVE.

wire A thin metal thread that bends easily. Dentists employ wires in various treatments and procedures. For example:

- oral or plastic surgeons use a network of internal suspension wires to connect the upper jaw to the cheekbone, stabilizing the bone so it can heal
- orthodontists use an arch wire to apply the force necessary to move teeth into a new position and a separating wire between two teeth to move the teeth apart
- prosthodontists use wrought wire (a wire formed by pulling a piece of metal through a mold or die) to make the strong clasps used to hold dentures in place

The arrangement of wires is known as wiring. For example, a list of dental wiring includes:

- circumferential wiring to connect the upper jaw to the bone at the side of the face
- continuous multiple loop wiring, also known simply as multiple loop wire, to hold the teeth in place after a fracture of the jawbone
- craniofacial wiring to connect the jawbone to facial bones not right next to the jaw
- ivy loop wiring to hold two teeth together
- perialveolar wiring to hold a splint to the upper jaw with wires passed through the bone from the cheek to the palate
- pyriform aperture wiring to stabilize a fracture of the upper jaw with a wire passed through the bone in the nose

wisdom teeth, impacted   The wisdom tooth is the third molar, the last back tooth on each side of the upper and lower JAW. Anecdotally, these teeth are known as "wisdom" teeth because they are the last to appear, usually in the late teens or early 20s, when a person is presumed to have acquired some "wisdom."

A wisdom tooth is characterized as *impacted* if its ability to erupt into the mouth is impeded by either soft or bony tissue. The impaction may be complete or partial, or it may be angular, which means that the tooth is sitting at an angle to the tooth in front of it. In an extreme case, a wisdom tooth or teeth may actually be lying horizontal in the jaw. Because these teeth cannot erupt straight up through the gum, they must be surgically removed to prevent them from disrupting the teeth in front of them or damaging the jawbone or the nerves around the teeth.

Symptoms and Diagnostic Path

The most common symptoms of an impacted wisdom tooth (or teeth) are pain and swelling of the gum tissue atop the tooth. Wisdom teeth that erupt partway are more difficult to clean, which makes them more susceptible than other teeth to decay and the gum around them more susceptible to periodontal disease. When impaction is suspected, dental X-rays can provide conclusive proof one way or the other.

Treatment Options and Outlook

The treatment for an impacted wisdom tooth is EXTRACTION. Extracting a wisdom tooth is easier if done before the tooth has developed full roots in a dense jawbone. Removing a wisdom tooth that has partially erupted through the gum is a simple extraction. If the tooth is imbedded in the jawbone, however, the dentist or oral surgeon must make an incision in the gum, remove the bone over the tooth, and then remove the tooth, a more complicated procedure that may require breaking the tooth into small pieces to get it out of the jaw.

Risk Factors and Preventive Measures

There is no way to prevent impaction of a wisdom tooth. The only known risk factor is a jaw too small to accommodate all the teeth in an adult mouth.

women's dental associations   The first professional organization for women dentists, the Women's Dental Association of the United States, was founded in 1892 in Philadelphia by Mary

Stillwell-Kuesel with 12 women dentist members: Helen Addenbrook, Anna Burmeister, Kate A. Doherty, Mary Halsey, Mary Hastings, Vida Latham, Josephine Pfeifer, Katherine Prothero, Celia Rich, Mae Fontaine, Minnie Proctor, and MINNIE EVANGELINE JORDAN. A year later, there were 32 members; the roster eventually reached 100 before apparently disbanding around the turn of the 20th century. In 1921, the Federation of American Women Dentists was founded at the annual meeting of the AMERICAN DENTAL ASSOCIATION in Milwaukee with Jordon as its first president. The organization, known today as the American Association of Women Dentists, represents many of the women who account for about 14 percent of the general dentists currently practicing in the United States.

See DENTISTRY; HOBBS, LUCY BEAMAN; JONES, EMELINE ROBERTS; PARMLY, LEVI SPEAR; SCHOOLS OF DENTISTRY.

X

xerostomia A medical condition in which the salivary glands do not secrete sufficient amounts of SALIVA, resulting in excessive dryness ("cotton mouth") that can make speech and swallowing difficult, increase the risk of CAVITIES (because the teeth are no longer continuously bathed in mineral-rich saliva), raise the risk of oral infection, increase the likelihood of HALITOSIS (bad breath), and damage oral tissues.

Symptoms and Diagnostic Path
The lack of moisture in the tissues inside the mouth is clearly visible on physical examination.

Treatment Options and Outlook
If the underlying cause of the dryness cannot be eliminated, treatment is designed to reduce the incidence of cavities and infection by:

- prescribing fluoride supplements
- avoiding medicines such as decongestants and antihistamines that increase dryness
- keeping the mouth moist by drinking sufficient quantities of sugar-free liquids
- using a commercial SALIVA SUBSTITUTE mouthwash
- keeping the mouth as clean as possible to reduce the risk of infection in dry tissues

Risk Factors and Preventive Measures
Xerostomia may be a symptom of a systemic disease such as diabetes or SJÖGREN'S SYNDROME (dryness of the membranes in eyes, nose, and mouth), it may be due to an injury to the salivary glands, it may be a side effect of anticholin-

ergic medicines (products such as antihistamines or decongestants that decrease the secretions of the mucous membranes), or it may be a result of radiation therapy in the area of the salivary glands.

Preventive measures include treating the underlying illness (when possible) and/or limiting the medicines to the smallest effective dose.

X-ray examination Noninvasive diagnostic tool using a form of radiation to create pictures of the body's solid internal structure; used in dentistry to detect cavities, track the progress of periodontal disease, and evaluate the fit and stability of dental restorations such as caps, CROWNS, and fillings.

There are two categories of dental X-rays: Intra-oral X-rays (pictures taken with the X-ray film positioned inside the patient's mouth) and extra-oral X-rays (pictures taken with the X-ray film sitting outside the patient's mouth).

Intra-oral X-rays This type of X-ray is routinely recommended to track tooth development, establish a baseline picture of the mouth when a patient visits a dentist for the first time, detect cavities, detail abnormalities in the jawbone, record the progress of damage due to PERIODONTAL DISEASE, or provide a picture of the mouth for a patient about to begin orthodontia. The specific types of intra-oral X-rays are:

- *Bite-wing X-rays:* Images of teeth in one area of the mouth, showing the teeth from the top (crown) to the place where the tooth meets the jawbone.

- *Periapical X-rays:* Images of teeth in one part of the mouth showing the entire length of the teeth, from the crown down to the area below the root where the tooth is set into the jawbone.
- *Occlusal X-rays:* Images of the entire dental ARCH; all the teeth in the upper or lower jaw.

Extra-oral X-rays These X-rays may include images of the teeth. These images are pictures of the jaw and skull BONES used to track the relative development of teeth and jaws, visualize impacted teeth, identify problems in the jawbones and the temporomandibular joint (the joint that connects the upper jaw on the temporal bone at the side of the face), provide a picture of the entire mouth at the start of orthodontia, and detect and/or diagnose abnormalities such as tumors. Specific types of extra-oral X-rays usually performed in a dentist's office are:

- *Cephalometric projection:* An image of one side of the head showing the teeth and jaw in relation to the other facial bones at the base of the skull. This X-ray image is useful in planning orthodontia.
- *Panoramic X-rays:* Images produced by a camera that circles the head to make one picture showing the entire mouth, including all the teeth in both the upper and the lower jaws. This X-ray image is used to show the position of teeth that have not yet erupted through the gum and to discover and diagnose tumors in the jaw.

Specific types of extra-oral dental X-rays commonly performed in a hospital or freestanding radiological facility are:

- *CT scans:* Three-dimensional images used to identify abnormalities such as tumors in the oral/facial bones.

- *Sialograms:* Images of the salivary glands created by injecting a dye to make the soft tissue of the gland visible on X-ray film; used to diagnose an abnormality or disorder of the salivary glands such as a blockage or a tumor.

A specialized technique called a *subtraction X-ray* enables the dentists to overlay two X-rays of the same area taken at different times, "subtracting out" everything that is the same in the two images to leave a clear image of only the portion that is different. As a result, the dentist can see small changes that might not have otherwise been visible.

Procedure

In the dentist's office, the patient is seated in front of or under the X-ray camera; the dentist or dental assistant positions the instrument holding the film against the teeth, covers the patient with a lead-lined apron to protect the thyroid gland and organs in the chest and abdomen, and then leaves the room and activates the X-ray camera from another area of the office.

In traditional X-ray procedures, the camera takes the picture and produces a set of negatives showing the patient's teeth and/or jaw. Modern X-ray cameras use digital imaging to send the image directly to a computer, enabling the dentist to access the image within seconds, enhance the image (for example, enlarge it to make the details more visible), and print out a picture or store the image in the computer. If necessary, the image may also be transmitted via e-mail to another computer. For example, after a ROOT CANAL RESTORATION, the endodontist may send an image of the tooth to the patient's regular dentist, who stores it in the patient's file.

Risks and Complications

X-rays are ionizing radiation, the form of radiation that breaks apart molecules and can damage body tissues. Depending on the part of the body exposed, excess exposure to X-rays may cause anemia, cataracts, skin irritation (X-ray dermatitis), burns, cancer, abnormal sperm production, testicular atrophy, male and female infertility, and fetal damage, including birth defects, mental retardation, and childhood leukemia.

Modern dental X-ray machines produce a picture so quickly that the risk of injury is minimal. To reduce the risk even further, dentists cover the patient with a lead-lined apron to shield the reproductive organs and the thyroid gland; also, digital imaging exposes the patient to significantly less radiation that does traditional X-ray imaging.

Outlook and Lifestyle Modifications
The process results in a clear picture of solid structures—bones—inside the body.

See also MAGNETIC RESONANCE IMAGING; SALIVARY GLANDS.

X-ray therapy See KELLS, C. EDMOND; RADIATION THERAPY.

yawn An involuntary physical reflex common to all mammals, including human beings; one consequence of a vasovagal reaction, the physical phenomenon involving the vagus nerve (a nerve that carries messages from the brain to the ear, tongue, throat, lungs, heart, stomach, and abdominal organs) in which the nerve signals blood vessels in these organs to expand, leading to falling blood pressure, slower heartbeat, dizziness, nausea, and, in severe reactions, fainting. The most common dental effect of a yawn is discomfort at the site of the temporomandibular joint.

The mechanics of the yawn are obvious: The mouth opens, the lower JAW drops, the yawning person inhales, the lungs expand and the abdominal muscles contract, pushing the diaphragm (the large muscle separating the chest cavity from the abdominal cavity) down, and finally the inhaled air is exhaled. The reasons for a yawn are less well understood. The most common explanation is that a yawn is a reflex triggered by falling levels of oxygen and rising levels of carbon dioxide (a waste product) in the blood. The suggests that a yawn is the body's attempt to bring in more oxygen so as to increase alertness or to pump up the alveoli, the small air sacs in the lung where the body exchanges carbon dioxide for fresh oxygen. However, controlled studies have shown that increasing the oxygen and reducing the carbon dioxide in the air does not affect the incidence of yawning. A second, more fanciful possibility is that yawning is an evolutionary maneuver, like grinning, designed to bare the teeth and intimidate an enemy.

Excessive yawning, defined as more than one or two yawns a minute, may indicate a disorder of the central nervous system such as epilepsy, a brain tumor, or a progressive form of palsy such as Parkinson's disease. Excessive yawning may also occur during withdrawal from opiates (barbiturates, cocaine, heroin), or as a side effect when taking medicines such as selective serotonin reuptake inhibitors (SSRIs) that affect neurotransmitters, the naturally occurring chemicals that enable nerve cells in the brain to send messages back and forth.

Z

zinc, dietary Mineral required for healthy growth; protects nerve and brain tissue, supports the immune system, and helps speed healing of injured tissues; a component of enzymes and hormones such as insulin that enable the body to digest and use the nutrients in food.

The best sources of dietary zinc are foods from animals: meat, liver, oysters, and eggs. Plant foods such as beans, nuts, seeds, and whole grains also provide zinc, but the zinc in plant foods is less easily absorbed by the body than is the zinc in animal foods.

VITAMINS and MINERALS often function in tandem. For example, the body needs vitamin D in order to absorb calcium. With regard to zinc, animal studies suggest that an excess of zinc in the diet may reduce the absorption of calcium leading to a deficiency that weakens the teeth. Whether this occurs in human beings remains to be seen.

zinc (Zn), elemental Elemental zinc is blue-white metal used in a number of dental compounds such as AMALGAMS and cements. Zinc oxide (a white or yellowish powder) may be mixed with silver and used as a dental amalgam to fill CAVITIES. Zinc oxide plus eugenol (ZOE), a compound that dries to a hard substance, may be used as a permanent or temporary filling during root canal work or as a material from which to make dental IMPRESSIONS. Other zinc compounds such as zinc oxyphosphate, zinc phosphate, and zinc polycarboxylate are employed as dental cements for restorations or appliances such as bridges, CROWNS, INLAYS, and orthodontic appliances.

zygoma The scientific name for the cheekbone; from the Latin and Greek root zygom-, meaning "to join." The zygoma is a paired bone (one on each side of the face) right above and to the side of the upper jaw (maxilla); the term zygomaticomaxillary refers to an area that overlaps cheekbone and the maxilla. A fracture of either the upper jawbone of the cheekbone may require wiring that penetrates both BONES so as to hold them in line as they heal.

The zygomatic ARCH is the point where the cheekbone joins the flat temporal bone that comes down the side of the face next to the eye. The zygomaticoorbital region is the area that includes the cheekbone and the orbit, the bony socket around the eye. The term zygomaticofacial refers to the cheekbone and the face; the term zygomaticofrontal refers to the cheekbone and the frontal bone (the bone over the eye); and the term zygomaticotemporal refers to the cheekbone and the temporal bone.

APPENDIXES

APPENDIX I
GOVERNMENT AGENCIES

Division of Oral Health, Centers for Disease Control and Prevention

www.cdc.gov/OralHealth

The goal of the CDC's Division of Oral Health is to "prevent and control oral diseases and conditions and reduce disparities by building the knowledge, tools, and networks that promote healthy behaviors and effective public health practices and programs."

The site has a superlative search engine for anyone interesting in the esoterica of dental/oral health statistics and studies. For example, typing "dental decay" into the search bar brings up reports such as "Water Fluoridation and Costs of Medicaid Treatment for Dental Decay—Louisiana, 1995–1996," as well as simple news releases ("Oral Health Improving for Most Americans, but Tooth Decay among Preschool Children on the Rise"). Consumers, however, are most likely to use the equally excellent Oral Health A-Z feature. Bring up the list, go to A, click on Adult Oral Health, and up comes the following:

Adult Oral Health

There are threats to oral health across the life span. Nearly one-third of all adults in the United States have untreated tooth decay. One in seven adults aged 35 to 44 years has gum disease; this increases to one in every four adults aged 65 years and older. In addition, nearly a quarter of all adults have experienced some facial pain in the past six months. Oral cancers are most common in older adults, particularly those over 55 years who smoke and are heavy drinkers.

More Information on Adult Oral Health

- Fact Sheets and FAQs
- MMWRs and Journal Articles
- Oral Cancer: Overview

Additional Resources
The Oral Health of Older Americans

A research brief produced by the National Center for Health Statistics in its Aging Trends series

There is a similar wealth of information through the rest of the alphabetical listings as well.

National Institute of Dental and Craniofacial Research (NIDCR)

www.nidcr.nih.gov

The National Institute of Dental and Craniofacial Research (NIDCR), a division of the National Institutes of Health created by President Harry Truman in 1948, aims to improve the dental, oral, and craniofacial (head and face) health of Americans through research, training, and dissemination of information.

Buttons at the top of the home page offer consumers five broad categories from which to choose. "Oral health" is the most useful, with lists of articles on dental and oral health conditions, plus offers for brochures and reports. "Clinical trials" describe current NIDCR research efforts along with information about how to enroll in a study. "Research" explains current projects and proposals for future investigations. "Grants and funding" is primarily for professionals, as is the fifth category, "Careers and training."

STATE AND REGIONAL DENTAL REGULATORY AGENCIES

The following state agencies issue licenses to dentists and, in some cases, other dental professionals such as dental hygienists. Their sites provide information about licensing requirements and, in most cases, offer a dental consumer in the United States a way to document and evaluate the credentials, affiliations, and performance for various practicing dentists and dental specialists.

Alabama Board of Dental Examiners
5346 Stadium Trace Parkway, Suite 112
Hoover, AL 35244
(205) 985-7267
http://www.dentalboard.org/index.htm

Alaska State Dental Board
P.O. Box 110806
Juneau, AK 99811-0806
(907) 465-2542
http://www.dced.state.ak.us/occ/pden.htm

Arizona Dental Examiners Board
5060 North 19th Avenue, Suite 406
Phoenix, AZ 85015
(602) 242-1492
http://www.azdentalboard.org

**Arkansas State Board of
     Dental Examiners**
101 East Capitol Avenue, Suite 111
Little Rock, AK 72201
(501) 682-2085
http://www.asbde.org

Dental Board of California
1432 Howe Avenue, #85
Sacramento, CA 95825
(916) 263-2300
http://www.dbc.ca.gov

Colorado Board of Dental Examiners
1560 Broadway, Suite 1310
Denver, CO 80202
(303) 894-7763
http://www.dora.state.co.us/DENTAL

Connecticut State Dental Commission
410 Capitol Avenue
Hartford, CT 06134-0308
(860) 509-7590
http://www.state.ct.us/dph

Delaware Board of Dental Examiners
861 Silver Lake Boulevard, Suite 203
Cannon Building
Dover, DE 19904
(302) 744-4500
http://www.dpr.delaware.gov/boards/dental/
     index.shtml

District of Columbia Board of Dentistry
717 14th Street NW, Suite 600
Washington, DC 20005
(877) 672-2174
http://www.dchealth.dc.gov/doh/cwp/view,a,1
     371,q,600666,dohNav_GID,1878,dohNav,%
     7C34427%7C34429%7C,.asp

Florida Department of Health—Dentistry
4052 Bald Cypress Way, Bin C08
Tallahassee, FL 32399-3256
(850) 245-4474
http://www.doh.state.fl.us/mqa

Georgia Board of Dentistry
237 Coliseum Drive
Macon, GA 31217-3858
(478) 207-1681
http://www.sos.georgia.gov/plb/dentistry

Hawaii State Board of Dental Examiners
Dept. of Commerce and Consumer Affairs
P.O. Box 3469
Honolulu, HI 96801
(808) 586-2711
http://www.hawaii.
     gov/dcca/areas/pvl/boards/dentist

Idaho State Board of Dentistry
P.O. Box 83720
Boise, ID 83720-0021
(208) 334-2369
http://www.2.state.id.us/isbd

Illinois State Board of Dentistry
Department of Professional Regulation and
    Education
320 West Washington Street, 3rd Floor
Springfield, IL 62786
(217) 782-0458
http://www.dpr.state.il.us

Indiana State Board of Dental Examiners
402 West Washington Street
Indianapolis, IN 46204
(317) 234-2010
http://www.state.in.us/hpb/isbde

Iowa Board of Dental Examiners
400 SW 8th Street, Suite D
Des Moines, IA 50309-4687
(515) 281-5157
http://www.state.ia.us/dentalboard

Kansas Dental Board
900 SW Jackson Street, Room 564S
Topeka, KS 66612
(785) 296-6400
http://www.kansas.gov/kdb

Kentucky Board of Dentistry
312 Whittington Parkway, Suite 101
Louisville, KY 40222
(502) 429-7280
http://dentistry.ky.gov

Louisiana State Board of Dentistry
365 Canal Street, Suite 2680
New Orleans, LA 70130
(504) 568-8574
http://www.lsbd.org

Maine Board of Dental Examiners
143 State House Station
Augusta, ME 04333
(207) 287-3333
http://www.mainedental.org

**Maryland State Board of Dental
    Examiners**
The Benjamin Rush Building
Spring Grove Hospital Center
55 Wade Avenue

Baltimore, MD 21228
(410) 402-8500
http://www.dhmh.state.md.us/dental

**Massachusetts Board of Registration in
    Dentistry**
239 Causeway Street, 5th Floor
Boston, MA 02114
(617) 727-0084
http://www.mass.gov/dph/boards.dn

Michigan Board of Dentistry
Capitol View Building
201 Townsend Street
Lansing, MI 48913
(517) 373-3740
http://www.michigan.gov/mdch/0,1607,7-132-
    27417_27529_27533---,00.html

Minnesota Board of Dentistry
2829 University Avenue SE, Suite 450
Minneapolis, MN 55414-3246
(612) 617-2250
http://www.dentalboard.state.mn.us

Mississippi Board of Dental Examiners
600 East Amite Street, Suite 100
Jackson, MS 39201-2801
(601) 944-9622
http://www.msbde.state.ms.us/msbde/msbde.
    nsf

Missouri State Dental Board
3605 Missouri Boulevard
P.O. Box 1367
Jefferson City, MO 65102-1367
(573) 751-0040
http://www.pr.mo.gov/dental.asp

Montana Board of Dentistry
301 South Park
P.O. Box 200513
Helena, MT 59620-0513
http://www.dentistry.mt.gov

Nebraska Board of Dentistry
P.O. Box 94986
Lincoln, NE 68509-4986

(402) 471-4915
http://www.hhs.state.ne.us

Nevada State Board of Dental Examiners
6010 South Rainbow Boulevard
Las Vegas, NV 89118
http://www.nvdentalboard.nv.gov

New Hampshire Board of Dental Examiners
2 Industrial Park Drive
Concord, NH 03301-8520
(603) 271-4561
http://www.state.nh.us/dental

New Jersey State Board of Dentistry
124 Halsey Street
P.O. Box 45005
Newark, NJ 07101
(973) 504-6405
http://www.state.nj.us/lps/ca/medical/dentistry.
　htm

New Mexico Board of Dental Health Care
P.O. Box 25101
Santa Fe, NM 87504-5101
(505) 476-4680
http://www.rld.state.nm.us/Dental/index.html

New York State Board of Dentistry
89 Washington Avenue, 2nd Floor–West Wing
Albany, NY 12234
(518) 474-3817
http://www.op.nysed.gov/dentbroch.htm

North Carolina State Board of Dental Examiners
507 Airport Boulevard, Suite 105
Morrisville, NC 27560-8200
(919) 678-8223
http://www.ncdentalboard.org

North Dakota State Board of Dental Examiners
P.O. Box 7246
Bismarck, ND 58507-7246
(701) 258-8600
http://www.nddentalboard.org

Ohio State Dental Board
Riffe Center
77 South High Street, 18th Floor
Columbus, OH 43215-6135
(614) 466-2580
http://www.dental.ohio.gov

Oklahoma Board of Dentistry
201 Northeast 38th Terrace, #2
Oklahoma City, OK 73105
(405) 524-9037
http://www.dentist.state.ok.us

Oregon Board of Dentistry
1600 Southwest 4th Avenue, Suite 770
Portland, OR 97201
http://www.oregon.
　gov/Dentistry/contact_us.shtml

Pennsylvania State Board of Dentistry
P.O. Box 2649
Harrisburg, PA 17105-2649
(717) 783-7162
http://www.dos.state.pa.us/bpoa/cwp/view.
　asp?a=1104&q=432687

Puerto Rico Board of Dental Examiners
P.O. Box 10200
San Juan, PR 00908
(787) 723-1617

Rhode Island State Board of Examiners in Dentistry
Three Capitol Hill, Room 205
Providence, RI 02908
(800) 942-7434
http://www.health.ri.gov/hsr/professions/
　dental_app.php

South Carolina State Board of Dentistry
Synergy Business Park/Kingstree Building
110 Centerview Drive, Suite 202
Columbia, SC 29210
(803) 896-4599
http://www.llr.state.sc.us/pol/Dentistry

South Dakota State Board of Dentistry
P.O. Box 1037
Pierre, SD 57501-1037
(605) 224-1282
http://www.sdboardofdentistry.com

Tennessee Board of Dentistry
Cordell Hull Building
425 Fifth Avenue North
Nashville, TN 37243
(615) 253-5515
http://www.health.state.tn.us/contact.htm

Texas State Board of Dental Examiners
333 Guadalupe, Tower 3, #800
Austin, TX 78701
(512) 463-6400
http://www.tsbde.state.tx.us

**Utah Board of Dentists and Dental
   Hygienists**
160 East 300 South
Salt Lake City, UT 84111
(801) 530-6628
http://www.dopl.utah.gov/licensing/dentistry.
   html

Vermont Board of Dental Examiners
Office of Professional Regulation
National Life Building, North floor 2
Montpelier, VT 05620-3402
(802) 828-1505
http://www.vtprofessionals.org/opr1/dentists

Virginia Board of Dentistry
Perimeter Center
9960 Mayland Drive, Suite 300
Richmond, VA 23233
(804) 367-4538
http://www.dhp.state.va.us/dentistry

**Virgin Islands (U.S.) Board of Dental
   Examiners**
48 Sugar Estate
Saint Thomas, VI 00802
(340) 774-0117

**Washington State Dental Health Care
   Quality Assurance Commission**
Washington State Department of Health Systems Quality Assurance
310 Israel Road
Tumwater, WA 98501
(360) 236-4700
http://fortress.wa.gov/doh/hpqa1/hps3/Dental/
   default.htm

West Virginia Board of Dental Examiners
1319 Robert C. Byrd Drive
P.O. Box 1447
Crab Orchard, WV 25827
(877) 914-8266
http://www.wvdentalboard.org

Wisconsin Dentistry Examining Board
1400 East Washington Avenue
P.O. Box 8935
Madison, WI 53708
(608) 266-2811
http://www.drl.wi.gov/boards/den/index.htm

Wyoming Board of Dental Examiners
1800 Carey Avenue, 4th Floor
Cheyenne, WY 82002
(307) 777-6529
http://www.plboards.state.wy.us/dental/index.
   asp

Source: American Association of Dental Boards, www.
aadexam.org/.

APPENDIX II
PROFESSIONAL ASSOCIATIONS AND ORGANIZATIONS

Searching the Web for information about dental and oral health can be risky. The open nature of the Internet encourages the exchange of anecdotal (and sometimes misleading) evidence. As a result, it may be difficult to vouch for the quality and reliability of the information on a specific site.

Not so with the Web sites listed here. Each deals with an aspect of dentistry, its practitioners, and its history. Furthermore, each is run by a thoroughly professional organization or individual posting only up-to-date and accurate information. And each makes clear that the best source for personal medical advice on this topic is one's own dental specialist.

GENERAL DENTISTRY

American Dental Association
211 East Chicago Avenue
Chicago, IL 60611
(312) 440-2500
http://www.ada.org

The American Dental Association, founded in 1859 in Niagara Falls, New York, is the world's oldest and largest professional dental organization with more than 155,000 members in the United States. Its Web site offers not only information about dental health and a link to a "find-a-dentist" page, but also a virtual tour of the ADA headquarters, library, and scientific laboratories in Chicago (Windows Media Player required), along with a complete e-store offering informational booklets and downloads for consumers. The home page also links to a page for the American Dental Association Seal of Acceptance. The seal, first awarded in 1931, has long been considered a symbol of safety and effectiveness. A complete list of the dental products (toothpaste, dental floss, manual and electric toothbrushes, mouth rinse, and chewing gum) carrying the seal as of October 2008 is available.

The state affiliates for the American Dental Association are:

Alabama Dental Association
836 Washington Avenue
Montgomery, AL 36104-3839
(334) 265-1684
http://www.aldaonline.org

Alaska Dental Society
9170 Jewel Lake Road, Suite 203
Anchorage, AK 99502-5381
(907) 563-3003
http://www.akdental.org

Arizona Dental Association
3193 North Drinkwater Boulevard
Scottsdale, AZ 85251-6491
(480) 344-5777
http://www.azda.org

Arkansas Dental Association
7480 Highway 107
Sherwood, AR 72120
(501) 834-7650
http://www.dental-asda.org

California Dental Association
1201 K Street
Sacramento, CA 95814

(800) 232-7645
http://www.cda.org

Colorado Dental Association
3690 South Yosemite, Suite 100
Denver, CO 80237-1808
(303) 740-6900
http://www.cdaonline.org

Connecticut State Dental Association
835 West Queen Street
Southington, CT 06489
(860) 378-1800
http://www.csda.com

Delaware State Dental Society
The Christiana Executive Campus
200 Continental Drive, Suite 111
Newark, DE 19713
(302) 368-7634
http://www.delawarestatedentalsociety.org

District of Columbia Dental Society
502 C Street, NE
Washington, DC 20002-5810
(202) 547-7613
http://www.dcdental.org

Florida Dental Association
1111 East Tennessee Street, Suite 102
Tallahassee, FL 32308-6913
(850) 681-3629
http://www.floridadental.org

Georgia Dental Association
7000 Peachtree Dunwoody Road NE, Suite 200
Building 17
Atlanta, GA 30328-1655
(404) 636-7553
http://www.gadental.org

Hawaii Dental Association
1345 South Beretania Street, Suite 301
Honolulu, HI 96814-1821
(808) 593-7956
http://www.hawaiidentalassociation.net

Idaho State Dental Association
1220 West Hays Street
Boise, ID 83702-5315

(208) 343-7543
http://www.isdaweb.com

Illinois State Dental Society
1010 South Second Street
P.O. Box 376
Springfield, IL 62705-0376
(217) 525-1406
http://www.isds.org

Indiana Dental Association
401 West Michigan Street, Suite 1000
Indianapolis, IN 46202-3233
(317) 634-2610
http://www.indental.org

Iowa Dental Association
5530 West Parkway, Suite 100
Johnston, IA 50131
(515) 986-5605
http://www.iowadental.org

Kansas Dental Association
5200 SW Huntoon Street
Topeka, KS 66604
(785) 272-7360
http://www.ksdental.org

Kentucky Dental Association
1920 Nelson Miller Parkway
Louisville, KY 40223-2164
(502) 489-9121
http://www.kyda.org

Louisiana Dental Association
7833 Office Park Boulevard
P.O. Box 261173
Baton Rouge, LA 70809-7604
(225) 926-1986

Maine Dental Association
P.O. Box 215
Manchester, ME 04351-0215
(207) 622-7900
http://www.medental.org

Maryland State Dental Association
6410 Dobbin Road, Suite F
Columbia, MD 21045-4774
(410) 964-2880

Massachusetts Dental Society
2 Willow Street, Suite 200
Southborough, MA 01745-1027
(508) 480-9797
http://www.massdental.org

Michigan Dental Association
230 Washington Square North, Suite 208
Lansing, MI 48933-1312
(517) 372-9070
http://www.smilemichigan.com

Minnesota Dental Association
1335 Industrial Boulevard, Suite 200
Minneapolis, MN 55413-4801
(612) 767-8400
http://www.mndental.org

Mississippi Dental Association
2630 Ridgewood Road, Suite C
Jackson, MS 39216-4903
(601) 982-0442
http://www.msdental.org

Missouri Dental Association
3340 American Avenue
Jefferson City, MO 65109
(573) 634-3436
http://www.modental.org

Montana Dental Association
17 1/2 South Last Chance Gulch
P.O. Box 1154
Helena, MT 59624
(406) 443-2061
http://www.mtdental.com

Nebraska Dental Association
3120 O Street
Lincoln, NE 68510-1533
(402) 476-1704
http://www.nedental.org

Nevada Dental Association
8863 West Flamingo Road, Suite 102
Las Vegas, NV 89147-8718
(702) 255-4211
http://www.nyda.org

New Hampshire Dental Society
23 South State Street
Concord, NH 03301
(603) 225-5961
http://www.nhds.org

New Jersey Dental Association
One Dental Plaza
P.O. Box 6020
North Brunswick, NJ 08902-6020
(732) 821-9400
http://www.njda.org

New Mexico Dental Association
9201 Montgomery Boulevard NE, Suite 601
Albuquerque, NM 87111
(505) 294-1368
http://www.nmdental.org

New York State Dental Association
20 Corporate Woods Boulevard, Suite 602
Albany, NY 12211
(518) 465-0044
http://www.nysdental.org

North Carolina Dental Society
P.O. Box 4099
Cary, NC 27519-4099
(919) 677-1396
http://www.ncdental.org

North Dakota Dental Association
P.O. Box 1332
Bismarck, ND 58502-1332
(701) 223-8870
http://www.nddental.com

Ohio Dental Association
1370 Dublin Road
Columbus, OH 43215-1009
(614) 486-2700
http://www.oda.org

Oklahoma Dental Association
317 NE 13th Street
Oklahoma City, OK 73104
(405) 848-8873
http://www.okda.org

Oregon Dental Association
P.O. Box 3710
Wilsonville, OR 97070-3710
(503) 218-2010
http://www.oregondental.org

Pacific Basin Dental Association
(American Samoa, Guam, Northern Marina
   Islands, Marshall Islands, Palau)
P.O. Box 16
Majuro, MH 96960
(692) 625-3355 x 2101

Pennsylvania Dental Association
P.O. Box 3341
Harrisburg, PA 17105-3341
(717) 234-5941
http://www.padental.org

**Colegio de Cirujanos Dentistas
   de Puerto Rico**
Avenida Domenech #200
San Juan, PR 00918
(506) 256-3100
http://www.ccdpr.org

Rhode Island Dental Association
200 Centerville Road, Suite 7
Warwick, RI 02886-4339
(401) 732-6833
http://www.ridental.com

South Carolina Dental Association
120 Stonemark Lane
Columbia, SC 29210-3841
(803) 750-2277
http://www.scda.org

South Dakota Dental Association
804 North Euclid, Suite 103
P.O. Box 1194
Pierre, SD 57501-1194
(605) 224-9168
http://www.sddental.org

Tennessee Dental Association
660 Bakers Bridge Avenue, Suite 300
Franklin, TN 37067

(615) 628-0208
http://www.tenndental.org

Texas Dental Association
1946 South IH-35, Suite 400
Austin, TX 78704
(512) 443-3675
http://www.tda.org

Utah Dental Association
1151 East 3900 South, Suite 160
Salt Lake City, UT 84124-1255
(801) 261-5315
http://www.uda.org

Vermont State Dental Society
100 Dorset Street, Suite 18
South Burlington, VT 05403-6241
(802) 864-0115
http://www.vsds.org

Virginia Dental Association
7525 Staples Mill Road
Richmond, VA 23228
(804) 261-1610
http://www.vadental.org

Virgin Islands Dental Association
Medical Arts Complex, Suite 10
Saint Thomas, VI 00802
(340) 777-5950

Washington State Dental Association
1001 Fourth Avenue, Suite 3800
Seattle, WA 98154
(206) 448-1914
http://www.wsda.org

West Virginia Dental Association
2016 1/2 Kanawha Boulevard East
Charleston, WV 25311-2204
(304) 344-5246
http://www.wvdental.org

Wisconsin Dental Association
6737 West Washington Street, Suite 2360
West Allis, WI 53214
(414) 276-4520
http://www.wda.org

Wyoming Dental Association
P.O. Box 40019
Casper, WY 82604
(307) 237-1186
http://www.wyda.org

Source: Health Guide USA, http://healthguideusa.
org/state_dental_associations.htm

DENTAL SPECIALTIES

American Academy of Cosmetic Dentistry (AACD)

5401 World Dairy Drive
Madison, WI 53718
(800) 543-9220
(608) 222-8583
http://www.aacd.com

AACD, founded in 1984, is the largest international association of cosmetic and reconstructive dentists, dental laboratory technicians, educators, researchers, students, and hygienists.

The academy's site explains modern cosmetic dentistry techniques and offers several interactive services. On the home page, click "For the Public" to bring up several quick links. The two most valuable are "How to Choose Your Dentist" and "Ask An AACD Member Dentist Your Dental Question." The first link sets out the obvious standards for professional care: Make sure the dentist belongs to AACD, ask for before-and-after pictures of the dentist's patients, get references from other dentists (and other patients), check to see that your dentist participates in continuing education courses to keep his knowledge and techniques up-to-date. The second link goes to a form you can use to e-mail or print and fax your question to the AACD. There is also an 800 number for patients who prefer to use the phone.

American Academy of Oral and Maxillofacial Pathology (AAOMP)

710 East Ogden Avenue, Suite 600
Naperville, IL 60563-8614
(888) 552-2667
http://www.aaomp.org

AAOMP represents oral and maxillofacial pathologists, dentists specializing in the diagnosis and management of diseases affecting the mouth and upper face, identifying the connection between oral health and systemic disease.

A link at the bottom of the AAOMP home page connects the patient to a list of oral and maxillary pathologists in the United States. A separate link ("Public") on the left side of the home page enables a patient to click on to one of five subjects: Introduction, Information on Oral Disease, Real Life Stories, FAQs, and Resources & Links.

American Academy of Oral and Maxillofacial Radiology (AAOMR)

P.O. Box 55722
Jackson, MS 39296
(601) 934-6060
http://www.aaomr.org

The American Academy of Oral Roentgenologists, founded in October 1949 at a meeting in San Francisco, was renamed the American Academy of Oral Roentgenology in 1951. The organization changed its name to the American Academy of Dental Radiology in 1967, changing that to the current name in 1986. As of this writing, the academy maintains a membership roster of approximately 400 dental professionals and members of the dental radiographic industry. AAOMR published reports and newsletters, some of which are available on the organization site.

American Academy of Pediatric Dentistry (AAPD)

211 East Chicago Avenue, Suite 700
Chicago, IL 60611-2663
(312) 337-2169
http://www.aapd.org

The American Academy of Pediatric Dentistry, founded in 1947, is the membership organization for more than 7,000 dentists specializing in the treatment of infants, children, and adolescents, as well as patients with special needs. The academy publishes two professional journals, *Pediatric Dentistry* and *Journal of Dentistry for Children*.

The AAPD Web site explains the organization's mission as advocates for dental health. Its FAQs page offers a guide for parents, answering questions such as what to use to clean a baby's teeth, when to schedule a child's first dental checkup, the importance of "baby teeth," and how to prevent tooth decay associated with baby bottles or nursing. There is, of course, a "How to Find a Pediatric Dentist" page.

American Academy of Periodontology (AAP)

737 North Michigan Avenue, Suite 800
Chicago, IL 60611
(312) 573-3256
http://www.perio.org

The American Academy of Periodontology, founded in 1914 as the American Academy of Oral Prophylaxis and Periodontology, adopted its current name five years later. In 1967, the academy merged with American Society of Periodontists. Today the AAP represents more than 8,000 dentists specializing in the diagnosis and treatment of periodontal disease.

The academy's Web site offers consumers a pathway to finding a periodontist, along with information about various forms of gum diseases and treatments, plus a media center with press releases detailing advances in periodontology and a page that encourages patients to sign up for the latest news bulletins.

American Association of Endodontists (AAE)

211 East Chicago Avenue, Suite 1100
Chicago, IL 60611-2691
(800) 872-3636
http://www.aae.org

AAE, founded in February 1943, is the professional organization for dentists specializing in conditions affecting the interior of the tooth, that is, the dental pulp. The American Dental Association classified endodontics as a dental specialty in 1963. Today, AAE sees its mission as "providing a single forum for exchange of information into an agency for education of the profession, formulation of educational policies and development of an educational system for its specialty. It is an advocate for endodontists and endodontics to both the dental profession and the public, promoting the highest quality endodontic care for all patients."

On the AAE home page, click onto "Patients and the Public" to reach a page with useful consumer information such as a link to an interactive map that enables patients to find a local AAE endodontist; news releases describing advances in endodontic dentistry; and interesting factoids such as: "22 million endodontic procedures are performed each year; nearly 15 million are root canals" possibly thanks to the welcome fact that "root canal treatment can be virtually painless thanks to advances in anesthesia and technology."

American Association of Oral and Maxillofacial Surgeons (AAOMS)

9700 West Bryn Mawr Avenue
Rosemont, IL 60018-5701
(847) 673-6200
http://www.aaoms.org

AAOMS represents more than 8,500 oral and maxillofacial surgeons in the United States. Its Web site offers a slew of patient-friendly features accessed simply by clicking the "Public Information" button at the top of the home page to open up the page with a definition of the specialty, an interactive feature enabling a patient to locate a specialist, patient information (brochures available from the site's e-store), press releases, and media kits.

American Association of Orthodontists (AAO)

401 North Lindbergh Boulevard
Saint Louis, MO 63141-7816
(314) 993-1700
http://www.aaortho.org

The AAO, founded in 1900 as the American Society of Orthodontists, adopted its present name in 1937. Today, the association has 15,000 members in the United States and Canada. Its well-designed Web site offers the usual useful features such as a find-a-specialist page and FAQs on orthodontics history and treatment. But a special attraction is a group of pages with coloring-book pictures (i.e., a jack-o-lantern picture for the month of October) designed to appeal to the younger patients who make up the majority of the orthodontics audience.

American Association of Public Health Dentistry (AAPHD)
3085 Stevenson Drive, Suite 200
Springfield, IL 62703
(217) 529-6941
http://www.aaphd.org

The AAPHD, founded in 1937, draws its membership list from a broad range of professionals and laypersons who share a common concern with improving the oral health of the American public. The organization's goals include educating the public to the importance of oral health, promoting programs that reduce the incidence of oral disease, and expanding research and knowledge of dental public health. The association's site offers consumers information about the role of the public health dentist but is most useful for those planning a career in this branch of dentistry.

American College of Prosthodontists
211 East Chicago Avenue, Suite 1000
Chicago, IL 60611
(312) 573-1260
http://www.prosthodontics.org

The American College of Prosthodontists is the professional association of dentists whose postgraduate training concentrates on repairing or replacing teeth with such appliances as dental implants, dentures, veneers, and crowns as well as improving the appearance of the teeth with techniques such as dental whitening.

Consumers who click the "Public & Patients" button at the top of the home page are directed to a new screen on which they can read a definition of a prosthodontist, find clear, consumer-friendly explanations of prosthodontic procedures, use an interactive tool to find a prosthodontist, run through the customary useful FAQs page, and enter a "Press Room" that makes available the latest news about this dental specialty.

APPENDIX III
ACCREDITED DENTAL SCHOOLS, UNITED STATES

The following schools are accredited in the United States. The list is expected to grow.

ALABAMA

University of Alabama School of Dentistry
1530 3rd Avenue South, SDB 406
Birmingham, AL 35294-0007
(205) 934-4720
http://www.dental.uab.edu

ARIZONA

A.T. Still University Arizona School of Dentistry and Oral Health
5850 East Still Circle
Mesa, AZ 85206
(480) 219-6000
http://www.atsu.edu/asdoh

Midwestern University College of Dental Medicine
19555 North 59th Avenue
Glendale, AZ 85308
(623) 572-3800
http://www.midwestern.edu

CALIFORNIA

Loma Linda University School of Dentistry
Dental School
Loma Linda, CA 92350
(909) 558-4222
http://www.llu.edu/llu/dentistry

University of California at Los Angeles School of Dentistry
Center for Health Science, Room 53-038
Los Angeles, CA 90095-1668
(310) 206-6063
http://www.dent.ucla.edu

University of California at San Francisco School of Dentistry
513 Parnassus Avenue, S-630
San Francisco, CA 94143
(415) 476-1323
http://dentistry.ucsf.edu

University of Southern California School of Dentistry
925 West 34th Street
Los Angeles, CA 90089-6041
(213) 740-3124
http://www.usc.edu/hsc/dental

University of the Pacific Arthur A. Dugoni School of Dentistry
2155 Webster Street
San Francisco, CA 94115
(415) 929-6425
http://www.dental.pacific.edu

COLORADO

University of Colorado–Denver School of Dentistry
Lazzara Center for Oral-Facial Health
13065 East 17th Avenue
Aurora, CO 80045
(303) 724-7100
http://www.uchsc.edu/sod

CONNECTICUT

University of Connecticut School of Dental Medicine
263 Farmington Avenue
Farmington, CT 06030-3915
(860) 679-2808
http://sdm.uchc.edu

DISTRICT OF COLUMBIA

Howard University College of Dentistry
600 W Street NW
Washington, DC 20059
(202) 806-0440
http://www.howard.edu

FLORIDA

Nova Southeastern University College of Dental Medicine
3200 South University Drive
Fort Lauderdale, FL 33328
(954) 262-7311
http://dental.nova.edu

University of Florida College of Dentistry
1600 SW Archer Road, Room D4-6
Gainesville, FL 32610-0405
(352) 273-5802
http://www.dental.ufl.edu

GEORGIA

Medical College of Georgia School of Dentistry
1120 15th Street, Room AD 1119
Augusta, GA 30912-0200
(706) 721-2117
http://www.mcg.edu/SOD

IOWA

University of Iowa College of Dentistry
100 Dental Science Building
Iowa City, IA 52242
(319) 335-7145
http://www.dentistry.uiowa.edu

ILLINOIS

Southern Illinois University School of Dental Medicine
2800 College Avenue, Building 273/2300
Alton, IL 62002
(618) 474-7120
http://www.siue.edu/dentalmedicine

University of Illinois at Chicago College of Dentistry
801 South Paulina Street, Suite 102
Chicago, IL 60612
(312) 996-1040
http://dentistry.uic.edu

INDIANA

Indiana University School of Dentistry
1121 West Michigan Street
Indianapolis, IN 46202
(317) 274-7461
http://www.iusd.iupui.edu/default.aspx

KENTUCKY

University of Kentucky College of Dentistry
800 Rose Street, D 136 UKMC
Lexington, KY 40536-0297
(859) 323-1884
http://www.mc.uky.edu/Dentistry

University of Louisville School of Dentistry
501 South Preston Street
Louisville, KY 40292
(502)852-5295
http://www.dental.louisville.edu/dental

LOUISIANA

Louisiana State University School of Dentistry
1100 Florida Avenue
New Orleans, LA 70119-2799
(504) 619-8500
http://www.lsusd.lsuhsc.edu

MARYLAND

University of Maryland Baltimore College of Dental Surgery
650 West Baltimore Street, Suite 6402
Baltimore, MD 21201
(410) 706-7461
http://www.dental.umaryland.edu

MASSACHUSETTS

Boston University Goldman School of Dental Medicine
100 East Newton Street
Boston, MA 02118
(617) 638-4790
http://dentalschool.bu.edu

Harvard University School of Dental Medicine
188 Longwood Avenue
Boston, MA 02115
(617) 432-1401
http://www.hsdm.med.harvard.edu

Tufts University School of Dental Medicine
One Kneeland Street
Boston, MA 02111
(617) 636-6636
http://www.tuftSouthedu/dental

MICHIGAN

University of Detroit Mercy School of Dentistry
2700 Martin Luther King Jr. Boulevard, MB 98
Detroit, MI 48208-2576
(313) 494-6621
http://www.udmercy.edu/dental

University of Michigan School of Dentistry
1011 North University Avenue
Ann Arbor, MI 48109-1078
(734) 763-3311
http://www.dent.umich.edu

MINNESOTA

University of Minnesota School of Dentistry
515 Southeast Delaware Street, Room 15-209
  Moos Tower
Minneapolis, MN 55455
(612) 624-2424
http://www.dentistry.umn.edu

MISSISSIPPI

University of Mississippi School of Dentistry
Medical Center
2500 North State Street
Jackson, MS 39216-4505
(601) 984-6000
http://www.dentistry.umc.edu

MISSOURI

University of Missouri
Kansas City School of Dentistry
650 East 25th Street
Kansas City, MO 64108
(816) 235-2010
http://www.umkc.edu/dentistry

NORTH CAROLINA

University of North Carolina School of Dentistry
1090 Old Dental Building, UNC-CH CB 7450
Chapel Hill, NC 27599-7450
(919) 966-2731
http://www.dent.unc.edu

NEBRASKA

Creighton University School of Dentistry
2500 California Plaza
Omaha, NE 68178-0240
(402) 280-5060
http://www.cudental.creighton.edu

University of Nebraska Medical Center College of Dentistry
40th and Holdrege streets

Lincoln, NE 68583-0740
(402) 472-1344
http://www.unmc.edu/dentistry

NEVADA

University of Nevada–Las Vegas School of Dental Medicine
Shadow Lane Campus
1001 Shadow Lane
Las Vegas, NV 89106-4124
(702) 774-2500
http://www.dentalschool.unlv.edu

NEW JERSEY

University of Medicine and Dentistry of New Jersey
New Jersey Dental School
110 Bergen Street, Room B815
Newark, NJ 07103-2425
(973) 972-4633
http://www.dentalschool.umdnj.edu

NEW YORK

Columbia University College of Dental Medicine
630 West 168th Street, PH7 East Room 122
New York, NY 10032
(212) 305-4511
http://www.cpmcnet.columbia.edu/dept/dental

New York University College of Dentistry
345 East 24th Street
New York, NY 10010
(212) 998-9800
http://www.nyu.edu/dental

State University of New York at Buffalo School of Dental Medicine
315 Squire Hall
Buffalo, NY 14214-3008
(716) 829-2836
http://www.sdm.buffalo.edu

State University of New York at Stony Brook School of Dental Medicine
Health Sciences Center
154 Rockland Hall

Stony Brook, NY 11794-8700
(631) 632-8950
http://www.hsc.stonybrook.edu/dental

OHIO

Case Western Reserve University School of Dental Medicine
10900 Euclid Avenue
Cleveland, OH 44106-4905
(216) 368-3266
http://www.case.edu/dental/site/main.html

Ohio State University College of Dentistry
305 West 12th Avenue
Columbus, OH 43218-2357
(614) 292-9750
http://www.dent.ohio-state.edu

OKLAHOMA

University of Oklahoma College of Dentistry
1201 North Stonewall Avenue
Oklahoma City, OK 73117
(405) 271-6326
http://www.dentistry.ouhsc.edu

OREGON

Oregon Health and Science University School of Dentistry
611 Southwest Campus Drive
Portland, OR 97239
(503) 494-8801
http://www.ohsu.edu/sod/admissions

PENNSYLVANIA

Temple University
The Maurice H. Kornberg School of Dentistry
3223 North Broad Street
Philadelphia, PA 19140
(215) 707-2799
http://www.temple.edu/dentistry

University of Pennsylvania School of Dental Medicine
Robert Shattner Center

240 South 40th Street
Philadelphia, PA 19104-6030
(215) 898-8961
http://www.dental.upenn.edu

University of Pittsburgh School of Dental Medicine

3501 Terrace Street
Pittsburgh, PA 15261
(412) 648-1938
http://www.dental.pitt.edu

PUERTO RICO

University of Puerto Rico School of Dentistry

Medical Sciences Campus
Main Building–Office #A103B, 1st Floor
San Juan, PR 00936-5067
(787) 758-2525, ext. 1105
http://www.dental.rcm.upr.edu

SOUTH CAROLINA

Medical University of South Carolina College of Dental Medicine

171 Ashley Avenue
Charleston, SC 29425-1376
(843) 792-3811
http://academicdepartments.musc.edu/
   dentistry/about/index.htm

TENNESSEE

Meharry Medical College School of Dentistry

1005 D. B. Todd Blvd.
Nashville, TN 37208
(615) 327-6207
http://www.mmc.edu/education/dentistry

University of Tennessee College of Dentistry

University of Tennessee Health Science Center
875 Union Avenue
Memphis, TN 38163
(901) 448-6202
http://www.utmem.edu/dentistry

TEXAS

Baylor College of Dentistry

Texas A & M Health Science Center
3302 Gaston Avenue
Dallas, TX 75246
(214) 828-8300
http://www.tambcd.edu

University of Texas Health Science Center Houston Dental Branch

6516 M. D. Anderson Boulevard, Room 147
Houston, TX 77225-0068
(713) 500-4021
http://www.db.uth.tmc.edu

University of Texas Health Science Center San Antonio Dental School

7703 Floyd Curl Drive, Mail Code 7914
San Antonio, TX 78284-7914
(210) 567-3160
http://www.dental.uthscsa.edu

VIRGINIA

Virginia Commonwealth University School of Dentistry

520 North 12th Street, Box 980566
Richmond, VA 23298-0566
(804) 828-9184
http://www.dentistry.vcu.edu

WASHINGTON

University of Washington

Health Sciences School of Dentistry
D322 Health Sciences Building
1959 Northeast Pacific Street
Seattle, WA 98195
(206) 543-5982
http://www.dental.washington.edu

WEST VIRGINIA

West Virginia University School of Dentistry

Robert C. Byrd Health Science Center
1150 HSC North/Medical Center Drive
Morgantown, WV 26506-9400

(304) 293-2521
http://www.hsc.wvu.edu/sod

WISCONSIN

Marquette University School of Dentistry
1801 West Wisconsin Avenue
Milwaukee, WI 53233

(414) 288-7485
http://www.dental.mu.edu

Sources: The Dental Site.com, http://www.dentalsite.com/dentists/densch.html; Dentist.net, http://www.dentist.net/dentalschools.asp; Health Guide USA, http://healthguideusa.org/dental_schools.htm

APPENDIX IV
HEALTH-CARE FACILITY RATINGS

Routine dental procedures for healthy people rarely require a hospital visit, but some special-needs patients or patients undergoing complicated oral surgeries may benefit from an in-hospital setting. In that case, the following Web sites are useful when evaluating facilities.

American Association for Accreditation of Ambulatory Surgery Facilities (AAAASF)
http://www.aaaasf.org/consumers.php

The AAAASF accredits ambulatory surgery facilities to ensure that they meet local, state, and federal regulations including fire safety, sanitation, and building codes; follow all pertinent federal laws and regulations such as standards governing hazardous waste and the Americans with Disabilities Act; employ advanced techniques for patient safety during surgery and in the recovery period; permit only qualified surgeons, certified by the American Board of Medical Specialties and with access to an accredited hospital to perform surgery, and only board-certified or board-eligible physicians or certified registered nurse anesthetists to administer anesthesia; and certified or registers personnel to maintain the recovery room.

Accreditation Association for Ambulatory Health Care, Inc. (AAAHC)
http://www.aaahc.org

The AAAHC accredits ambulatory health-care organizations including (but not limited to) ambulatory and physician office-based surgery centers, managed-care organizations, and Native American and student health centers to make sure they meet all standards governing patients' rights, quality care, clinical record keeping, dissemination of health information, administration and governance, and facility maintenance.

Health Grades
http://www.healthgrades.com

Health Grades, a health-care ratings, information, and advisory services company, ranks more than 5,000 private, state, and city hospitals as one-star (poor), three-star (average), or five-star (excellent) based on their performance in 28 medical procedures and diagnoses in specialties such as cardiac surgery, cardiology, orthopedic surgery, neurosciences, pulmonary/respiratory treatment, vascular surgery, obstetrics, and women's health. The rankings, updated each year, are available free of charge at this site.

Five-star hospitals have significantly lower risk-adjusted mortality rates for three consecutive years and improve 21 percent more than the U.S. hospital average and 45 percent more than one-star hospitals. A typical patient would have, on average, a 65 percent lower chance of dying in a five-star hospital than in a one-star hospital, and a 45 percent lower chance of dying in a five-star rated hospital compared to the U.S. hospital average.

Joint Commission on the Accreditation of Healthcare Organizations (JCAHO)
http://www.jcaho.org

JCAHO, an independent not-for-profit organization created in 1951, evaluates and accredits health-care organizations including hospitals, hospice service, nursing homes, rehabilitation facilities, laboratories, home health care, and medical equipment services. To access the evaluations, click on to the home page, scroll down to the box on the bottom right labeled "Information For," and click "General Public." When the next page appears, click "Quality Check—Search for Joint Commission Accredited Organizations," then follow the directions to obtain a complete quality report including an evaluation of the facility and its individual services, plus its comparative standing in relation to other facilities in the area and across the country. To access this page directly, go to: www.qualitycheck.org/consumer/searchQCR.aspx.

Medicare

http://www.medicare.gov

In order to participate in Medicare- and Medicaid-funded programs, hospitals and other health-care facilities must meet government standards of care. To access information about a specific hospital from the home page, scroll down to "Search Tools," click on "Compare Hospitals in Your Area," then follow the prompts as the pages change. Note: When searching for a facility by name, you must have the exact name. For example, Mount Sinai Hospital, a major facility in New York City, is not accessible as "Mt. Sinai."

APPENDIX V
WEB RESOURCES

American Cancer Society

http://www.cancer.org

The American Cancer Society's 13 divisions and more than 3,400 local offices deliver cancer prevention, early detection, and patient services programs. Naturally, the site is devoted primarily to basic information about the various forms of cancer: prevention, warning signs, symptoms, diagnosis, treatment, and patient care. But typing "dentistry" or "oral cancer" into the search box on the home page produces a wealth of articles including (but not limited to) information on reconstructive oral surgery, oral adverse effects of cancer drugs or treatments, the importance of dental evaluation in treating oral cancers, and general advice about feeling well during or after cancer treatment (e.g., "Beauty Shown More than Skin Deep: Survivors with Attitude").

AnimatedTeeth.com

http://www.animated-teeth.com

This site is like a really big dental toy chest with quizzes, descriptions of common dental conditions, and explanations of treatments and procedures complete with animated teeth. It may sound too cute for words but the information is rock solid.

Answers.com

http://www.answers.com

An excellent site for general information on multiple topics, including dentistry and dental health, delivering multiple entries from a wide range of sources for each search. For example, typing "dental decay" into the search bar on the home page brings up 32 pages of material with six definitions and scientific descriptions of the decay process, documented with 85 footnotes and accompanied by eight print and 72 additional Web sources, making this site the ultimate layperson's research reference.

eMedicine

http://www.emedicine.com

This online medical library is one of three sites maintained by WebMD. eMedicine's distinguishing feature is its willingness to accept questions posed in slang terms as well as medical language. The articles, drawn from a variety of professional journals, are sophisticated in content but written so as to be accessible to the informed reader. To use this site the reader must register, but registration is free.

Intelihealth.com

http://www.intelihealth.com/IH/ihtIH/c/408/ 408.html

A reliable, well-organized and useful site, produced as a collaboration between Aetna and its "content partner," the Harvard Medical School; on the Dental Health page, the attribution reads, "featuring consumer information from the Columbia University College of Dental Medicine." Enter the site, go to the list in the left column, then click on "Dental Health." When the page changes, you might choose "Understand Conditions" for a complete alphabetical list of dental problems or "Explore Treatments" for a guide to professional remedies. The only drawback? Ads for insurance plans.

MedicineNet.com

http://www.medicinenet.com

This online health-care/medical publishing company, run by board-certified professionals, is one of three sites maintained by WebMD.

The site provides access to an extraordinary range of articles on health subjects from medical journals, medical institutions such as the Cleveland Clinic, government agencies, and MedicineNet's own roster of experts. For example, typing the words "dental decay" into the search bar brings up nine articles on diseases and conditions, eight articles on medications, 16 articles on tests and procedures, 25 pieces on health features, tips, and recipes, and 11 articles on health news related to dental decay. The only problematic feature on the site is "Sponsored Links," a list of paid advertisements for individual practitioners and people selling over-the-counter dental products.

Online Etymology Dictionary

http://www.etymonline.com

This site, created by Lancaster, Pennsylvania, historian, author, journalist, and lecturer Douglas Harper, is invaluable for those who enjoy decoding compound words and identifying their origin in language. The site uses a long list of sources, including *The Oxford English Dictionary*, *Klein's Comprehensive Etymological Dictionary of the English Language*, and Robert L. Chapman's *Dictionary of American Slang* to track the evolution of common and uncommon words, including many familiar dental terms. For example, the entry for the word *orthodontia* reads: "Orthodontics, 1909, from Mod. L. [modern Latin] *orthodontia* (1849), from *ortho-* (q.v.) + *odon* (gen. *odontos*) 'tooth.' *Orthodontist* is attested from 1903."

Online Metrics Conversion

http://www.sciencemadesimple.net/length.php

Given the fact that virtually all modern medical measurements, including the length of incisions and the diameter of surgical sutures, are commonly presented in metric terms, a conversion chart is a necessity. This site's "Metric Conversion Chart" is a handy tool for quick reference; for more information check out any of 14 categories, each of them exhaustive. For example, click "Length/ Height," and you get a chart with 49 different measurements starting at *angstrom* and ending at *yard*, with stops in between for such esoterica as *bolts, chains, lines, palms, skeins,* and *spans.*

WebMD

http://www.webmd.com

WebMD, the company that also owns and operates eMedicine.com and MedicineNet.com, produces and publishes original articles on health subjects written by experts in the relevant fields. As with articles in print journals, WebMD's pieces are vetted by independent reviewers. In addition, this site offers access to articles from standard journals and other sources, including reliable scientific Web sites.

Typing "dental decay" into this site's search bar brings up 138 health reference articles, 94 news features, and five comments from dental experts, which are then divided into categories that include 67 pieces on overviews and facts, 19 on preventing dental problems, 15 on treatment, eight on risk factors, 138 on oral health, eight on baby and child health, and four devoted to parenting for good health and so on. As with eMedicine, the only problematic category is "Sponsored Links," which for dentistry means ads for individual dentists and over-the-counter products.

Who Named It?

http://www.whonamedit.com

This site is a biographical dictionary of scientific eponyms including diseases, conditions, or procedures named for the person who identified or invented them, including many entries relevant to dental and oral health. From the home page, it is possible to access the eponyms by letter of the alphabet, scientific category (e.g., abscess), geographical location (Argentina, Australia, etc.), or gender, with male entries in the main list and a separate category for female entries.

GLOSSARY

ablate   From the Latin *ab-* and *latus*, meaning "to take away." In dentistry or medicine, to remove a body part or destroy its function; for example, the use of radiation therapy to ablate a tumor of the gum, jaw, or tongue.

abscess   An infection in a closed space; for example, under the gum at the base of an infected tooth.

abutment   The teeth remaining on either side of the space left by a missing tooth.

acellular   Without living cells; for example, an acellular matrix, a meshlike sheet of material used as a base on which new body cells can grow.

acid   In chemistry, a compound that releases a molecular fragment called a hydrogen ion (symbol: H+) when dissolved in water; the chemical opposite of a base, a compound that releases a hydroxyl ion (symbol: OH-).

acid etch   Dental procedure during which the dentist applies a weak acid to the surface of the tooth, creating very small crevices that increase the ability of dental/orthodontic appliances to stick to the tooth.

acrylic   A synthetic plastic material widely used on dental appliances such as false teeth.

adhesive   Material that enables one surface to stick to another; a glue or paste. Dental adhesives are products used to form a bond between a dental restoration and a tooth.

adverse effect   Uncommon, unexpected, and unusual reaction to a specific medicine, as opposed to a side effect, which is a common, expected, and ordinarily mild reaction. For example, tenderness at the site of a novocaine injection is a common side effect; the potentially fatal allergic reaction known as anaphylaxis is a rare adverse effect.

aerobic   From the Latin *aer-*, meaning "air," and the Greek *bios*, meaning "life." Oxygen-dependent, as in aerobic bacteria—bacteria that require oxygen to live.

afferent   From the Latin *afferens*, meaning "bringing to," as in an afferent nerve, a nerve that carries impulses to the central nervous system (brain and spinal cord).

agenesis   From the Greek *a-*, meaning "without," and *genesis*, meaning "formation." Failure of a fetal body part to develop.

alginate   A plasterlike material obtained from seaweed; commonly used to create dental impressions (models of a patient's teeth).

alloy   A mixture of two metals. For example, dental amalgam is an alloy of mercury and another metal, most commonly silver, used to fill the space left by a cavity.

alveolus   A small cavity; in dentistry, the socket in which a tooth sits.

anaphylaxis   A potentially fatal allergic reaction to a chemical substance such as a food or drug.

anatomy   The arrangement of bones in the skeleton; the dental anatomy is the arrangement of teeth in the jaw.

anesthetic   Any substance or technique that produces pain relief accompanied by a loss of consciousness, a state known as *anesthesia*, which is the interruption of one or more of the chemical reactions by which the body transmits pain messages form the site of an injury to the brain. General anesthesia causes loss of consciousness; local anesthesia numbs a specific area without causing loss of consciousness.

anodontia   From the Greek *an-*, meaning "not," and *dont*, meaning "teeth." Partial or complete congenital absence of teeth due to failed dental development.

anomaly   A variation from what is generally considered normal. In dentistry, an abnormal structure such as extra teeth or teeth missing at birth.

antero-, anterior   From the Latin *anteus*, meaning "front," as in the anterior teeth (the six upper and six lower front teeth).

antibiotic   From the Greek *an*, meaning "not," and *bios*, meaning "life." Medical drug that destroys or inhibits the growth of disease-causing organisms. A broad-spectrum antibiotic is a drug considered effective against the two main classifications of bacteria, gram-negative bacteria and gram-positive bacteria.

antibiotic prophylaxis   The practice of giving antibiotics before surgery to reduce the risk of subsequent infection.

antibody   A molecule released by the cells of the immune system in response to the introduction of an antigen, a substance such as an allergen or a bacteria or foreign tissue (e.g., a transplanted organ).

anticoagulant   A compound such as warfarin (Coumadin) that reduces the ability of blood platelets to stick together to form a blood clot, thus reducing the risk of a blocked artery.

antigen   Any substance or organism such as an allergen, bacteria, or transplanted tissue that triggers the release of an antibody when introduced into the body.

antiseptic   A chemical used to destroy disease-causing organisms such as bacteria, fungi, and viruses on living tissues.

apex   Tip, as in apex of the nose.

arch   The curved bone forming the base of either the top or the bottom jaw. The shape of the bone—the arch form—may be curved ("horseshoe") or more straight-edged ("v-shape").

argyria   In dentistry, a localized blue coloring of the gum caused by the presence of silver amalgam in gum tissue.

artery   From the Latin and Greek *arteria*, meaning "pipe." A blood vessel that carries oxygenated blood from the heart to the tissues and organs of the body, as opposed to a vein, which carries blood from tissue and organs back to the heart. A small artery is called an *arteriole*.

articulator   A device that hold models of the teeth in position so that an orthodontist can evaluate the patient's bite.

artificial   Not natural; in medicine, a material or device that does not arise from natural cell growth; for example, a denture or an artificial tooth. Some artificial materials and/or devices such as dental implants remain separate and intact inside the body. Others, such as the porous materials used to replace bone, including the jawbone, act as a base for new cell growth and are ultimately absorbed into the body. Artificial materials and devices are widely used in dental surgery.

asepsis   The process of destroying or removing disease-causing organisms so as to reduce the risk of infection.

aspirator   A hollow tube used to suction saliva and other fluids from the mouth during a dental procedure; the process of using the aspirator is called *aspiration*.

atrophy   From the Greek *a*, meaning "not," and *trophe*, meaning "nourishment." Tissue shrinkage or wasting, such as the gum recession common in periodontal disease.

augmentation   From the Latin *augmentare*, meaning "to make bigger." In dental surgery, an enlargement such as tissue used to augment gum so that the gum covers the bottom of the teeth.

auto-   From the Greek *autos*, meaning "self."

autogenous   From the Greek *autos*, meaning "self," and *gen*, meaning "born." In dentistry, tissue such as bone cells taken directly from the jaw of the person for whom it will be used.

autologous   From the Greek *autos*, meaning "self," and *logos*, meaning "place." Term used to describe tissue.

avulsion, evulsion From the Latin *avulsio*, meaning rip, tear; the accidental tearing away of a body part such as an avulsed tooth ("knocked out tooth").

axon From the Greek *axon*, meaning "axis." The part of the nerve cell that sends impulses out from the cell.

bacteria From the Greek *bakterion*, meaning "small rod." Member(s) of a family of one-cell microorganisms; some beneficial, others pathogenic (disease causing).

bandage Material applied to a wound to stop bleeding, to keep out dirt and debris, to prevent drying or to absorb liquid drainage, or to hold a dressing in place.

base In chemistry, a compound that when dissolved in water releases a molecular fragment called a hydroxyl ion (symbol: OH-), the chemical opposite of an acid, a compound that when dissolved in water releases a molecular fragment called a hydrogen ion (symbol: H+).

baseline In medicine and dentistry, a standard against which to measure future developments, such as a baseline X-ray of the teeth or an X-ray of the jaw showing the state of the bone beneath the gum.

base metal A metal such as copper or tin that is not resistant to chemical reactions such as corrosion.

beam In medicine, a straight line of light or radiation, such as the light from a flashlight or the radiation from an X-ray machine.

beeswax A natural substance secreted by bees in building a hive; an ingredient in dental waxes; also known simply as *wax*.

behavior modifiction Use of an technique such as biofeedback; reinforcement (rewarding good behavior) or aversion therapy (punishing bad behavior) to change a person's responses to various stimuli, such as dental treatment.

benign From the Latin *benignus*, meaning "kind." Mild, as in a benign illness; nonmalignant, as in a benign (noncancerous) tumor.

bi- From the Latin *bi*, meaning "two."

bicuspid From the Latin *bi*, meaning "two," and *cuspis*, meaning "point"; one of eight teeth, four on top and four on the bottom, with two points (cusps).

B.I.D. From the Latin *bis in die*, meaning "twice a day"; instruction on a prescription.

bifid From the Latin *bifidus*, meaning "cut in two." Separated into two parts, as a bifid (cleft) tongue.

bilateral From the Latin *bi-*, meaning "two", and *latus*, meaning "side." Two sided, as in bilateral cleft lip, a lip with a cleft on each side.

binder In dentistry, a sticky substance that holds solid particles together in a mixture such as an amalgam.

biocompatible Able to interact with a biological system without triggering an adverse reaction; for example, the material used to fill defects in a tooth.

biodegradable Able to be broken down quickly and safely by biological means, such as bacterial action, and then to be absorbed safely into the environment (e.g., the soil).

biofilm A thin, sticky layer of microorganisms and bodily material such as saliva, mucus, or blood that forms on a body surface such as the teeth or on the surface of a medical device on or in the body, such as a contact lens, a heart valve replacement, or a urinary catheter (a tube leading from the urinary bladder to the surface of the body). The biofilm on teeth is called *plaque*.

biopsy From the Greek *bio-*, meaning "life," and *opsis-*, meaning "view." Diagnostic examination of tissue samples.

birth defect Abnormality, such as extra or missing teeth, present at birth.

block Term used to describe anesthesia that numbs a specific area of the body, such as one side of the face. Also known as regional anesthesia.

blood Liquid that transports essential nutrients such as oxygen, vitamins, minerals, hormones, and other biochemicals to every living body cell while carrying away waste materials such as carbon dioxide.

blood gases Dissolved oxygen (O_2) and carbon dioxide (CO_2) in the blood and dissolved bicarbonate (HCO_3^-) in the blood plasma.

bloodstream The blood flowing through the blood vessels.

blood vessel Component of the circulatory system; tube through which blood flows to and from all body organs and tissues.

bonding In dentistry, a technique for attaching orthodontic appliances to the teeth or for attaching covers to the teeth so as to produce a uniform and pleasing effect.

border An edge; in dentistry, the edge of a denture.

brace A device to support a body part; in dentistry, an orthodontic appliance.

calculus From the Latin *calculus* meaning pebble; a hardened deposit of minerals, bacteria, and other oral debris on the surface of the tooth, commonly at the gum line; also known as *dental tartar*.

carcinoma From the Greek *karkinos,* meaning "cancer," and *oma,* meaning "tumor." The most common type of cancer; malignant tumor arising from epithelial cells, such as carcinoma of the tongue.

caries Tooth decay; commonly, the term *cavity* describes a small depression or hole in the tooth caused by tooth decay.

cauterize From the Greek word *kauterion*, meaning "branding iron." In medicine and dentistry, to cut or burn body tissues with electric current (electrocautery), or with ultrasound waves, or with a caustic substance such as an acid, or with a cold substance such as liquid nitrogen (cryosurgery), or with heat as in a hot iron poker.

cavity From the Latin *cavus,* meaning "hollow." Any natural or acquired open space in the body such as the oral cavity (the inside of the mouth) or a hole in the tooth due to dental decay.

cell From the Latin word *cella*, meaning "chamber." The smallest unit of a living structure capable of independent life; a nucleus (center) surrounded by protoplasm (cellular fluid) enclosed within a cell membrane.

cementum Heavily mineralized connective tissue that covers the root of the tooth and anchors ligaments in the gum to the tooth.

cheilo- From the Greek *cheilos,* meaning "lip."

chin The lower jaw and its covering layers of fat, muscle, and skin.

chisel From the Latin word *caedare,* meaning "to cut." Surgical instrument used to chip away excess bone.

chromosome From the Greek word *chroma,* meaning "color," and soma, meaning "body." Threadlike structures in the cells of all living organisms, composed of DNA (deoxyribonucleic acid), the material that contains an individual's genetic code (inherited characteristics). Human beings normally have 46 chromosomes (23 pairs, one from each parent); each chromosome carries an estimated 20,000 to 30,000 different genes, the basic units of heredity.

clamp In dentistry, a device used to hold things together during a dental procedure; for example, a *gingival clamp* is a device used to pull back gum tissue during periodontal surgery.

clasp In dentistry, a device attached to a removable denture that links to a device attached to a tooth, to hold the denture in place.

cleft An opening in a body structure, either normal (such as the cleft between the buttocks) or abnormal (as in a cleft lip or palate).

clot Soft mass of gelled material, as in a blood clot.

cohesion From the Latin word *cohaero,* meaning "to stick together"; the ability of molecules in a material to stick together so as to form a mass, as in a paste.

complication In medicine or dentistry, an often unexpected problem that occurs during illness or after a treatment or a surgical procedure; for example, sensitivity to heat and/or cold after a dental crown is put in place.

compound A mixture of ingredients held together with chemical bonds. Dental compounds include amalgam, a compound used to fill teeth, and the material used to make impressions of the teeth.

compress From the Latin *com-*, meaning "together," and *pressus*, meaning "press." Dressing such as a gauze pad placed over the site of an extraction so as to prevent swelling and/or to stop bleeding after removal of a tooth.

concrescence From the Latin words *con*, meaning "together," and *crescere*, meaning "to grow"; fusion of the roots of two teeth after the teeth have emerged and/or after the roots have developed.

congenital From the Latin word *congenitus*, meaning "present at birth"; a cleft lip is a congenital defect.

corona From the Greek *korone*, meaning "crown." In anatomy, the top of a structure, such as the corona dentis (top of a tooth).

craniofacial From the Greek *cranion*, meaning "skull"; relating to both the skull and the face. For example, a cleft palate is a craniofacial defect.

crescent, sublingual The U-shape area of the mouth under the tongue.

crevice From the Greek word *crevis*, meaning "groove" or "space." A narrow opening due to a crack in a surface. In dentistry, a crack in a tooth, or a gingival crevice, which is a separation between the tooth and the gum caused by periodontal disease.

crevicular fluid In dentistry, crevicular fluid is an anti-inflammatory liquid produced in the space between the tooth and the free gingiva (gum that is not firmly attached to the tooth).

cross contamination The spread of microorganisms from one patient to another when the dentist/physician uses unclean or poorly sterilized instruments or recycled products.

crown A dental restoration that covers the entire top of the tooth and extends at least partway down the sides. An artificial replacement for the natural enamel covering of a tooth.

cryo- From the Greek *kryos*, meaning "cold."

cure In dentistry, a procedure that hardens materials such as composite fillings and restorations.

curettage Surgery performed with an instrument called a curet or curette; in dentistry, a periodontal technique to remove calculus or dead tissue from the surface of a tooth.

curing A chemical reaction that hardens a plastic material; for example, exposing the material used to make dental caps to high-intensity light emitted by a curing light.

cusp From the Latin *cuspis*, meaning "point"; a high point on the chewing surface of a tooth.

cyst From the Greek *kystis*, meaning "bladder." A saclike membrane filled with liquid, gas, or solid material; may be found on or in any tissue or organ in the body, such as a dental cyst at the base of a tooth.

dam A barrier against fluid; in dentistry, a rubber or plastic device used to keep an area of the mouth dry, most commonly during surgery.

debridement, nonsurgical Scaling; the removal of debris from the teeth and under the gums during periodontal treatment.

decalcification Loss of calcium from teeth and/or bones due to a disease or medical condition such as osteoporosis.

deformity Malformation of a body part; for example, a cleft palate.

dehydration Abnormal loss of moisture from body tissues.

dentin, dentine The hard, ivorylike material under the enamel surface of the tooth; the major bulk of the tooth, enclosing the pulp chamber and the canals in the root(s) of the tooth.

dentition The arrangement of the teeth in the upper and lower jaw.

dentogenesis   From the Latin words *dens*, meaning "tooth," and the Greek word *genesis*, meaning "origin." The creation of dentin, the connective tissue around the root of a tooth.

denture   An artificial replacement for missing teeth.

detritus   From the Latin word *detero-*, meaning "to wear away"; in dentistry, fragments of material such as food that cling to the surface of a tooth.

diagnosis   From the Greek word *diagnosis*, meaning "distinguishing or separating out"; the process by which a doctor or dentist identifies the cause and/or nature of a disease or medical condition.

diastema   Space between two teeth, most commonly between the two central front teeth.

die   In dentistry, a hard metal or plaster reproduction of a tooth.

direct restoration   A restoration such as a filling for a cavity that is prepared and put in place in one visit. The opposite is an indirect restoration such as an inlay, which require two visits, one to prepare the tooth and one to insert the laboratory-made restoration.

disinfection   A process that eliminates most microorganisms on the surface of inanimate objects such as a dental tool or a dental chair.

distal   From the Latin word *distalis*, meaning "away from the center"; behind. In dentistry, toward the back of the mouth. For example, the second molar is distal to the first molar.

distraction   Term used to describe teeth or parts of the jaw that are farther than normal from an imaginary line drawn down the center of the jawbone.

dowel   In dentistry, a metal pin (commonly gold) inserted into a root canal to lend stability to a crown.

drift   An unplanned and unwanted movement of teeth, for example, after an extraction leaves a space in the jaw.

dys-   From the Greek prefix *dys-*, meaning "not" or "bad"; the opposite of *eu-*, meaning "good."

dysplasia   From the Greek *dys*, meaning "bad," and *plassos*, meaning "mold or form." Abnormal benign or malignant proliferation of cells that interrupts the normal shape/structure of body cells.

ecto-   From the Greek word *ektos*, meaning "outside." The opposite of *endo-*, meaning "inside."

-ectomy   From the Greek word *ektomia*, meaning "cut out."

edentulus   Toothless; from the Latin prefix *e-*, meaning "out", and *dent*, meaning "tooth."

efferent   From the Latin word *efferens*, meaning "taking out"; for example, an efferent nerve is a nerve that carries impulses from the central nervous system (brain and spinal cord) to the body.

elastic cartilage   From the Greek word *elastos*, meaning "to push." Stretchable connective tissue containing elastin (a network of elastic fibers), the tissue in expandable body structures such as muscles and the walls of blood vessels; also known as yellow cartilage.

elastin   From the Greek word *elastos*, meaning "to push." The stretchable protein that enables body tissues such as muscles and the walls of blood vessels to expand.

electroplating   A chemical reaction that applies a metal coating to an object. The object is immersed in a solution containing particles of a metal, and then an electrical current is passed through the solution to force the particles to adhere as a thin coating on the surface of the object. Electroplating is used in dentistry to create metal-coated impressions and to coat dentures with a thin layer of gold.

embolism   From the Greek word *embolisma*, meaning "something pushed in." An obstruction, commonly a blood clot, in a blood vessel. An air embolism is a bubble of air in a blood vessel.

endo-   From the Greek word *endon*, meaning "within," as in endodontics, the branch of dentistry dealing with the interior of the tooth. The opposite of *exo-* or *ecto-* meaning "outside."

epidermis From the Greek prefix *epi-*, meaning "on," and *dermis*, meaning "skin." Collectively, the epithelium, the top layers of skin cells.

erosion From the Latin word *erosion*, meaning "to chew away." In dentistry, the destruction of tissue on the surface of the tooth that creates smooth, nondecayed indentations at the point where the enamel covering the tooth meets the cementum covering the tooth root.

erythoplakia, erythroplasia Flat or slightly raised red, smooth or bumpy, potentially precancerous spots on the mucous membrane lining of the mouth.

evulsion From the Latin word *evulsio*, meaning "to tear out"; in dentistry, the sudden loss of a tooth due to an injury.

excise From the Latin word *excidere*, meaning "cut out"; for example, to excise a tumor.

excursion Movement of a body part in one direction and then back to the original position, such as lateral excursion (movement of the lower jaw from side to side), protrusive excursion (forward movement of the lower jaw), or retrusive excursion (backward movement of the lower jaw).

exo-, ecto- From the Greek prefix *exo-*, meaning "outside"; for example, exogenous, something from outside the body. The opposite of *endo-*, meaning "inside." The similar prefix *ecto-* means "on the outside."

extra- From the Latin word *extra*, meaning "outside." For example, *extraoral* means outside the oral cavity (mouth).

extraction Dental surgery to remove a tooth.

extrinsic From the Latin word *extra*, meaning "outside." In medicine and dentistry, originating outside the body.

extrusion The upward movement of a tooth that is erupting through the gum or the movement of a tooth upward or downward and out of its place in the jaw after the tooth above or below it is extracted.

exudate From the Latin prefix *ex-*, meaning "out," and *sudo* meaning "sweat"; any fluid flowing out of a body tissue; for example, gingival exudates, the liquid flowing out of inflamed gum tissue.

face From the Latin word *facies*, meaning "face." Front part of the head, including the forehead, eyes, nose, cheeks, mouth, and chin. Note: Ears are not considered part of the face.

factor From the Latin word *fascere*, meaning "to make." Any one of several components that produce a specific result; for example, in dentistry, failure to keep the teeth clean is a factor leading to the buildup of plaque on the tooth surface.

festoon From the Latin word *festum*, meaning "festival decoration." Carved surface of the base of a denture to simulate the natural tissues replaced by the denture.

fiber optics The process of transmitting light along very fine glass or plastic fibers; for example, via a fiber optic light attached to a dental handpiece used to visualize the interior of cavities and other hollow structures inside the mouth.

fissure From the Latin word *fissure*, meaning "a deep divide/cleft," such as the opening in a cleft lip or palate.

fistula From the Latin word *fistula*, meaning "tube." An abnormal opening from one body surface to another; for example, a salivary fistula opening directly from the salivary gland to the surface of the skin.

fit In dentistry, the way a denture, false tooth, or filling adapts to the place in which it sits.

fix From the Latin *figo*, meaning "to fasten." To make stable; in dentistry, to attach securely a replacement such as a filing or a crown or a denture. The material used to make a secure attachment is called a *fixative*.

fluorine An element included in public water supplies (as sodium fluoride) to harden teeth and prevent tooth decay.

foramen, *pl.* foramina From the Latin word *forare*, meaning "to pierce." An opening such as the mental foramen, a opening in the lower jaw through which blood vessels and nerves pass.

forceps   From the Latin *forceps,* meaning "tongs." Any instrument used to grasp and remove an object; for example, a dental forceps is a tool used to grasp and remove a tooth.

fracture   From the Latin *fractura,* meaning "break." A break in a body part such as a tooth or the mandible (lower jawbone).

frenum   From the Latin *frenum,* meaning "bridle." In dentistry, a fold of mucous membrane between the lips or cheek and each jaw that limits the movement of the lips.

function   From the Latin *function,* meaning "to perform." In physiology, the normal behavior or a body part; for example, normal dental function, a.k.a. normal occlusion, is the normal position and movement of the teeth when a person is chewing.

fungus   From the Latin *fungus,* meaning "mushroom." Microscopic organism such as yeast and mold, some known to cause a fungal infection such as oral candidiasis (thrush).

furcation   On a tooth with more than one root, the groove between the branches of the roots.

fusion   From the Latin *fusio,* meaning "melting, pouring." In medicine, a joining of body structure, for example, a birth defect such as the fusion of the roots of two adjoining teeth.

gauze   Loosely woven material, commonly cotton, used to cover wounds; for example, a pad pressed against the site of an extracted tooth to reduce bleeding.

gel   A semisolid material, such as a fluoride tooth gel used as a dentifrice to increase mineralization and reduce the risk of cavities.

gene   A unit on a chromosome; genes contain DNA determining specific hereditary characteristics such as *dentinogenesis imperfecta,* a disorder of normal tooth development that leads to weakened, discolored teeth.

gnatho-, gnath-   From the Greek *gnathos,* meaning "jaw."

groove   Any natural hollow or depression on an internal or external body surface such as the indentation between the cusps—the linear, troughlike depression between the raised points on top of a tooth.

handpiece   Instrument used to hold rotating pieces such as a drill in a dental engine.

hardener   Material that solidifies and strengthens a mixture of other materials; for example, the mercury used in some dental fillings or the acrylic used in making some dental models. The process of solidifying and strengthening the mixture is called *hardening.*

hardness   The degree to which a substance resists damage such as scratching or breakage; for example, dental enamel is the hardest mineralized tissue in the mammalian body.

headgear   A dental appliance that circles the head and serve as an anchor for an intraoral (inside the mouth) device.

hem-, hema-, hemato-, hemo-   From the Greek *haima,* meaning "blood."

hemi-   From the Greek *hemisus,* meaning *half.*

hemorrhage   From the Greek *haima,* meaning "blood," and *rheos,* meaning "flow." Bleeding, commonly uncontrolled bleeding.

hereditary   From the Latin *heres,* meaning "heir." The transmission of characteristics from one generation to the next through the material in genes and chromosomes.

hetero-, heter-   From the Greek *heteros,* meaning "other." Different; as in heterograft, a transplant of tissue from one person to another.

histology   From the Greek *histos,* meaning "web," and *logos,* meaning "knowledge." The study of body tissues; for example, a biopsy is an histological test.

homo- , homeo-   From the Greek *homos,* meaning "same," as in homograft, the transfer of tissue from one part of a person's body to another or from one genetically identical person to another.

hydr-, hydra-, hydro-   From the Greek *hydro-* meaning "liquid." Prefix meaning *moisture* or *water,* as in hydration, a medical technique such as the intravenous injection of liquids to maintain the proper fluid balance in the body.

hyper- From the Greek *hyper*, meaning "over." Higher amount or degree.

hyperplasia From the Greek *hyper*, meaning "over," and *plasis*, meaning "formation." Abnormal increase in the number of cells in a body tissue/part.

hyperthermia From the Greek *hyper* meaning "over," and *therme-*, meaning heat. Fever.

hypertrophy From the Greek *hyper*, meaning "large," and *trophe*, meaning "nutrition, nourishment." Abnormal growth in body cells leading to enlargement of a body tissue/part.

hypo- From the Greek *hypo*, meaning "under." Lesser quantity or degree, as in hypocalcification (less than normal hardness of the dental enamel) or hypodermic injection, an injection of material under the skin.

hypoplasia From the Greek *hypo*, meaning "under, lesser," and *plasis*, meaning "formation." The incomplete or underdevelopment of a part of the body, such as dental hypoplasia, the lack of a normal amount of enamel on the surface of the teeth.

I and D Abbreviation for *incision and drainage*.

iatrogenic From the Greek *iatros*, meaning "physician," and *gen*, meaning "producing." The result, commonly an adverse reaction, of a medical treatment.

idiopathic From the Greek *idios*, meaning "one's own." Of unknown origin, as in an idiopathic disease, an illness for which there is no known cause.

imaging Noninvasive diagnostic tool used to produce a picture of the body's internal structures; for example, CT (computer assisted tomography) scan, MRI (magnetic resonance imaging), sonography, X-ray.

impacted Wedged in place; in dentistry, an impacted tooth is one wedged in place against another tooth in the jaw under the gum so that it cannot erupt out of the gum into its normal position.

implant Mechanical or cosmetic device inserted into the body; for example, a base for a false tooth inserted into and permanently attached to the jawbone.

impression The pattern left when a patient bites into a tray filled with a soft plastic material that hardens to create a mold of the teeth; used most commonly in orthodontia.

incisal biting edge of your centrals and laterals.

incision From the Latin *incidere*, meaning "cut into." Intentional surgical cut through body tissues, most commonly used to describe a cut through the skin.

indirect restoration A restoration such as an inlay that requires two visits, one to prepare the tooth and one to insert the laboratory-made restoration. The opposite is a direct restoration such as a filling for a cavity that is prepared and put in place in one visit.

infection In medicine, presence in the body of disease-causing microorganisms (bacteria, fungi, viruses) that multiply, injure tissues and cells, and trigger inflammation and/or fever and/or tissue death.

inferior From the Latin *infra*, meaning "below." Below, under; for example, the mouth is situated inferior to the nose.

inflammation A reaction to an injury, usually involving pain, swelling, heat, and redness at the site. The inflammatory response is the process of inflammation.

infra- From the Latin *infra*, meaning "below."

injection From the Latin *injicere*, meaning "thrusting in." Introduction of medicine or nutrients under the skin (subcutaneous), into the muscle (intramuscular), into a blood vessel (intravenous/intrarterial), or into a body cavity.

injury From the Latin *in*, meaning "not," and *jus*, meaning "right/law." Damage done to body tissues.

inlay A dental restoration that sits inside the cusps of the tooth. Also any material put into a tooth to repair a cavity.

intensity From the Latin *tensus*, meaning "stretch out." A measure of the strength of energy, as in the high-intensity curing light used to harden some dental mixtures.

inter- From the Latin *inter*, meaning "between."

intercoronal The spaces between the tips (corona) on top of a tooth.

interdental Between the teeth; for example, the interdental gingival is the soft tissue filling the space between two adjacent teeth.

intermaxillary Between the upper (maxilla) and lower (mandible) jaw; for example, an intermaxillary anchorage is an orthodontic anchorage used to exert traction on two teeth, one in the upper jaw and one in the lower.

interocclusal Between the occlusal surfaces of the teeth, the surfaces that meet in chewing; for example, the interocclusal distance is any space between these surfaces.

interproximal The space between adjacent surfaces; in dentistry, between adjoining teeth.

intra- From the Latin *intra*, meaning "within." For example, orthodontic braces are an intraoral (inside the mouth) appliance, and an intravenous injection is an injection of a medical substance into a vein.

intrinsic From the Latin *intrinsecus*, meaning "inside." Naturally occurring, inherent.

ion From the Greek *ion*, meaning "leaving, going out." An electrically charged atom, group of atoms, or fragment of a molecule.

ionizing radiation Radiation that damages body tissues by breaking apart cells and separating molecules into electrically charged fragments called ions that can link to other molecular fragments to form potentially damaging components.

ipse- From the Latin *ipse*, meaning "same." For example, in medicine, ipsilateral means on the same side of the body.

irradiation Exposure to any form of radioactivity, including radiation from any medical diagnostic technique such as a CT scan (computerized axial tomography) or an X-ray.

irrigate To clean a wound or body cavity, such as the mouth, by flushing with copious amounts of fluid, generally a saline solution or Ringer's solution.

isogenic From the Greek *iso*, meaning "the same." From the same source.

joint From the Latin *jungere*, meaning "to join." The point where two or more bones come together, such as the temporomandibular joint, which connects the large temporal bone at the side of the skull with the ends of the mandible (lower jaw) on each side of the face.

joule, J Unit of energy named for the British physicist James P. Joule (1818–89). One calorie equals 4.2 joules; one joule equals 0.23 calories.

junction, junction- From the Latin *jungere*, meaning "to join." The surface or site where two bones or pieces of cartilage meet, as in a joint.

juxtaposition From the Latin *juxta*, meaning "near," and *posito*, meaning "place." Side-by-side positioning, as in the edges of a wound closing; correct juxtaposition is important to reducing the visibility of a scar after surgery.

kaolin A fine ground white clay used in making porcelain restorations (dentures, teeth).

labio- From the Latin *labium*, meaning "lip." As in labiodental, meaning relating to the lips and teeth.

laceration From the Latin *lacerare*, meaning "tear to pieces." A jagged wound.

lateral From the Latin *latus*, meaning "side." In anatomy, the side of the body or a body part that is farther from the center of the body. For example, the lateral side of the jawbone is the outer side, the one farthest from the center of the mouth.

lesion From the Latin *laedere*, meaning "to injure." Any injured or diseased area of body tissue; for example, a canker sore is an oral lesion.

ligament From the Latin *ligamentum*, meaning "band." Fibrous tissue that connects two or more tissues such as two bones or ties a muscle to a bone.

ligature Thread used to tie off a bleeding blood vessel during surgery.

lingual From the Latin *lingua*, meaning "tongue." Related to the tongue; for example, the lingual surface of the tooth is the side nearest to the tongue.

local In medicine, used to describe an anesthetic that affects the immediate area around the site of the injection.

luxation From the Latin *luxatio*, meaning "dislocate."

macro- From the Greek *macros*, meaning "large."

mal- From the Latin *malus*, meaning "bad."

malformation Deformity, usually congenital; failure of a body structure to develop normally; for example, a cleft palate.

malfunction Abnormal function of an organ or system; for example, the failure of the teeth to meet so that a person can chew effectively.

malignant From the Latin *malignere*, meaning "to behave maliciously." Describing a disease that resists treatment.

mandible The curved bone forming the lower jaw.

maneuver From the Latin *manu*, meaning "hand," and *operare*, meaning "to work." In medicine and dentistry, a plan or more commonly a treatment procedure.

margin From the Latin *margo*, meaning "edge." Border, as in the margin of a cavity, the place where the filling meets the tooth.

masticate From the Latin *masticare*, meaning "to chew." Mastication is the act of grinding food and mixing it with saliva so that it is easy to swallow.

maxilla The upper jawbone; a bone that supports the upper teeth, includes the hard palate, and is part of the nasal cavity and the orbit (the circular bones enclosing the eyeball).

maxillofacial Referring to the maxilla (upper jaw) and the face, as in maxillofacial surgery.

medical device Defined by the Food Drug and Cosmetic Act as an "article intended to diagnose, cure, treat, prevent, or mitigate a disease or condition, or to affect a function or structure of the body, that does not achieve its primary effect through a chemical action, and is not metabolized."

membrane Thin, flexible tissue surrounding or covering a body structure; for example, the cell membrane (outer covering of an individual cell) or the membrane lining the mouth.

mental In dentistry, from the Latin *mentum*, meaning "chin." In dentistry, relating to the chin.

meso-, mesial From the Greek *mesos*, meaning "middle." In dentistry, a term meaning nearer to the front of the mouth. For example, a cuspid is mesial to a bicuspid, and the mesial surface of the bicuspid is the part of the bicuspid closest to the cuspid.

meta- From the Greek *meta*, meaning "over, above," as in meta-analysis, a study consisting of the analysis of many studies.

metabolism From the Greek *metabole*, meaning "change." The sum of all the chemical and physical changes required for life including anabolism (building up) and catabolism (taking apart) of molecules in body tissues, the conversion of food into energy, and the production of waste in body cells.

micro- From the Greek *micros*, meaning "small."

midline In dentistry, an imaginary plane drawn through the center of the mouth perpendicular to the nose; that is, between the two middle front teeth.

milli- From the Latin *mille*, meaning "one-thousandth." One thousandth, as in a millimeter, which is one thousandth of a meter.

mixed dentition The presence of both primary teeth and permanent teeth in the mouth at the same time.

morbidity From the Latin *morbidus*, meaning "disease." State of ill health or complications following medical treatment.

mucocele   From the Greek *muco*, meaning "mucus," and *kele*, meaning "tumor." Swelling due to mucus collected in a gland, usually due to an injury that has damaged a duct (the small tube that carries a secretion, such as saliva, out of the gland).

mucosa, mucous membrane   From the Latin *mucosus*, meaning "mucous." The tissue lining various body cavities such as the mouth, characterized by the secretion of a clear, sticky liquid called mucus.

nano-   From the Greek *nanos*, meaning "dwarf." In metric measurements, one-billionth, as in a nanometer equaling 1,000,000th of a meter.

necrosis   From the Greek *nekrosis*, meaning "death." For example, in dentistry, necrotizing ulcerative periodontitis, an acute episode of periodontal disease characterized by the loss of gum and bone tissue.

neo-   From the Greek *neos*, meaning "new, young." For example, neoplasm, a new growth of tissue.

noble metal   A metal such as gold or platinum that is resistant to chemical reactions such as corrosion.

norm   The expected and usual behavior; for example, the ability of the teeth to break food into easily swallowed pieces.

notch   An indentation; for example, an indentation in a denture to accommodate a membrane on the inside of the mouth.

obdurator   In dentistry, a device that covers and closes an opening in the hard palate (the roof of the mouth).

occlusion   From the Latin word *occludare*, meaning "to close." The physical relationship between the upper and lower teeth when the jaws are closed.

odontalgia   From the Greek *odont*, meaning "tooth," and algos, meaning "pain." Toothache.

odontogenisis   From the Greek words *odont*, meaning "tooth," and *gen-*, meaning "to produce or give birth." The formation of teeth.

odontoma   A formation composed of enamel, dentin, and cementum that resembles a tooth.

onlay   A dental restoration that covers at least one cusp of a tooth.

opportunistic infection   An infectious illness that does not pose a serious threat to a healthy body but may prove fatal to a person with a compromised immune system.

oro-   From the Latin *oris*, meaning "mouth, opening." Referring to the oral cavity, as in orofacial (mouth/face) surgery.

orthodontia, orthodontics   From the Greek *ortho*, meaning "straight" and *dont*, meaning "teeth." The branch of dentistry dealing with malformations in the dental structure; e.g., realigning the teeth to correct a malocclusion.

os-, osteo-   From the Latin and Greek *os*, meaning "bone," as in osteoporosis (porous, weakened bones).

packing   Process of filling a natural body cavity or wound with absorbent sterile material to slow or stop bleeding or, in dentistry, to fill a cavity.

pad   In medicine, a soft dressing used to relieve pressure or to fill a cavity so that a bandage fits more snugly; in anatomy, a thick piece of body tissue such as the fat pad under the skin of the face that rounds out the cheek.

papilla   From the Latin *papula*, meaning "pimple." Small, round, fingerlike projection, such as one of the tiny bumps on the upper surface of the tongue.

para-   From the Greek *para-* or *par-*, meaning "next to."

patch   In medicine, a small, usually round area of skin or mucous membrane with a color or texture different from the surrounding tissue; for example, a mucous patch, the pale yellow, gray, or white spot on the lining of the mouth that may be a sign of syphilis.

path-, patho-   From the Greek *pathos*, meaning "suffering disease." For example, pathology is the study of abnormal tissues, and pathogens are disease-causing microorganisms (bacteria, fungi, viruses).

pedodontist From the Greek *pais*, meaning "child," and *odous*, meaning "tooth." In dentistry, a person who specializes in treating children's teeth.

percutaneous From the Latin *per*, meaning "through," and *cutis*, meaning "skin." Through the skin; for example, a percutaneous medication (a drug that passes through the skin into the body).

peri- From the Greek *peri*, meaning "around"; for example, in dentistry, a periapical X-ray is a picture of the area around the root (apex) of the tooth.

perineural From the Greek *peri-*, meaning "around," and *neuron*, meaning "nerve." Around the nerve, as in a perineural block, a form of anesthesia that numbs a large area around a specific nerve.

periodontics From the Greek *peri-*, meaning "around," and *dont-*, meaning "tooth"; the branch of dentistry dealing with the treatment of conditions affecting the gums, the tissue surrounding the teeth.

philtrum From the Greek *philtron*, meaning "love potion." The depression in the center of the upper lip that forms the cupid's bow, the twin-peaked center of the upper lip.

plaque From the French *plaque*, meaning "flat plate." An area of tissue that is different in texture or color from the surrounding skin or mucous membrane; also, commonly, a deposit of cholesterol inside an artery.

-plasty From the Greek *plastos*, meaning "formed."

post- From the Latin *post*, meaning "behind or after."

posterior In dentistry, a term used to describe the back of the mouth or the back teeth.

probe From the Latin *probere*, meaning "to test." In dentistry, a very thin rod or instrument used to examine the pockets formed when the gum is loosened by periodontal disease.

prosthesis From the Greek *prosthesis*, meaning "addition." An artificial substitute for a body part missing due to a birth defect or destroyed by illness or injury; for example, a denture or a false tooth. A dentist who specializes in the replacement of missing teeth is called a *prosthodontist*.

proximal From the Latin *proximo*, meaning "next to." In dentistry, the surfaces of a tooth close to or touching the next tooth in the jaw; the space between adjacent teeth is the *interproximal space*.

pulp Dental pulp; the center part of the tooth, composed of blood vessels, nerves, and cells that produce dentin, the primary building block of teeth.

pus Thickened, sometimes smelly yellow-white fluid, a sign of infection; composed of phagocytes (white blood cells in the immune system that attack and engulf invading microbes).

Q.D. From the Latin *quaque*, meaning "each," and *die*, meaning "day"; every day; direction on a prescription.

Q.I.D. From the Latin *quater in die*, meaning "four times a day"; direction on a prescription.

quadrant From the Latin *quadrans*, meaning "one quarter." One quarter of a circle; in dentistry, a fourth the total of the top and bottom dental arches (the jawbone and teeth). For example, one half of the arched jaw and teeth is one quarter of the dental arches.

Q.V. From the Latin *quantin* meaning "as much," and *vis*, meaning "wish." As much as desired; direction on a prescription.

RDH Registered dental hygienist.

reaction From the Latin *reagere*, meaning "acting back." Response of a body tissue to a stimulus; for example, slight swelling at the site of an injection of anesthetic into the gum prior to dental surgery.

recession From the Latin *recessus*, meaning "withdrawing." In dentistry, shrinkage of gum or bone tissue measured by the distance of the top of the gum from the cementoenamel junction, the place where the enamel covering the top of the tooth meets the cementum covering the tooth root.

recycling In dentistry, an unacceptable practice in which an orthodontist reuses appliances such as wires and bands taken from one patient's mouth and inserted into another's.

regeneration From the Latin *regene-*, meaning "to reproduce." In medicine, the regrowth of tissue, such as the body's replacement of bone tissue to fill in the cavity left when a tooth is extracted.

reimplantation, replantation The surgical reattachment of an organ or body part to its original site; for example, the reimplantation of a tooth knocked out in an accident.

rejection From the Latin *reicere*, meaning "discard." A response of the immune system; the body's refusal to integrate foreign tissue, such as a transplanted organ or blood of a type different from the patient's.

repositioning In plastic surgery, a procedure to move organs or tissues to improve their function; for example, to correct a protruding jaw by shortening the jawbone and/or moving it backward.

resect, resection From the Latin word *sextus*, meaning "cut off." In surgery, to remove part or all of an organ or tissue such as the tip of the root of a tooth.

resin Natural substance derived from plants or synthetic substances such as silicone that are solid when cool, pliable when warm; used in pharmaceutical products and dental appliances such as dentures.

resorption Natural physiological process leading to the loss of body tissue and, under normal circumstances, its replacement by new tissue; for example, the resorption of bone in the jaw that occurs after an injury or infection.

rest A dental extension inserted into a tooth to help support another appliance such as a partial denture.

restoration From the Latin *restaurare*, meaning "to repair." In dentistry, a device such as a bridge, false tooth, or filling used to repair a dental defect or replace missing tooth/teeth.

retainer A orthodontic appliance worn periodically, most commonly at night, to hold the repositioned teeth in place as the jawbone hardens around them and the teeth become firmly implanted after orthodontic treatment.

retractor Surgical instrument used to hold the edges of an incision apart so as to give the surgeon a clear view of the operating field.

retro- From the Latin *retro*, meaning "back." Backward; previous.

revascularization Establishment of a blood supply to body tissue; for example, after the transplant of a piece of skin from one part of the body to another.

ridge In anatomy, an elevation such as the bony ridge left in the jaw after teeth are removed.

rim Margin or border.

Ringer's solution Liquid that provides water and nutrients to the body via an intravenous (IV) needle, commonly after surgery.

rongeur From the French *ronger*, meaning "gnaw." Surgical forceps used to chisel away bone.

root The part of a tooth that is below the gum, covered with cementum rather than enamel and attached with ligaments to the jawbone.

root canal An extension of the pulp (the material in the center of a tooth) down through the root, connecting with the gum tissue via an opening at the bottom of the root through which the tooth's nerves and blood vessels enter. The term *root canal* is sometimes used as shorthand for any dental procedure performed inside this part of the tooth.

rubor From the Latin *rubor*, meaning "red." Redness of the skin or mucous membrane, one sign of irritation or infection.

sagittal plane From the Latin *sagitta*, meaning "arrow." The imaginary line that divides the body in half, right and left, from the top of the head to the bottom of the feet. In dentistry, the imaginary line dividing the mouth into two halves, left and right, from front to back.

saline From the Latin *salis*, meaning "salt." A saline solution is a liquid used to flush a body cavity, such as the mouth, during surgery or administered intravenously to maintain the body's fluid balance.

scaffold In surgery, a piece of collagen or absorbable synthetic mesh implanted to provide a base on which to grow new body cells, forming new tissue.

sealant Material used to seal irregularities on the surface of a tooth so as to reduce the risk of decay.

secondary In medicine, a condition or illness arising as the result of an existing condition or illness; for example, in dentistry, a second cavity in a tooth resulting from the first.

sectioning The process of cutting a tooth into sections to facilitate extraction.

semi- From the Latin word *semis*, meaning "half."

sensitizer A natural or artificial substance that, after repeated exposure, increases the risk of an allergic reaction to itself or to another substance. Formaldehyde is a common allergic sensitizer.

separator An instrument used to separate tissue during surgery; in dentistry, an instrument used to wedge teeth apart when examining adjacent surfaces or preparing a denture or restoration.

socket In dentistry, the alveolus, the hollow in the jaw into which a tooth fits.

soft tissue Body tissue that joins or supports body structures and organs; for example, the connective tissue that joins teeth to the gum and jawbone.

sordes From the Latin word *sordeo*, meaning "filth." Material consisting of bits of food, skin, and microorganisms that forms a whitish crust on the tongue, gums, teeth, and lips of a person who is running a fever or is dehydrated.

space maintainer A gadget used to maintain a space when a tooth is lost. For example, when a primary tooth falls out, a space maintainer keeps the space between the abutting teeth open until a permanent tooth erupts, thus preventing the teeth from shifting out of position.

sponge Gauze covered materials or nonwoven lint-free fabric used to absorb blood and other fluids during surgery.

sterile Treated with chemical agents, bombarded with electrons, or exposed to heat, steam, or radiation (ultraviolet light) so as to destroy all microorganisms.

sterilization A process in which a medical material is treated to remove all microorganisms.

sub- From the Latin prefix *sub-*, meaning "under." For example, subgingival (under the edge of the gum, or gingiva).

sulcus From the Latin word *sulcus*, meaning "furrow." Long, narrow groove such as the groove(s) or depressions on the surface of a tooth, or the gingival sulcus, the space between the tooth and the circle of gum surrounding it.

superinfection A second infection at the same site, usually due to an organism's becoming resistant to the antibiotic used to treat the first infection.

supernumerary From the Latin *super*, meaning "above," and *numerus*, meaning "number." More than the normal amount; in dentistry, supernumerary teeth (more than the normal number of teeth).

suppuration From the Latin *suppuro-*, meaning "form," and *pur*, meaning "pus."

supra-, super From the Latin *supra*, meaning "on the higher position."

surgery From the Greek *cheir*, meaning "hand," and *ergon*, meaning "work." The branch of medicine that treats with an operation, a procedure that physically cuts, repairs, or manipulates various parts of the body. A dental surgeon is a physician who specializes in surgery on the teeth; a maxillofacial surgeon is a physician who specializes in surgery on the face and jaw.

symmetry From the Greek prefixes *sym-* or *syn-*, meaning "together" and *metron*, meaning "measure." Even positioning of parts around a center line; for example, the position of teeth around the right and left sides of the upper and lower jaw.

syndrome From the Greek word *syndromis*, meaning "running together." A group of symptoms or effects characteristic of a medical disease or inherited disorder.

system   A group of related organs; for example, in dentistry, the masticatory (chewing) system: jaws, teeth, tongue, lips, temporomandibular joint, and their various nerves, muscles, and glands.

tartar   A synonym for calculus.

taurodontism   From the Greek word *tauros*, meaning "bull." A condition in which the chamber inside the tooth is very long and the roots (and root canals) are short; the name derives from the similarity to cow teeth.

technique   From the Greek word *techne*, meaning "skill." In medicine, a method of enacting a treatment or procedure; for example, the technique for extracting a tooth.

tempering   From the Latin word *tempera*, meaning "to moderate." A method of hardening material, usually metal, by exposing it to heat.

template   A pattern; in dentistry, a mold used to make a model of the teeth.

temporo-   From the Latin word *temporalis*, meaning "temple," as in the temporal bones, the two bones that form part of the base of the skull and the sides of the face.

temporomandibular joint (TMJ)   The joint on either side of the face connecting the mandible (lower jaw) to the temporal bone at the base of the skull.

therapy   From the Greek word *therapeia*, meaning "treatment."

therm-, thermo-   From the Greek word *therme*, meaning "heat," as in thermoplastic, a material that softens when warmed and hardens when cooled.

thrombo-   From the Greek word *thrombus*, meaning "clot."

tissue   In anatomy, a grouping of similar cells forming material that behaves in a specific way; for example, gum tissue.

-tomy   From the Greek word *tome*, meaning "incision."

trauma   The Greek word meaning "wound, damage." Physical or psychological injury.

trench mouth   Obsolete term for Vincent disease, a virulent form of periodontal disease, the name "trench mouth" comes from the fact that soldiers in the trenches in France during World War I were likely to develop this condition.

typodont   A model of the jaws and teeth used for teaching dental technique.

ulcer   A sore characterized by a loss of the epithelium (top layer) of the skin or mucous membrane accompanied by damage to and, if untreated, eventual death of the tissue underneath.

ultra   From the Latin word *ultra*, meaning "beyond." Excessive, above, more than, as in ultrasonic, sound comprised of very–high frequency waves of energy.

ultrasonic   From the Latin words *ultra*, meaning "beyond," and *sonus*, meaning "sound"; term used to describe energy in the form of sound waves whose frequency is above 20,000 cycles per second (20,000 Hertz [Hz]), the highest frequency the human ear can hear.

undercut   In dentistry, either the part of a tooth between the top of the tooth and the gum or the part of a prepared cavity (a cavity that has been cleaned out and is ready for the filling) that enables the filling to "lock"—that is, to hold securely in place.

ut dict   From the Latin words *ut dictum*, meaning "as directed." A term used in writing a prescription.

varnish, dental   A solution of natural plant compounds (resins or gums) applied as a thin protective coating over the teeth.

veneer   Thin top layer; in dentistry, a layer of material (usually porcelain or acrylic) colored to look like a tooth and affixed over a crown or over a tooth itself.

vermilion border   Also known as the *vermilion margin* or the *carmine margin*, it is the edge of the lip, the dividing line between the skin of the face and the *vermilion zone*, the pink external surface of the lips.

vestibule From the Latin word *vestibulum*, meaning "a small space." In dentistry, the space between the teeth and jaw and the inside of the cheek or the lips.

viewbox A box with a light source inside that enables a dental professional to view X-rays.

vital From the Latin word *vita*, meaning "life." Alive, as in vital tissue, tissue with an adequate blood supply.

working end The section of a dental instrument used to accomplish a specific purpose; for example, the sharp end of a dental probe used to find cavities in the enamel surface of the tooth.

working occlusion The surfaces of the upper and lower teeth that meet when biting or chewing.

working side The side of teeth or a denture toward which the lower jaw moves when biting or chewing.

xeno- From the Greek word *xenos*, meaning "stranger." In medicine, something from a person other than the patient. For example, a xenograft is a graft of tissue from another person's body.

xero- From the Greek word *xeros*, meaning "dry." For example, xerochilia (dry lips).

zero variance Normal; no deviation from the expected norm.

zone From the Latin word *zona*, meaning "an area or space." For example, in dentistry, the neutral zone, an area between the lips and cheeks on one side and the tongue on the other in which the teeth are equally affected by the muscles on either side.

BIBLIOGRAPHY

BOOKS/REPORTS

ADA Council on Scientific Affairs. "ADA Positions & Statements, Statement on Lasers in Dentistry." Posted April 2009. Available online. URL: www.ada.org/prof/resources/positions/statements/lasers_final.asp.

American Board of Dental Public Health. "Informational Brochure." Reviewed July 17, 2007. Available online. URL: www.aaphd.org/docs/ABDPHbrochure.doc. Accessed October 28, 2008.

Ammar, Hany, Mohamed Abdel-Mottaleb, and Anil Jain. "Automated Dental Identification System (ADIS)." *ACM International Conference Proceeding Series* 228(2007). Available online. URL: portal.acm.org/citation.cfm?I d=1248460.1248503&coll=&dl=. Accessed December 9, 2008.

Berardi, Rosemary R., Edward M. DeSimone, Gail D. Newton, Michael A. Oszko, Nicholas G. Popovich, Carol J. Rollins, Leslie A. Shimp, and Karen J. Tietze. *Handbook of Nonprescription Drugs.* 13th ed. Washington, D.C.: American Pharmaceutical Association, 2002.

Brown, David L., and Gregory H. Borschel. *Michigan Manual of Plastic Surgery.* Philadelphia: Lippincott, Williams & Wilkins, 2004.

Center for Drug Evaluation and Research, U.S. Food and Drug Administration. "FDA Alert: Information on Bisphosphonates (marketed as Actonel, Actonel+Ca, Aredia, Boniva, Didronel, Fosamax, Fosamax+D, Reclast, Skelid, and Zometa)." Available online. URL: www.fda.gov/cder/drug/infopage/bisphosphonates/default.htm. Accessed July 17, 2007.

Center for Drug Evaluation and Research, U.S. Food and Drug Administration. "Summary of Proposed Rule on Pregnancy and Lactation Labeling." Available online. URL: www.fda.gov/cder/regulatory/pregnancy_labe ling/summary.htm. Accessed October 18, 2008.

Centers for Disease Control and Prevention. *The Burden of Oral Disease: Tool for Creating State Docu-ments.* Atlanta, Ga.: U.S. Department of Health and Human Services, 2005. Available online. URL: www.cdc.gov/oralheal th/library/burdenbook. Accessed September 4, 2008.

Dental Board of California. "The Facts about Fillings." Sacramento, Calif.: California Department of Consumer Affairs, May 2004. Available online. URL: www.dbc. ca.gov/formspubs/pub_dmfs2004.pdf. Accessed August 6, 2008.

Griffith, H. Winter. *Complete Guide to Prescription & Nonprescription Drugs.* Revised and updated by Stephen Moore. New York: Penguin, 2007.

Handbook of Diagnostic Tests. 2d ed. Springhouse, Penn.: Springhouse Corporation, 1999.

Handbook of Signs & Symptoms. 2d ed. Philadelphia: Lippincott, Williams & Wilkins, 2002.

The International Classification of Sleep Disorders. Westchester, Ill.: American Academy of Sleep Medicine, 2001. Available online. URL: www.abs m.org/PDF/ICSD.pdf.

Knight, Joseph. "Stomatitis." My Optum Health. Available online. URL: www.myoptumhealth.com/portal/ADAM/ite m/Herpetic+stomatitis. Updated August 14, 2006. Accessed November 4, 2007.

Lehman, Richard A. *Handbook of Clinical Dentistry.* Hudson, Ohio: Lexi-Comp, 2005.

McPhee, Stephen J., and Maxine A. Papadakis, eds., and Lawrence M. Tierney, senior ed. *Current Medical Diagnosis and Treatment.* 47th ed. New York: McGraw Medical, 2008.

The Merck Manual of Diagnosis and Therapy. 18th ed. Whitehouse Station, N.J.: Merck Research Laboratories, 2006.

Mosby's Dental Dictionary. St. Louis, Mo.: Mosby, 2004.

Moslehzadeh, Kaban, ed. "OHI-S (Simplified)." World Health Organization Oral Health Country/Area Profile Programme. Available online. URL: www.whocollab.od.mah.se/expl/ohisgv64.html. Accessed July 17, 2009.

———. "Oral Hygiene Index." World Health Organization Oral Health Country/Area Profile Programme. Available online. URL: www.whocollab. od.mah.se/expl/ohigv60.html.

———. "Oral Hygiene Indices." World Health Organization Oral Health Country/Area Profile Programme. Available online. URL: www.whocollab. od.mah.se/expl/ohiintr od.html. Accessed July 17, 2009.

National Cancer Institute. "Lip and Oral Cavity Cancer Treatment." Available online. URL: www. cancer.gov/cancertopics/pdq/treatment/lip-and-oral-cavity/Patient/page1. Last modified on September 20, 2007. Accessed February 23, 2008.

———. SEER State Fact Sheet. "Cancer: Oral Cavity and Pharynx." National Cancer Institute. Available online. URL: seer.cancer.gov/statfacts/html /oral-cav.html. Accessed November 8, 2008.

National Center for Chronic Disease Prevention and Health Promotion. "Oral Health, Preventing Cavities, Gum Disease, and Tooth Loss at a Glance, 2010." Available online. URL: www.cdc.gov/ chronicdisease/resources/publications/AAG/doh. htm. Accessed March 21, 2010.

National Organization for Rare Disorders. "Amelogenesis Imperfecta, 2006." Available online. URL: www.raredi seases.org/search/rdbdetail_abstract. html?disname=Amelogenesis%20Imperfecta. Accessed February 11, 2008.

New York State Department of Environmental Conservation. "Managing Dental Mercury." Available online. URL: www.dec.ny.gov/chemical/8513. html. Accessed June 23, 2008.

NIDCR/CDC Dental, Oral and Craniofacial Data Resource Center. "Annual Report—Oral Health U.S., 2002." Available online. URL: drc.hhs.gov/ report.htm. Accessed September 14, 2008.

Rinzler, Carol Ann. *The Encyclopedia of Cosmetic and Plastic Surgery.* New York: Facts On File, 2009.

———. *Heartburn and Reflux for Dummies.* Hoboken, N.J.: Wiley, 2004.

———. *Nutrition for Dummies.* 4th ed. Hoboken, N.J.: Wiley, 2006.

Sims, Ron. Guide to the G. V. Black Manuscripts and Photographs in the Galter Health Sciences Library, Northwestern University. Available online. URL: www.galter.northwestern.edu/gvblack/testgv4. htm. Accessed November 17, 2008.

Stedman's Medical Dictionary. 28th ed. Philadelphia: Lippincott, Williams & Wilkins, 2005.

The Visual Dictionary of the Human Body. New York: Dorling Kindersley, 1991.

Weinzweig, Jeffrey. *Plastic Surgery Secrets.* Philadelphia: Hanley & Belfus, 1999.

U.S. Department of Health and Human Services. "National Call to Action to Promote Oral Health." Available online. URL: www.surgeongeneral. gov/topics/oralhealth/nationalcalltoaction.htm. Accessed July 17, 2009.

U.S. Department of Health and Human Services. "Oral Health in America: A Report of the Surgeon General—Executive Summary." Available online. URL: www.surgeongener al.gov/library/oralhealth/. Accessed July 17, 2009.

U.S. Environmental Protection Agency. "State Mercury Medical/Dental Waste Programs." Available online. URL: www.epa.gov/epaoswer/hazwaste/ mercury/medical.htm. Updated December 5, 2007. Accessed June 23, 2008.

Walsh, J.J. "Bartolomeo Eustachius," New Advent. Availableonline.URL:www.newadvent.org/cathen/ 05626d.htm. Accessed September 5, 2008.

PERIODICALS/PRESS RELEASES/ BROCHURES

Aas, Jorn A., Ann L. Griffen, Sara R. Dardis, Alice M. Lee, Ingar Olsen, Floyd E. Dewhirst, Eugene J. Leys, and Bruce J. Paster. "Bacteria of Dental Caries in Primary and Permanent Teeth in Children and Young Adults." *Journal of Clinical Microbiology* 46, no. 4 (April 2008): 1,407–1,417. Available online. URL: jcm.asm.org/cgi/content/abstract /46/4/1407.

Amaechi, Bennett T., and Sudan M. Higham. "Diagnosis of Dental Caries Using Quantitative Light-induced Fluorescence." *Proceedings SPIE* 4432 (October 2001): 110–117. Available online. URL: adsabs.harvard. edu/ab s/2001SPIE.4432.110A. Accessed November 28, 2008.

American Association for Cancer Research. "Saliva Proteins Could Help Detection of Oral Cancer" (press release). Newswise. Available online. URL: www.newswise.com/p/articles/view544615. Posted September 23, 2008. Accessed September 25, 2008.

American Dental Association. "ADA Seeks Clarification on FDA Dental Amalgam Statement." Available online. URL: www.ada.org/public/ media/releases/0806_release03.asp. Posted June 17, 2008. Accessed June 21, 2008.

———. "ADA Statement on Intraoral/Perioral Piercing and Tongue Splitting." Available online. URL:

www.ada.org/prof/resources/positions/statements
/piercing.asp. Updated March 15, 2005. Accessed
October 11, 2008.

American Society on Aging, "CDC Aims to Prevent Oral
Diseases Among Older Americans," March 21, 2005.
Available online. URL: www.asaging.org/media/
pressrelease.cfm?id=85. Accessed April 5, 2010.

Baharav, Haim, Irit Kupershmit, Michal Oman, and
Harold Cardash. "Comparison between Incisal
Embrasures of Natural and Prosthetically Restored
Maxillary Anterior Teeth." *Journal of Prosthetic Dentistry*, 101, no. 3 (March 2009): 200–204.

Balderas-Dizon, Judica. "Bolton Tooth Size Analysis of Filipinos Ages 13 to 22 in Baguio City."
Philippine Journal of Orthodontics, 6, no. 1 (August
2007):17–31. Available online. URL: www.apo.
com.ph/legacy/journal/bolton%20analysis.pdf.
Accessed November 26, 2008.

Barnes, C.M., C.M. Russell, R.A. Reinhardt, J.B.
Payne, and D.M. Lyle. "Comparison of Irrigation
to Floss as an Adjunct to Tooth Brushing: Effect on
Bleeding, Gingivitis, and Supragingival Plaque."
Journal of Clinical Dentistry, 16, no. 3 (2005): 71–77.
Available online. URL: www.ncb i.nlm.nih.gov/
sites/entrez. Accessed December 7, 2008.

Becker, Marshall Joseph. "Etruscan Gold Dental
Appliances: Three Newly 'Discovered' Examples."
American Journal of Archaeology 103, no. 1 (January
1999): 103–111. Available online. URL: www.jstor.
org/pss/506579. Accessed January 13, 2009.

Bio-Oss (package insert). Osteohealth Company, New
York. Available online. URL: www.osteohealth.
com/Bio-Oss.html. Accessed June 21, 2008.

Cartsos, Vassiliki M., Shao Zhu, and Athanasios
I. Zavras. "Bisphosphonate Use and the Risk
of Adverse Jaw Outcomes: A Medical Claims
Study of 714,217 people." *Journal of the American Dental Association* 139 (January 2008): 23–30.
Available online. URL: jada.ada.org/cgi/conten t/
abstract/139/1/23. Accessed July 17, 2009.

Center for Devices and Radiological Health, U.S. Food
and Drug Administration. "Questions and Answers
on Dental Amalgam." Available online. URL: www.
fda.gov/cdrh/consumer/amalgams.htm.l. Accessed
June 12, 2008.

Centers for Disease Control and Prevention. "Bone
Allografts." Available online. URL: www.cdc.gov/
Oralhealth/infectioncontrol/faq/allografts.htm.
Accessed January 30, 2008.

———. "Guidelines for Infection Control in Dental
Health-Care Setting—2003." *Weekly Morbidity and
Mortality Report* 52, RR-17 (December 2003). Available online. URL: www.ada.org/prof/resources/
topics/cdc/index.asp. Accessed June 6, 2007.

———. "Standard Precautions." Available online.
URL: www.cdc.gov/ncidod/dhqp/gl_isolation_
standard.html. Accessed November 19, 2007.

———. "Surveillance for Dental Caries, Dental Sealants, Tooth Retention, Edentulism, and Enamel
Fluorosis—United States, 1988–1994 and 1999–
2002." *MMWR Surveillance Summaries* 54, no. 3
(August 26, 2005): 1–44. Available online. URL:
www.cdc.gov/MMWR/preview/mmwrhtm.l/
ss5403a1.htm. Accessed February 29, 2008.

Centers for Disease Control and Prevention, Division
of Healthcare Quality Promotion (DHQP), National
Center for Preparedness, Detection, and Control of
Infectious Diseases. "Fact Sheet: Universal Precautions for Prevention of Transmission of HIV and
Other Bloodborne Infections." Available online.
URL: www.cdc.gov/ncidod/dhq p/bp_universal_
precautions.htm.l. Accessed May 31, 2007.

Cheifetz, Andrew T., Stavroula K. Osganian, Elizabeth
N. Allred, Howard L. Needleman. "Prevalence of
Bruxism and Associated Correlates in Children as
Reported by Parents." *Journal of Dentistry for Children* 72, no. 2 (May 2005): 67–73(7). Available
online. URL: www.ingentaconnect.com/content/
aapd/jodc/2005./00000072/00000002/art00006.
Accessed January 25, 2008.

Chernin, D., and G. Shklar. "Levi Spear Parmly:
Father of Dental Hygiene and Children's Dentistry in America." *Journal of the History of Dentistry* 51, no. 1 (March 2003): 15–18. Available
online. URL: www.ncbi.nlm.nih.gov/p ubmed/
12641168?dopt=Abstract. Accessed December 6,
2008.

Ciancio, Sebastian. "Electric Toothbrushes—For Whom
Are They Designed?" *Advances in Dental Research* 16,
no. 1 (2002): 6–8. Available online. URL: adr.sagepub.com/c gi/content/full/16/1/6. Accessed February 7, 2009.

Crespi, Roberto, Paola Cappare, Isabel Toscanelli
Enrico Gherlone, and George E. Romano. "Effects
of ER: Yag Laser Compared to Ultrasonic Scaler in
Periodontal Treatment: A 2-Year Follow-Up Split-
Mouth Clinical Study." *Journal of Periodontology* 78
(2007): 1,195–1,200.

"Dental Product Spotlight: Injectable Local Anesthetics." *Journal of the American Dental Association* 134, no. 5 (2003): 628–629. Available online. URL: jada.ada.org/cgi/content/full/134/5/628. Accessed November 25, 2008.

de Vicente, J.C., L. de Villalaín, A. Torre, and I. Peña. "Microvascular Free Tissue Transfer for Tongue Reconstruction after Hemiglossectomy: A Functional Assessment of Radial Forearm versus Anterolateral Thigh Flap." *Journal of Oral and Maxillofacial Surgery* 66, no. 11 (November 2008): 2,270–2,275. Available online. URL: www.ncbi.nlm.nih.gov/pubmed/18940491. Accessed February 2, 2009.

Dhiman, R., P. Singh, S.K. Toy Chowdhury, and N.K. Singla. "Complete Mouth Rehabilitation of Sub Total Congenital Anodontia with Indigenous Implant Supported Prosthesis." *Journal of Indian Prosthodontic Society* 6, no. 2 (2006): 90–94. Available online. URL: www.jprosthodont.com/article.asp?issn=09724052;year=2006.;volume=6;issue=2;spage=90;epage=94;aulast=Dhiman. Accessed February 2, 2008.

Doruk, Cenk, Ali Altug Bicakci, and Hasan Babacan. "Orthodontic and Orthopedic Treatment of a Patient with Incontinentia Pigmenti." *The Angle Orthodontist* 73, no. 6 (December 2003): 763–768. Available online. URL: www.angle.org/anglonline/?request=get-document&issn=0003-3219&volume=073&issue=06&page=0763. Accessed February 2, 2008.

Douglass, Alan B., and Joanna M. Douglass. "Common Dental Emergencies." *American Family Physician* 67 (February 1, 2003): 511–516. Available online. URL: www.aafp.org/afp/2003.0201/511.html. Accessed June 17, 2007.

Dudlicek, Laura L., Elizabeth A. Gettig, Kenneth R. Etzel, and Thomas C. Hart. "Status of Genetics Education in U.S. Dental Schools." *Journal of Dental Education* 68, no. 8 (2004): 809–818. Available online. URL: www.jdentaled.org/cgi/content/abstract/68/8/809. Accessed August 12, 2008.

El-Gheriani, A.A., B.S. Maher, A.S. El-Gheriani, J.J. Sciote, F.A. Abu-shahba, R. Al-Azemi, and M.L. Marazita. "Segregation Analysis of Mandibular Prognathism in Libya." *Journal of Dental Research* 82, no. 7 (2003): 523–527. Available online. URL: jdr.iadrjournals.org/cgi/content/full/82/7/523#BROADBENT-ETAL-1975. Accessed November 26, 2008.

Enestrom, S., and P. Hultman. "Does Amalgam Affect the Immune System? A Controversial Issue." *International Archives of Allergy and Immunology* 106, no. 3 (March 1995): 180–203. Available online. URL: www.ncbi.nlm.nih.go v/entrez/query.fcgi?cmd=Retrieve&db=PubMed&list_uids=7888781&dopt=Abstract. Accessed May 22, 2007.

Fox, Margalit W. "Dorwin Teague, 94, Industrial Designer, Is Dead." *New York Times* (September 26, 2004). Available online. URL: www.nytimes.com/2004/09/26/obituaries/26teague.html?_r=1&oref=slogin. Accessed November 10, 2008.

Fox, P.C., and M.J. Cummins. "Use of Orally Administered Anhydrous Crystalline Maltose for Relief of Dry Mouth." *Journal of Alternative and Complementary Medicine* 7, no. 1 (February 2001): 33–43. Available online. URL: www.ncbi.nlm.nih.gov/pubmed/11246934. Accessed June 29, 2008.

Gaspirc, Boris, and Uros Skaleric. "Clinical Evaluation of Periodontal Surgical Treatment with an ER: YAG Laser: 5 Year Results," *Journal of Periodontology* 78 (2007): 1,864–1,871.

Gift, H.C., S.T. Reinine, and D.C. Larach. "The social impact of dental problems and visits." *American Journal of Public Health* 82, no. 12 (1992): 1663–1668. Available online. URL: www.ncbi.nlm.nih.gov/pubmed/1456343. Accessed September 13, 2008.

Greenwood, M., and J.G. Meechan. "General medicine and surgery for dental practitioners. Part 6: The endocrine system." *British Dental Journal* 195, no. 3 (2003): 129–133.

Griffin, S.O., B.F. Gooch, S.A. Lockwood, and S.L. Tomar. "Quantifying the diffused benefit from water fluoridation in the United States." *Community Dentistry and Oral Epidemiology* 29, no. 2 (April 2001): 120–129. Available online. URL: www.ncbi.nlm.nih.gov/pubmed/11300171. Accessed July 17, 2009.

Heytac, M. Cenk, Turan Cetin, and Gulash Seydaoglu. "The Effects of Ovulation Induction during Infertility Treatment on Gingival Inflammation." *Journal of Periodontology* 75, no. 6 (June 2004): 805–810. Available online. URL: www.joponline.org/doi/abs/10.1902/jop.2004.75.6.805. Accessed August 22, 2008.

Hujoell, P.P., and J. Cunha-Cruz, D.W. Banting, W.J. Loesche. "Dental Flossing and Interproximal Caries: A Systematic Review." *Journal of Dental Research*, 85, no. 4 (2006): 298–305. Available online. URL: jdr.sagepub.com/cgi/content/full/85/4/298. Accessed December 18, 2009.

Hyson, John M. "Women Dentists: The Origins." *Journal of the California Dental Association* (June 2002). Available online. URL: www.cda.org/liibrary/cda_member/p ubs/journal/jour0602/hyson.html. Accessed July 17, 2009.

Hyson, John M., and Audrey B. Davis. "Basil Manly Wilkerson: Dental Inventor Extraordinaire." *Journal of the History of Dentistry* 41, no. 1 (July 1999): 61–64. Available online. URL: www.fauchard.org/publications/history/Journal_99_47_2p61.html. Accessed November 10, 2008.

The Identalloy Council. "Helping Your Patients Understand the Long-lasting Value of Gold in Restorative Dentistry." Available online. URL: www.utilisegold.com/uses_ applications/dental. Accessed August 5, 2008.

"In Memoriam: B. Holly Broadbent, D.D.S." *The Angle Orthodontist* 48, no. 2 (1978): 172–173. Available online. URL: www.angle.org/pdfserv/i0003-3219-048-02-0172.pdf. Accessed November 26, 2008.

Inspektor Research Systems BV. "Quantitative Light-induced Fluorescence." Available online. URL: www.inspektor.nl/dental/qlfmain.htm. Accessed October 3, 2008.

"Invisalign," Align Technology. Available online. URL: www.invisalign.com/WhatIs/Pages/WhatIs.aspx. Accessed January 19, 2009.

Karts, Matthias, Michael Winterhalter, Sinikka Münte, Boris Francki, Apostolos Hondronikos, Andre Eckardt, Ludwig Hoy, Hartmut Buhck, Michael Bernateck, and Matthias Fink. "Auricular Acupuncture for Dental Anxiety: A Randomized Controlled Trial." *Anesthesia and Analgesia* 104, no. 2 (February 2007): 295–300. Available online. URL: www.anesthesiaanalgesia.org/cgi/reprint/104/2/295.pdf. Accessed June 15, 2008.

Kaufman, Eliezer, Joel B. Epstein, Eitan Naveh, Meir Gorsky, Anat Gross, and Galit Cohen. "A Survey of Pain, Pressure, and Discomfort Induced by Commonly Used Oral Local Anesthesia Injections." *Anesthesia Progress* 52, no. 4 (Winter 2005): 122–127. Available online. URL: www.pubmedcentral.nih.gov/articlerender.fcgi?artid=1586799. Accessed June 20, 2007.

Keel, Pamela K., David J. Dorer, Kamryn T. Eddy, Debra Franko, Dana L. Charatan, and David B. Herzog. "Predictors of Mortality in Eating Disorders." *Archives of General Psychiatry* 60 (2003): 179–183. Available online. URL: archpsyc.ama-assn.org/cgi/content/full/60/2/179. Accessed September 14, 2008.

King, Elizabeth Neber. "Women in Dentistry." *Washington University Dental Journal* (August–November 1945). Available online. URL: beckerexhibits.wustl.edu/mowihsp/health/women indentistry.htm. Accessed October 23, 2009.

Klages, Ulrich, Andreas Gorder Weber, and Heinrich Wehrbein. "Approximal Plaque and Gingival Sulcus Bleeding in Routine Dental Care Patients: Relations to Life Stress, Somatization and Depression." *Journal of Clinical Periodontology* 32, no. 6 (June 2005): 575–582(8). Available online. URL: www.ingentaconnect.com/search/artic le?title=Approximal+plaque+and+gingival+sulcus+bleeding+in&title_type=tka&year_from=1998&year_to=2009&database=1&pageSize=20&index=1. Accessed July 17, 2009.

Kolata, Gine. "Drug for Bones Is Newly Linked to Jaw Disease." *New York Times* (June 2, 2006).

Kretzcshmar, James L., and Jerry E. Peters. "Nerve Blocks for Regional Anesthesia of the Face." *American Family Physician* (April 1997). Available online. URL: www.findarticles.com/p/articles/mi_m3225/is_n5_v55/ai_19347021 Accessed April 24, 2007.

LaGravere, Manuel O., and Carlos Flores-Mor. "The Treatment Effects of Invisalign Orthodontic Aligners: A Systematic Review." *Journal of the American Dental Association* 136, no. 12 (2005): 1724–1729. Available online. URL: jada.ada.org/cgi/content/full/136/12/1724. Accessed January 18, 2009.

Leonelli de Moraes, Mari Eli, Luiz Cesar de Moraes, Gustavo Nogara Dotto, Patrícia Pasquali Dotto, and Luis Roque de Araújo dos Santos. "Dental Anomalies in Patients with Down Syndrome." *Brazilian Dental Journal*, 18, no. 4 (May 2007). Available online. URL: www.scielo.br/scielo.php?pid=S0103-64402007000400014&script=sci_arttext. Accessed December 4, 2009.

Longden, Tom. "Naughton, John." *Des Moines Register*. Available online. URL: www.desmoinesregister.com/art icle/99999999/FAMOUSIOWANS/41217032/-1/famousiowans. Accessed November 10, 2008.

"Loud and Clear on Oral Cancer." *USA Today* (November 26, 2007). Available online. URL: www.intelihealth.com/IH/ihtIH/WSIHW000/333/24129/650624.htm.l. Accessed December 6, 2007.

Malamed, Stanley F. "All about Vasoconstrictors." *Dimensions of Dental Hygiene* 3, no. 9 (September

2005): 22, 24–25. URL: www.dimensionsofdental hygiene.com/print.asp?id=614. Accessed November 8, 2009.

Marshall, Steven D., Matthew Caspersen, Rachel R. Hardinger, Robert G. Franciscus, Steven A. Aquilino, and Thomas E. Southard. "Development of the Curve of Spee." *American Journal of Orthodontics and Dentofacial Orthopedics* 134, no. 3 (2008): 344–352. Available online. URL: www.biomedexperts.com/Abstract.bme/18774080/Development_of_the_curve_of_Spee. Accessed January 21, 2009.

Mavrodisz, K., N. Rózsa, M. Budai, A. Soós, I. Pap, and I. Tarján. "Prevalence of Accessory Tooth Cusps in a Contemporary and Ancestral Hungarian Population." *European Journal of Orthodontics Advance Access* 29, no. 2 (2007): 166–169. Available online. URL: www.ejo.oxfordjournals.org/cgi/content/full/cjl084v1. Accessed December 13, 2008.

"Methamphetamine Use and Oral Health." *Journal of the American Dental Association* 136 (October 2005): 1491. Available online. URL: www.ada.org/goto/jada.

Milgrom, Peter, Susan E. Coldwell, Tracy Getz, Philip Weinstein, and Douglas S. Ramsay. "Four Dimensions of Fear of Dental Injections." *Journal of the American Dental Association* 128, no. 6 (June 1997): 756–766. Available online. URL: www.jada.ada.org/cgi/content/abstract/128/6/756. Accessed May 21, 2007.

Molinari, John A. "Infection Control: Its Evolution to the Current Standard Precautions." *Journal of the American Dental Association* 134, no. 5 (May 2003): 569–574. Available online. URL: jada.ada.org/cgi/reprint/134/5/569. Accessed June 6, 2007.

Nathoo, S. A. "The chemistry and mechanisms of extrinsic and intrinsic discoloration." *Journal of the American Dental Association* 128 (November 1997): 6S–10S. Available online. URL: jada.ada.org/cgi/content/abstract/128/Suppl/6S. Accessed February 6, 2009.

National Institutes of Health. "Repair of Orthodontically-Induced Tooth Root Resorption by Ultrasound." Clinical Trials.gov. Available online. URL: www.Clinicaltrials.gov/ct2/show/NCT00423956?cond=%22Root+Resorption%22&rank=1. Accessed October 6, 2008.

"Natrol." *Drug Store News* (June 25, 2001). Available online. URL: findarticles.com/p/articles/mi_m3374/is_8_23/ai_76 334993. Accessed June 30, 2008.

Obayon, Maurice M., Kasey K. Li, and Christian Guilleminault. "Risk Factors for Sleep Bruxism in the General Population." *Chest* 119 (2001): 53–61. Available online. URL: www.chestjournal.org/cgi/content/fu ll/119/1/53. Accessed January 26, 2008.

Obisesan, Olanrewaju. "Drug-Induced Bruxism." *U.S. Pharmacist* 1 (2005): HS21–26. Available online. URL: www.uspharmacist.com/index.asp?show=article&page=8_1418.htm. Accessed January 26, 2008.

Olivan-Rosas, G., J. López-Jiménez, M.J. Giménez-Prats, and M. Piqueras-Hernández. "Considerations and Differences in the Treatment of a Fused Tooth." *Medicina Oral, Patología Oral, Cirugía Bucal* 9, no. 3 (May–July 2004): 224–228. Available online. URL: www.ncbi.nlm.nih.gov/pubmed/15122124?dopt=Abstract. Accessed July 17, 2009.

Oliver, R., G.J. Roberts, and L. Hooper. "Penicillins for the Prophylaxis of Bacterial Endocarditis in Dentistry." PubMed. Available online. URL: www.ncbi.nlm.nih.gov/pubmed/15106220?dopt=Citation. Accessed September 8, 2008.

Oong, Ella M., Susan O. Griffin, William G. Kohn, Barbara F. Gooch, and Page W. Caufield. "The Effect of Dental Sealants on Bacteria Levels in Caries Lesions." *Journal of the American Dental Association* 139, no. 3 (2008): 271–278. Available online. URL: jada.ada.org/cgi/content/full/139/3/271. Accessed July 17, 2009.

"Oral Moisturizers." *Journal of the American Dental Association* 138 (July 2007): 1,044. Available online. URL: www.ada.org/prof/resources/pubs/jada/patient/patient_76.pdf. Accessed June 26, 2008.

Parker-Pope, Tara. "Dentists Back Sealants, Despite Concerns." *New York Times* (October 21, 2008).

Patnaik, V.V.G., K. Singla Rajan, and Sanju Bala. "Anatomy of 'A Beautiful Face & Smile.'" *Journal of the Anatomical Society of India* 52, no. 1 (2003): 74–80. Available online. URL: www.sld.cu/galerias/pdf/sitios/prot esis/anatomy_of_a_beautiful_face_&_smile.pdf. Accessed November 28, 2008.

Peck, Sheldon, "A Biographical Portrait of Edward Hartkey Angle, the First Specialist in Orthodontics, Part 1." *The Angle Orthodontist*, 79, no. 6 (November 2009): 1,021–1,027.

Peretz, B., and G.M. Gluck. "Assessing an Active Distracting Technique for Local Anesthetic Injection in Pediatric Dental Patients: Repeated Deep Breathing and Blowing Out Air." *Journal of Clinical Pediatric Dentistry* 24, no. 1 (Fall 1999): 5–8. Available online. URL: www.ncbi.nlm.nih.gov/entrez/query.fcgi?cmd=Retrieve&db=PubMed&list_uids=10709535&dopt=Abstract. Accessed May 21, 2007.

Piccione, Anthony, Thomas J. Coates, June M. George, David Rosenthal, and Peter Karzmark. "Nocturnal Biofeedback for Nocturnal Bruxism." *Journal of Applied Psychophysiology and Biofeedback* 7, no. 4 (December 1982): 405–419. Available online. URL: www.springerlink.com/index/W7256K2372974N28.pdf. Accessed July 17, 2009.

Pollack, Andrew. "Bacteria Enlisted for New Trials on Dental Health." *New York Times* (November 30, 2004). Available online. URL: www.query.nytimes.com/gst/fullpage.html?res=9507EEDE113EF933A05752C1A9629C8B63&sec=&spon=&pagewanted=all. Accessed July 17, 2009.

Putnins, E.E., D. DiGiovanni, and A.S. Bhullar. "Dental Unit Waterline Contamination and Its Possible Implications during Periodontal Surgery." *Journal of Periodontology* 72, no. 3 (March 2001): 393–400. Available online. URL: www.ncbi.nlm.nih.gov/entrez/query.fcgi?cmd=Retrieve&db=PubMed&list_uids=11327068&dopt=Abstract. Accessed May 25, 2007.

Al-Qahtani, K., V. Brousseau, D. Paczesny, G. Domanowski, Q. Hamid, M. Hier, M. Black, E. Franco, and K. Kost. "Koilocytosis in Oral Squamous Cell Carcinoma: What Does It Mean?" *Otolaryngology* 36, no. 1 (February 2007): 26–31. Available online. URL: www.ncbi.nlm.nih.gov/pubmed/17376347. Accessed February 4, 2009.

Reagan, S.E., and T.M. Dao. "Oral Rehabilitation of a Patient with Congenital Partial Anodontia Using a Rotational Path Removable Partial Denture." *Quintessence International* 26, no. 3 (March 1995): 181–185. Available online. URL: www.ncbi.nlm.nih.gov/pubmed/7568733. Accessed February 2, 2008.

Ring, Malvin E. "Behind the Dentist's Drill." *Invention and Technology Magazine* 11, no. 2 (Fall 1995). Available online. URL: www.americanheritage.com/articles/magazine /it/1995/2/1995_2_24.shtml. Accessed February 17, 2009

———. "A Minnesota Dental Laboratory of 100 Years Ago." *Northwest Dentistry* 83, no. 2 (March–April 2004). Available online. URL: www.mndental.org/archive/3_04/feat ures/article_2. Accessed June 25, 2008.

Ring, Malvin E. and Neal Hurley. "James Beall Morrison: The Visionary Who Revolutionized the Practice of Dentistry." *Journal of the American Dental Association* 131, no. 8 (August 2000): 1,161–1,167. Available online. URL: jada.ada.org/cgi/content/full/131/8/1161. Accessed July 17, 2009.

Russo, R., and N. Scarborough. "Inactivation of Viruses in Demineralized Bone Matrix: FDA Workshop on Tissue Transplantation and Reproductive Tissue." Available online. URL: www.cdc.gov/Oralhealth/infectioncontrol/faq/allografts.htm. Accessed July 17, 2009.

Salama, Fouad S., Mosleh Al Shamrani, and Omar Bawazir. "Macrodontia of Maxillary Central Incisor: Case Report." *Pakistan Journal of Orthodontics, Pediatric and Community Dentistry* 1, no. 2 (December 2002): 93–95. Available online. URL: www.pakmedinet.com/3638. Accessed November 11, 2009.

Schoorm, Robert S., Harold I. Sussman, and Gregory K. Kazandjian. "Acupuncture: A Unique Effort to Treat Periodontal Disease." *Journal of the American Dental Association* 132, no. 12 (December 2001): 1,705–1,706. Available online. URL: jada.ada.org/cgi/content/abstract /132/12/1705. Accessed June 15, 2008.

Sedghizadeh, R.P., S.K. Kumar, and A. Gorur. "Identification of Microbial Biofilms in Osteonecrosis of the Jaws Secondary to Bisphosphonate Therapy." *Journal of Oral and Maxillofacial Surgery* 66, no. 4 (April 2008): 767–775. Available online. URL: www.ncbi.nlm.nih.gov/pubmed/18355603. Accessed February 1, 2009.

Shah, Geeta, and Tina S. Alster. "Treatment of an Amalgam Tattoo with a Q-Switched Alexandrite (755 nm) Laser." *Dermatologic Surgery* 28, no. 12 (December 2002): 1,180–1,181. Available online. URL: www.blackwell-synergy.com/doi/abs/10.1046/j.1524-4725.2002.02121.x?cookieSet=1&journalCode=dsu. Accessed June 21, 2008.

Slayton, R.L., L. Williams. J.C. Murray, J.J. Wheeler, A.C. Lidral, and C.J. Nishimura. "Genetic Association Studies of Cleft Lip and/or Palate with Hypodontia outside the Cleft Region." *Cleft Palate—Craniofacial Journal* 40, no.3 (May 2003): 274–279. Available online. URL: www.ncbi.nlm.nih.gov/pubmed/12733956. Accessed December 4, 2009.

Terézhalmy, G.T., and R.D. Bartizek. "Plaque-Removal Efficacy of Four Types of Dental Floss." *Journal of Periodontology* 79, no. 2 (February 2008): 245–251. Available online. URL: www.ncbi.nlm.nih.gov/pubmed/18251638. Accessed May 15, 2008.

Tezal, Mine, Maureen A. Sullivan, Mary E. Reid, James R. Marshall, Andrew Hyland, Thom Loree, Cheryl Lillis, Linda Hauck, Jean Wactawski-Wende, and Frank A. Scannapieco. "Chronic Periodontitis and the Risk of Tongue Cancer." *Archives of Otolaryngology: Head and Neck Surgery* 133 (May 2007): 450–454. Available online. URL: archotol.ama-assn.org/cgi/content/short/133/5/450. Accessed May 22, 2007.

Thayer, M.L. "The Use of Acupuncture in Dentistry." *Dental Update* 34, no. 4 (May 2007). Available online. URL: www.ncbi.nlm.nih.gov/pubmed/17580824. Accessed May 30, 2008.

Wade, Tamsin, and Alison Gammon. "Ingestion of Mouthwash by Children: Child Proof Caps Are Needed to Prevent Deaths." *British Medical Journal* 318 (April 1999): 1,078. Available online. URL: www.pubmedcentral.nih.gov/articlerender.fcgi?artid=1115472. Accessed October 27, 2007.

Wahl, Norman, "Orthodontics in 3 Millennia. Chapter 6: More Early 20th-century Appliances and the Extraction Controversy." *American Journal of Orthodontics and Dentofacial Orthopedics* 128, no. 6 (September 2005): 795–800.

White, D.J. "Dental Calculus: Recent Insights into Occurrence, Formation, Prevention, Removal and Oral Health Effects of Supragingival and Subgingival Deposits." *European Journal of Oral Science* 105, no. 5, Part 2 (October 1997): 508–522. Available online. URL: www.ncbi.nl m.nih.gov/pubmed/9395117. Accessed November 18, 2008.

Wynn, Richard L., and Timothy F. Meiller. "Artificial Saliva Products and Drugs to Treat Xerostomia." *General Dentistry* 48, no. 6 (November–December 2000): 630–635. Available online. URL: www.ncbi.nlm.nih.gov/pubmed/12004.654. Accessed June 24, 2008.

Xie, Hua, Guy S. Cook, J. William Costerton, Greg Bruce, Timothy M. Rose, and Richard J. Lamont. "Intergeneric Communication in Dental Plaque Biofilms." *Journal of Bacteriology* 182, no. 23 (December 2000): 7,067–7,069. Available online. URL: www.pubmedcentral.nih.gov/articlerender.fcgi?artid=94835. Accessed November 28, 2008.

INTERNET

Note: Some Internet address do not use the designation "www."

"The ABFO Identification Guidelines." Forensic Dentistry Online. URL: www.forensicdentistryonline.org/Forensic_pages_1/ident_guidelines.htm. Accessed December 11, 2008.

"About External Radiotherapy," CancerHelpUK. URL: www.cancerhelp.org.uk/help/default.asp?page=3595#imrt. Accessed September 28, 2008.

Academy of General Dentistry. "Why Is Oral Health Important for Men?" AGD Oral Health Resources. URL: www.agd.org/support/articles/?ArtID=1266. Accessed March 3, 2008.

———. "Why Is Oral Health Important for Women?" URL: www.agd.org/support/articles/?ArtID=1369. Accessed March 3, 2008.

Academy of Osseointegration. "Dental Implants, FAQS." URL: www.oseo.org/resources/implant_faqs.htm. Accessed May 15,2007.

Aetna Dental Plans. "Gingivectomy and Gingivoplasty." Simple Steps to Dental Health. URL: www.simplestepsdental.com/SS/ihtSS/r.WSIHW000/st.32576/t.32603/pr.3.htm.l. Accessed August 23, 2008.

Aguiar, Ara. "Periodontal Disease Recognition: A Review Course for Dental Hygienists." Periodontics Information Center. URL: www.dent.ucla.edu/pic/members/pdr/classifications.html. Accessed July 17, 2009.

"Air Abrasion (Drill-less Dentistry)," WebMD. URL: www.WebMD./oral-health/guide/air-abrasion. Accessed September 23, 2008

"Amalgam." iVillage. URL: oral.health.ivillage.com/common/articleprintfriendly.cfm?artid=3114. Accessed October 14, 2007.

American Academy of Dermatology. "Lichen Planus." URL: www.aad.org/public/publications/pamphlets/common_lichen.htm.l. Accessed February 24, 2008.

American Academy of Periodontology. "Gum Disease and Pregnancy Problems." Perio.org. URL: www.perio.org/consumer/mbc.baby.htm. Accessed September 4, 2008.

———. "Types of Gum Disease." Perio.org. URL: www.perio.org/consumer/2a.html. Accessed October 11, 2008.

American Association of Endodontists. "Cracked Teeth." URL: www.aae.org/patients/patientinfo/faqs/cracksum.htm. Accessed April 8, 2007.

———. "Endodontic Retreatment." URL: www.aae.org/patients/patientinfo/faqs/retxsum.htm. Accessed April 8, 2007.

———. "Root Canal Treatment." URL: www.aae.org/patients/patientinfo/faqs/rootcanals.htm. Accessed April 8, 2007.

American Association of Orthodontics. "Orthodontic Facts." URL: www.braces.org/pressroom-html/facts/index.html. Accessed January 12, 2009.

American Association of Women Dentists. "History of AAWD." URL: www.aawd.org/aboutus/history/. Accessed December 31, 2008.

American Cancer Society. "Detailed Guide: Oral Cavity and Oropharyngeal Cancer. What Are the Key Statistics about Oral Cavity and Oropharyngeal Cancers?" URL: www.cancer.org/docroot/cri/content/cri_2_4_1x_what_are_the_key_statistics_for_oral_cavity_and_oropharyngeal_cancer_60.asp?sitearea=cri. Accessed November 9, 2008.

———. "Detailed Guide: Oral Cavity and Oropharyngeal Cancer. How Are Oral Cavity and Oropharyngeal Cancers Staged?" URL: www.cancer.org/docroot/CRI/content/CRI_2_4_3X_How_is_oral_cavity_and_oropharyngeal_cancer_staged_60.asp. Accessed February 1, 2009.

American Dental Association. "ADA Seal of Acceptance: Frequently Asked Questions (FAQ)." URL: www.ada.org/ada/seal/faq.asp. Accessed January 20, 2009.

———. "ADA Statement on Toothbrush Care: Cleaning, Storage and Replacement." URL: www.ada.org/prof/resources/positions/statements/toothbrush.asp. Accessed October 30, 2007.

———. "Amalgam (Silver-Colored) Fillings." URL: www.ada.org/public/topics/fillings_faq.asp. Accessed October 11, 2007.

———. "Dental Emergencies and Injuries." URL: www.ada.org/public/manage/emergencies.asp. Accessed April 12, 2007.

———. "Disorders of the Mouth." URL: www.ada.org/public/topics/oral_changes_faq.asp. Accessed September 24, 2007.

———. "Fluoride and Fluoridation," URL: www.ada.org/public/topics/fluoride/fluoride_article01.asp. Accessed December 16, 2008.

———. "Forensics in Dentistry." URL: www.ada.org/public/topics/forensics_faq.asp. Accessed December 9, 2008.

———. "Gender and Gingiva: Study Finds Infertility Treatment Affects Periodontal Health." URL: www.ada.org/prof/resources/pubs/adanews/adanewsarticle.asp?articleid=951. Accessed August 23, 2008.

———. "History of Dentistry." URL: www.ada.org/public/resources/history/timeline_20cent.asp. Accessed April 8, 2007.

———. "Infective Endocarditis." URL: www.ada.org/prof/resources/topics/infective_endocarditis.asp. Accessed April 25, 2007.

———. "Methamphetamine Use (Meth Mouth)." URL: www.ada.org/prof/resources/topics/methmouth.asp. Accessed October 18, 2007.

———. "Mouthguards." URL: www.ada.org/public/topics/mouthguards_faq.asp#3. Accessed August 28, 2008.

———. "Oral Changes with Age." URL: www.ada.org/public/topics/oral_changes_faq.asp. Accessed September 24, 2007.

———. "Potential Salivary Biomarkers Identified for Detecting Primary Sjögren Syndrome." URL: www.ada.org/prof/resources/topics/science_sjogran.asp. Accessed November 16, 2007.

———. "Root Canal (Endodontic) Treatment." URL: www.ada.org/public/topics/root_canal_faq.asp. Accessed September 30, 2008.

———. "Sealants." URL: www.ada.org/public/topics/sealants.asp. Accessed October 29, 2008.

———. "Tooth Extractions." URL: www.ada.org/public/topics/extractions.asp. Accessed April 12, 2007.

American Society for Therapeutic Radiology and Oncology. "Radiation Therapy for Head and Neck Cancer." RTAnswers. URL: www.rtanswers.org/treatment/disease/head_neck.htm#internal. Accessed September 27, 2008.

"Anemia." MedLine Plus. URL: www.nlm.nih.gov/medlineplus/ency/article/000560.htm. Accessed September 10, 2007.

Animated Teeth. "Bad Breath." URL: www.animated-teeth.com/bad_breath/t1_halitosis.htm. Accessed December 1, 2009.

———. "Dental Sealants/Sealing Teeth/Tooth Sealants." URL: www.animated-teeth.com/tooth_sealants/t1_sealing_teeth.htm. Accessed October 29, 2008.

———. "The Evolution of the Electric Toothbrush." URL: www.animated-teeth.com/electric_toothbrushes/t3_sonic_toothbrushes.htm. Accessed February 10, 2009.

———. "Mouth Guards: Sports Mouthguards/Football Protectors /Athletic Mouthpieces." URL: www.animated-teeth.com/mouthguards/a3-mouthguards-types.htm. Accessed August 29, 2008.

———. "The Root Canal Treatment Procedure: What Steps Are Involved with Endodontic Therapy?" URL: www.animated-teeth.com/root_canal/t5_root_canal_ treatment.htm. Accessed August 6, 2008.

———. "Tooth Decay." URL: www.animated-teeth.com/tooth_decay/t2_tooth_decay_caries.htm. Accessed February 13, 2009.

———. "Tooth Extractions/Oral Surgery/Dental Surgery." URL: www.animated-teeth.com/tooth_extractions/t2_teeth_extractions.htm. Accessed September 10, 2008.

Archwired. "A Brief History of Braces." URL: www.archwired.com. Accessed July 17, 2009.

Bartels, Cathy L. "Helping Patients with Dry Mouth." Oral Cancer Foundation. URL: www.oralcancerfoundation.org/dental/xerostomia.htm. Accessed June 25, 2008.

Bellis, Mary. "History of Dentistry." About.com. URL: inventors.about.com/library/inventors/bldental.htm. Accessed April 8, 2007.

———. "Toothbrush, Toothpaste, Dental Floss & Toothpicks." About.com. URL: inventors.about.com/od/dstartinventions/a/dentistry_2.htm. Accessed February 9, 2009.

"Bisphosphonates Used to Treat Osteoporosis May Come with Risks." Healthwyse. URL: healthwyse.wordpress.com/2008/02/17/bisphosphonates-used-to-treat-osteoporosis-may-come-with-risks. Accessed July 17, 2009.

"Blood Disorders." Colgate World of Care. URL: www.colgate.com/app/Colgate/US/OC/Information/OralHealthBasics/MedCondOralHealth/PhysDisorderOralEffects/BloodDisorders.cvsp. Accessed October 10, 2007.

Bouissac, Paul. "The Visual Role of the Sclera and the Teeth in Facial Interactions." Open Semiotics Resource Center. URL: www.semioticon.com/people/articles/interactions.htm. Accessed November 29, 2008.

Breiner, Mark. "History: Amalgam (Mercury) Fillings." Whole-Body Dentistry. URL: www.wholebodymed.com/historypolit.php. Accessed November 17, 2008.

"Bruxism." MedlinePlus. URL: www.nlm.nih.gov/medlineplus/ency/article/001413.htm. Accessed January 22, 2008.

"Bruxism/Teeth Grinding." MayoClinic.com. URL: www.mayoclinic.com/health/bruxism/DS00337. Accessed January 22, 2008.

Cadena, Christine. "Gingivitis and the PMS Connection." Associated Content. Posted February 20, 2007. URL: www.associatedcontent.com/article/139 141/gingivitis_and_the_pms_connection_.html?page=2&cat=70. Accessed July 20, 2009.

"Canker Sores." MayoClinic.com. URL: www.mayoclinic.com/health/canker-sore/DS00354. Accessed November 12, 2007.

Coleman, Grant Gordon. "Lip Profile Preferences in Varying Sagittal Mandibular Positions." Virginia Commonwealth University Digital Archive. URL: digarchive.library.vcu.edu/handle/10156/2134. Accessed July 20, 2009.

"Concussion Prevention and Athletic Mouthguards." Sports Dentistry Online. URL: www.sportsdentistry.com/concussion.html. Accessed August 29, 2008.

"Definition of Dental Drill." WebMD. URL: www.medterms.com/script/main/art.asp?articlekey=16046. Accessed July 6, 2008.

Dental Board of California. "Candidate Handbook: California Restorative Technique Examination 2009." URL: www.dbc.ca.gov/formspubs/pub_examguide.pdf. Accessed March 20, 2010.

———. "The Facts about Fillings." URL: www.dbc.ca.gov/formspubs/pub_donts200.pdf. Accessed March 20, 2010.

"Dental Care and Diabetes: Guide to a Healthy Mouth." MayoClinic.com. URL: www.mayoclinic.com/health/diabetes/DA00013. Accessed June 8, 2007.

"Dental Care during Pregnancy." Cleveland Clinic Health Information. URL: my.clevelandclin ic.org/healthy_living/Pregnancy/hic_Dental_Care_During_Pregnancy.aspx. Accessed October 17, 2006.

"Dental Crowns." WebMD. URL: www.webmd./oral-health/dental-crowns. Accessed November 22, 2008.

"Dental Drill." How Products Are Made. URL: www.madehow.com/Volume-3/Dental-Drill.html.

"Dental Erosion on Rise in U.S." MedicineNet. URL: www.medicinenet.com/script/main/art.asp?articlekey=87788. Accessed September 22, 2008.

"Dental Examination." iVillage. URL: yourtotalhealth. ivillage.com/dental-examination.html. Accessed September 25, 2008.

"Dental Health: Braces and Retainers." WebMD. URL: www.webmd/oral-health/guide/braces-and-retainers. Accessed July 20, 2009.

"Dental Health: Dental Bonding." WebMD. URL: www.WebMD./oral-health/guide/dental-bonding. Accessed January 22, 2008.

"Dental Health: Dentures." WebMD. URL: www. webmd.com/oral-health/guide/dental-health-dentures. Accessed February 25, 2009.

"Dental Implant Surgery." MayoClinic.com. URL: www.mayoclinic.com/print/dental-implants/HA00026/METHOD=print. Accessed June 10, 2007.

"Dental Plaque Identification at Home." MedlinePlus. URL: www.nlm.nih.gov/medlineplus/ency/article/003426.htm. Accessed October 13, 2008.

"Dentist Links Fosomax-type Drugs to Jaw Necrosis." Newswise. URL: newswise.com/articles/view/547657. Accessed July 20, 2009.

"Dentists Need Tools to Improve Brushing and Flossing Behavior." Newswise. URL: www.newswise.com/articles/view/529019/?sc=mwtr. Accessed April 29, 2007.

"Does Treating Periodontitis Help Control Diabetes?" Newswise. URL: www.newswise.com/articles/view/544265/?sc=mwtr;xy=5003042. Accessed September 15, 2008.

"Edward Hartley Angle." Who Named It? URL: www.whonamedit.com/doctor.cfm/239.html. Accessed July 12, 2008.

Eustice, Carol, and Richard Eustice. "Guide to Temporomandibular Disorders (TMD)." About.com. URL: arthritis.about.com/od/tmj/ss/guidetotmdtmj.htm. Accessed January 27, 2009.

"The Evolution of Mouthwash." Contemporary Dental Assisting. URL: www.contemporarydentalassisting.com/issues/articles/2006.-09_09.asp. Accessed October 16, 2007.

"FDA Declares Mercury Fillings to Be Perfectly Safe for Human Health." Natural News. URL: www.naturalnews.com/020310.html. Accessed October 11, 2007.

Federal Bureau of Investigation. "Privacy Impact Assessment, National Dental Image Repository." FBI.gov. URL: foia.fbi.gov/ndirpia.htm. Accessed December 9, 2008.

"Fewer Heart Patients Need Antibiotics before Dental Procedures." Newswise. URL: www.newswise.com/articles/view/529199/?sc=mwtr. Accessed April 25, 2007.

"Fluoridated Water Benefits Older Adults More than Kids." Newswise. Posted December 4, 2007. URL: www.newswise.com/p/articles/view/535912/. Accessed December 6, 2007.

"Gastroesophageal Reflux Disease (GERD)." WebMD. URL: www.webmd./heartburn-gerd/guide/reflux-disease?print=true. Accessed March 3, 2008.

Golonka, Debby. "Teething Products and Remedies." WebMD. URL: www.webmd.com/hw-popup/teeth-ing-products-and-remedies. Accessed July 20, 2009.

Grummons, Duane, and Terry Sellke. "Remembering an Orthodontic Giant, Robert M. Ricketts, D.D.S., M.S., N.M.D, May 5, 1920–June 18, 2003." URL: www.rmortho.com/bins/site/templates/ricketts Books.asp?_resolutionfile=templatespath%7CricckettsBooks.asp&area_1=rickettsBooks/navigation&area_2=rickettsBooks/sellke. Accessed December 4, 2008.

Haake, Susan Kinder. "Microbiology of Dental Plaque." Periodontics Information Center. URL: www.dent.ucla.edu/pic/members/microbio/mdphome.html. Accessed October 13, 2008.

"History of Crest." Procter and Gamble. URL: www.pg.com/company/who_we_are/crest_history.shtml. Accessed February 28, 2009.

Hoyle, Joe. "Oral Bacteria Could Point toward Cancer Diagnosis: Study." American Dental Association. URL: www.ada.org/prof/resources/pubs/adanews/adanewsarticle.asp?. Accessed January 30, 2008.

"Instrument Sterilization Protocols, Washington (State) Industrial Safety and Health Act." University of Washington School of Dentistry. URL: www.dental.washington.edu/hazards/chapter-2/instrument-sterilizati on-protocols.htm. Accessed November 16, 2007.

"The Intellidrug Tooth Implant." Gizmag Emerging Technology Magazine. URL: www.gizmag.com/g o/6778/. Accessed February 28, 2009.

Jahan-Parwar, Babak, and Keith Blackwell. "Facial Bone Anatomy." eMedicine. URL: www.emedicine.com/ent/topic9.htm. Accessed January 30, 2008.

———. "Lips and Perioral Region." eMedicine. URL: www.emedicine.com/Ent/topic7.htm. Accessed July 20, 2009.

Johnson, Romaine F. "Oral Cavity Reconstruction." *Grand Rounds Archives*, Baylor College of Medicine, Bobby T. Alford Department of Otolaryngology—Head and Neck Surgery. URL: www.bcm.edu/oto/grand/110720 02.htm. Accessed December 23, 2008.

Keim, Samuel M., and Douglas Smith. "Broken Jaw." eMedicine. URL: www.emedicinehealth.com/broken_jaw/article_em.htm. Accessed December 14, 2008.

Lubin, Edward. "Trigeminal Neuralgia." WebMD. URL: www.emedicinehealth.com/trigeminal_neuralgia_facial_nerve_pain/article_em.htm. Accessed July 20, 2009.

"Malocclusion of Teeth." MedlinePlus. URL: www.nlm.nih.gov/medlineplus/ency/article/001058.htm. Accessed July 20, 2009.

Marinho, V.C.C., J.P.T Higgins, S. Logan, and A. Sheiham. "Fluoride Varnishes for Preventing Dental Caries in Children and Adolescents." The Cochrane Collaboration. URL: www.cochrane.org/reviews/en /ab002279.html. Accessed July 20, 2009.

Massachusetts Department of Environmental Protection. "Dental Amalgam/Mercury Recycling." URL: www.mass.gov/dep/service/dentists.htm. Accessed July 19, 2008.

McElfish, Dr. Charles. "C. Edmund Kells Pioneered Electricity and Dental X-rays." Allegany College of Maryland. URL: www.ac.cc.md.us/dental/98-1newsletter/EdmundKells.html. Accessed July 26, 2008.

Moore, Shelley. "Who Invented the Electric Toothbrush?" eHow.com. URL: www.ehow.com/about_4598206_who-invented-electric-toothbrush.html. Accessed February 13, 2009.

"More U.S. Teeth Susceptible to Silent Enamel-eating Syndrome." Newswise. URL: www.newswise.com/articles/view/538380/?sc=mwtr. Accessed September 21, 2008.

"Mouthwash." How Products Are Made. URL: www.madehow.com/Volume-6/Mouthwash.html. Accessed October 16, 2007.

"Natal Health: Hormones and Oral Health." WebMD. URL: www.webmd.com/oral-health/guide/hormones-oral-health. Accessed July 25 2008.

National Cancer Institute, "Internal Radiation Therapy." URL: www.cancer.gov/cancertopics/radiation-therapy-and-you/page4. Accessed September 26, 2008.

National Eating Disorders Association. "Dental Complications of Eating Disorders: Information for Dental Practitioners." URL: www.edap.org/p.asp?WebPage_ID=286&Profile_ID=73512. Accessed April 12, 2007.

"National Geographic's Dr. Brady Barr's Bite Pressure Tests (Dangerous Encounters: Bite Force)." Dog Facts. URL: dogfacts.wordpress.com/2008/02/03/national-geographics-dr-brady-barrs-bite-pressure-tests. Accessed October 20, 2008.

National Institute of Dental and Craniofacial Research. "The Story of Fluoridation." URL: www.nidcr.nih.gov/OralHealth/Topics/Fluoride/TheStoryofFluoridation.htm. Accessed July 20, 2009.

———. "Studies Evaluate Health Effects of Dental Amalgam Fillings in Children." URL: www.nidcr.nih.gov/NewsAndReports/NewsReleases/NewRelease04182006.htm. Accessed October 11, 2007.

National Institute on Deafness and Other Communication Disorders. "Taste Disorders." URL: www.nidcd.nih.gov/health/smelltaste/taste.asp. Accessed January 20, 2009.

National Organization for Rare Disorders. "Amelogenesis Imperfecta." URL: www.rarediseases.org/search/rdbdetail_abstract.htm.l?disname=Amelogenesis%20Imperfecta. Accessed February 11, 2008.

"New Clinical Study Finds Waterpik Dental Water Jet Is an Effective Alternative to Traditional Flossing." Dental Compare. URL: www.dentalcompare.com/news.asp?newsid=100739. Accessed December 9, 2008.

"Noma." MedlinePlus. URL: www.nlm.nih.gov/medlineplus/ency/article/001342.htm. Accessed February 26, 2008.

"Oral Cancer." MedlinePlus. URL: ww.nlm.nih.gov/medlineplus/ency/article/001035.htm. Accessed November 9, 2008.

"Oral Cancer Treatment." Omni Medical Search. URL: www.omnimedicalsearch.com/conditions-diseases/oral-cancer-treatment-options.html. Accessed July 20, 2009.

Oral Health Center. "Dental Health Dental X-Ray." WebMD. URL: www.WebMD./oral-health/guide/dental-x-rays. Accessed June 2, 2007.

———. "Dental Health: Mouth Guards." WebMD. URL: www.WebMD./oral-health/mouth-guards. Accessed August 28, 2008.

———. "Weighing Your Toothpaste Options." WebMD. URL: www.webmd.com/oral-health/

weighing-your-toothpaste-options. Accessed February 27, 2009.

"Osteoporosis Drugs Linked to Jaw Infection, Study Shows." Dentist.com. URL: dentist.com.wordpress.com/2008/05/10/osteoporosis-drugs-linked-to-jaw-infection-study-shows. Accessed July 20, 2009.

"Pain Management: Temporomandibular Disorders." WebMD. URL: www.webmd.com.pain-management/guide/temporomandibular-disorders. Accessed January 24, 2009.

"Philippe-G. Woog, Ph.D." Broxo. URL: www.broxo.com/en/about_us/default.aspx. Accessed February 15, 2009.

Pierre Fauchard Academy. "Dr. G. V. Black" (updated 03); "Dr. Harvey J. Burkhart" (updated August 8, 2003); "Frederick S. McKay" (updated November 2, 2004). URL: www.fauchard.org/awards/hall_of_fame/. Accessed July 12, 2008.

Pizzorno, Joseph, and Lara Pizzorno. "Strong Bones for Life—Naturally (Part I)." WebMD. URL: blogs.webmd.com/integrative-medicine-wellness/2008/10/strong-bones-for-life-naturally.html. Accessed October 23, 2009.

Pretty, Iain A., and David Sweet. "Identification." Forensic Dentistry Online. URL: www.forensicdentistryonline.org/Forensic_pages_1/identguide.htm. Accessed December 11, 2008.

Radiological Society of North America. "Stereotactic Radiosurgery." Radiology Info. URL: www.radiologyinfo.org/en/info.cfm?pg=stereotactic&bhcp=1. Accessed October 7, 2008.

Renz, A., M. Ide, T. Newton, P.G. Robinson, and D. Smith. "Psychological Interventions to Improve Adherence to Oral Hygiene Instructions in Adults with Periodontal Diseases." The Cochrane Collaboration. URL: www.cochrane.org/reviews/en/ab005097.htm.l. Accessed April 30, 2007.

Ring, Malvin E. "Our Daily Thread: Dental Floss Is a Great Underappreciated Invention." American Heritage. URL: www.americanheritage.com/articles/magazine/it/2006/3/2006_3_32.shtml. Accessed December 6, 2008.

Sakuraba, Minoru, Takayuki Asano, Shimpei Miyamoto, Ryuichi Hayashi, Mitsuo Yamazaki, Masakazu Miyazaki, Toru Ugumori, Hiroyuki Daiko, and Yoshihiro Kimat. "A New Flap Design for Tongue Reconstruction after Total or Subtotal Glossectomy in Thin Patients." ScienceDi-

rect. URL: www.sciencedirect.com/science?_ob=ArticleURL&_udi=B7XNJ-4SD1KV8-1&_user=10&_rdoc=1&_fmt=&_orig=search&_sort=d&view=c&_acct=C000050221&_version. Accessed July 20, 2009.

"Scientists Re-grow Dental Enamel from Cultured Cells." Science Daily. URL: www.sciencedaily.com/releases/2007/03/070323171639.htm. Accessed September 18, 2008.

Scottish Executive Health Department Chief Scientist Office. "A Systematic (Cochrane) Review of Psychotherapy for Dental Anxiety." URL: www.sehd.scot.nhs.uk/cso/Publications/ExecSumms/Jan-Feb04/Adair.pdf. Accessed June 23, 2008.

"Tartar (Dental Calculus) Overview." WebMD. URL: www.WebMD.com/oral-health/tartar-dental-calculus-overview?page=2. Accessed November 18, 2008.

"Teething—Topic Overview." WebMD. URL: children.webmd.com/tc/teething-topic-overview. Accessed January 22, 2009.

"Teeth Whitening." WebMD. URL: www.webmd.com/oral-health/guide/teeth-whitening. Accessed December 25, 2008.

"Thrush," Medline Plus. URL: www.nlm.nih.gov/medlineplus/ency/article/000626.htm. Accessed December 17, 2008.

Todar, Kenneth. "The Bacterial Flora of Humans." Todar's Online Textbook of Bacteriology. URL: textbookofbacteriology.net/normalflora.html. Accessed November 27, 2008.

"Tooth Abrasion and Tooth Erosion." Simple Steps to Better Dental Health. URL: www.simplestepsdental.com/SS/ihtSSPrint/r.WSIHW000/st.32219/t.35262/pr.3/c.364288.html. Accessed September 22, 2008.

"Tooth Transplants." Dental Care Advice. URL: www.dentalcareadvice.com/dental-surgery-procedures/tooth-transplants.php. Accessed February 16, 2009.

Torma, Sami. "Finnish Patient Gets New Jaw from Own Stem Cells." Reuters Health. URL: www.reutershealth.com/en/index.htm.l. Accessed February 4, 2008.

University of Maryland Medical Center. "Amelogenesis Imperfecta." URL: www.umm.edu/ency/article/001578trt.htm. Accessed February 15, 2008.

University of North Carolina, School of Dentistry, Department of Pediatric Dentistry. "Amelogenesis Imperfecta." URL: www.dent.unc.edu/research/defects/ai. cfm. Accessed February 10, 2008.

"What Makes Us Yawn?" How Stuff Works. URL: www.howstuffworks.com/question572.htm. Accessed June 1, 2007.

"William Thomas Green Morton." Answers.com. URL: www.answers.com/topic/william-t-g-morton?cat= technology. Accessed July 16, 2008.

Wilwerding, Terry. "History of Dentistry 2001." Creighton University School of Dentistry. URL: cudental.creighton.edu/htm./history2001.pdf. Accessed July 16, 2008.

"Wisdom Teeth." MedicineNet. URL: www.medi-cinenet.com/script/main/art.asp?articlekey=4310 0&pf=3&page=1. Accessed December 30, 2008.

W.L. Gore and Associates. "Guided Bone Regen-eration." Gore Medical Products. URL: www.gore medical.com/en/file/AG5104.pdf. Accessed August 28, 2008.

"Women's Overall Health and Oral Health." Colgate World of Health. URL: www.colgate.com/app /Col-gate/US/OC/Information/OralHealthAtAnyAge/ Adults/WomensHealth/WomensOralHealthand OverallHealth.cvsp. Accessed July 24,2008.

Zwillach, Todd. "Safety of Dental Fillings Questioned." WebMD. URL: www.medicinenet.com/script/main/ art.asp?articlekey=63986. Accessed October 11, 2007.

INDEX

Note: **Boldface** page numbers indicate extensive treatment of a topic.

For Reference

Not to be taken from this room